Weaning from Mechanical Ventilation

Antuani Rafael Baptistella • Daniel Lago Borges
Luis Felipe da Fonseca Reis
Editors

Weaning from Mechanical Ventilation

A State-of-the-Art Approach

Springer

Editors
Antuani Rafael Baptistella
University of Western Santa Catarina (Unoesc)
Joaçaba, Santa Catarina, Brazil

Luis Felipe da Fonseca Reis
Augusto Motta University Center (UNISUAM)
Rio de Janeiro, Rio de Janeiro, Brazil

Daniel Lago Borges
Hospital Universitário of Maranhão Federal University (HUUFMA)
São Luís, Maranhão, Brazil

ISBN 978-3-032-01144-2 ISBN 978-3-032-01145-9 (eBook)
https://doi.org/10.1007/978-3-032-01145-9

This Springer imprint is published by the registered company Springer Nature Switzerland AG
The registered company address is: Gewerbestrasse 11, 6330 Cham, Switzerland

For Joaquim and Otávio.

Antuani

To my children, Ana Laura, Mateus, and Clarice.

Daniel

To my wife, Clara Diniz, and my children, Pedro and Maria.

Luis Felipe

Foreword

It is a privilege to write in place of my widely admired and close friend, the late Prof. Luciano Gattinoni. To my knowledge, this book, *Weaning from Mechanical Ventilation: A State-of-the-Art Approach*, may be a unique contribution in pulling together in one place virtually every important aspect of this problem's complexity. The chapter authors, each a noted expert, have together provided a detailed and comprehensive reference that will prove invaluable to those who seek to practice at the highest level in the ICU environment.

The subject of ventilator withdrawal and discontinuation is highly nuanced and of clear clinical importance. For a small but important fraction of patients receiving mechanical ventilation, protracted dependence on the ventilator entails serious hazard, disability, and economic cost. Many such patients have life-altering acute illnesses, underlying lung disease, or neuromuscular impairment. Their need for respiratory assistance may stem from multiple sources, including psychological distress, refractory hypoxemia and cardiovascular dysfunction. But perhaps the most common pathway is an imbalance between the level of ventilation demanded by the patient and the ability of the respiratory system to respond. An effective response requires an adequate central stimulus to breathe (ventilatory drive) and muscular endurance. Insufficient ventilatory drive is seldom the primary or isolated reason for an ongoing need for respiratory assistance. Instead, ventilator-dependent patients are often malnourished or otherwise deconditioned. Frequently, impaired diaphragmatic functioning, or hyperinflation of lungs and chest wall compromise respiratory efficiency. Moreover, many critically ill patients who receive sustained mechanical assistance experience forms of ICU-acquired neuromyopathy that may go unrecognized and are still incompletely explained.

The respiratory workload is jointly determined by the impedance of the respiratory system and the intensity and pattern of ventilation. For a given level of ventilation, energy output is minimized by increasing the frequency of respirations while limiting the depth of each breath; rapid spontaneous breathing, therefore, can be a useful adaptation to avoid fatigue. Unfortunately, as the tidal volume decreases, its dead space fraction increases and ventilatory efficiency falls. This obliges the patient with tachypnea to either increase minute ventilation, inflation work and power or allow hypercapnia to develop. Whether rapid shallow breathing proves physiological adaptive or maladaptive depends on whether gas exchanging inefficiency overwhelms the benefit of reduced effort.

Extensive investigation and debate have come closer to consensus on several weaning-related therapeutic issues. For example, there is general agreement that the respiratory muscles must not be overtaxed because recovery from established fatigue may require 24 h or longer to recover. Important questions, however, have not been resolved. Whereas well-moderated muscular activity is clearly desirable, the value of training the respiratory muscles remains unclear. Furthermore, the superiority of any one weaning strategy has not been demonstrated convincingly when each method is properly used, nor have standardized guidelines been established for the optimal pace of withdrawing machine assistance.

The abrupt removal of mechanical ventilation works well for most patients with rapidly resolving illness and ample respiratory reserve. Yet, the hours immediately after abrupt withdrawal can impose an immediate overload. The physiologic instability of this period suggests that a modest imbalance between respiratory capability and ventilatory requirement should be reversed stepwise by more gradual discontinuation of mechanical support. Such a graded transition from mechanical to spontaneous ventilation seems advisable for patients who experience panic reactions, congestive heart failure or cardiac ischemia, and for those confronted by unusually large breathing workloads. For these patients a fine line must be drawn between proceeding too quickly or too slowly. How best to monitor readiness for independent breathing, and even the advisability of graded withdrawal of machine assistance itself, are still questions in flux. As with many challenging medical problems, the best approach often requires personalized care rooted in close observation and a firm grasp of underlying physiology. I congratulate the editors and chapter authors for providing an excellent basis for making those bedside decisions.

John J. Marini

Professor of Medicine
University of Minnesota
St. Paul, MN, USA

Preface

Mechanical ventilation (MV) is a cornerstone of life support in intensive care medicine, yet it remains one of the most complex and challenging interventions. While MV serves as a temporary replacement for a patient's vital respiratory function, improper settings or prolonged use can lead to complications, including lung injury and diaphragm dysfunction. Therefore, weaning from MV should begin as soon as the underlying cause of acute respiratory failure (ARF) is resolved or adequately controlled.

Weaning, the process of discontinuing or withdrawing MV and restoring the patient's natural respiratory function, is a critical and universally important aspect of care for critically ill patients. Its complexity and impact on patient outcomes make it one of the most crucial phases of critical care management.

Weaning from Mechanical Ventilation: A State-of-the-Art Approach is the first book entirely dedicated to exploring the multifaceted process of weaning from mechanical ventilation. It provides a comprehensive examination of topics ranging from fundamental concepts, epidemiology, and weaning criteria to predictive tests, pathophysiology of failure, and strategies for effective management. This book also addresses emerging areas in the field, such as the role of nutrition, artificial intelligence, ultrasound, noninvasive ventilation, high-flow nasal cannula, inspiratory muscle training, diaphragm dysfunction, and airway clearance. It also addresses the specific challenges of weaning in unique patient populations, including those with COPD, neurological and cardiac conditions, COVID-19, and those in palliative care.

Written by experts with extensive experience and diverse perspectives, this book serves as a global reference, providing evidence-based insights and practical guidance. It aims to fill a critical gap in the literature and equip the multidisciplinary critical care team with the knowledge needed to make the weaning process safer, more efficient, and better tailored to individual patient needs. We hope that *Weaning from Mechanical Ventilation: A State-of-the-Art Approach* will become an invaluable resource for all professionals dedicated to improving outcomes for critically ill patients.

Joaçaba, Brazil — Antuani Rafael Baptistella
São Luís, Brazil — Daniel Lago Borges
Rio de Janeiro, Brazil — Luis Felipe da Fonseca Reis

Competing Interests

The editors declared no competing interests.

Acknowledgments

I would like to thank my dear wife Shaline for her support and encouragement in this project, and my sons Joaquim and Otávio, who make everything I do in my life even more meaningful.

I would also like to thank my loving family: especially my parents Valdir and Nayr, my sisters Carli and Alessandra, and my niece Helena, you are my base and my security.

On behalf of a very special patient, Odalides dos Santos, I would like to thank all the patients I have seen during my career.

On behalf of a special colleague, Dr. Carlos Alexandre Romero de Souza, I would like to thank all my colleagues with whom I have learned over the last 20 years, not only about intensive care and mechanical ventilation but also about how to make work a good place to build an important part of my life.

Finally, I would like to thank all the authors who gave their time and knowledge to write this book.

Antuani Rafael Baptistella

I want to sincerely thank my wife, Mayara, for her patience and support through every step of my professional journey, including this project.

To my parents, Rui and Elisa, my eternal gratitude for believing in my education, even in the face of challenges, and for making it possible for me to get here.

I'm also grateful to all the teachers who crossed my path, at every level of education, for helping shape my knowledge.

And finally, to every patient who teaches me, day after day, the true meaning of being human—thank you so much.

Daniel Lago Borges

I would like to thank my beloved wife Clara for her support and encouragement in this work and to my children Maria and Pedro, who, through their unconditional love, drive us forward.

I would also like to thank my dear family: my parents Adilson (In Memoriam) and Irene, my sister Andréa, and my nephews Ana Beatriz and João Victor.

I also thank Dr. Christina Maeda Takiya and Professors Dr. Agnaldo José Lopes and Fernando Silva Guimarães, who taught me about the foundations of research and its nonnegotiable ethics. And I would like to thank all my colleagues with whom I have divided the ICUs over the last 25 years, learning to place the patient at the center of care and that intensive care units are places of life and not death.

and

Finally, I would like to reinforce that Diagnosis is not destiny!

Luis Felipe da Fonseca Reis

Contents

About the Editors and Contributors

About the Editors

Antuani Rafael Baptistella, PT, PhD. Physiotherapist at the Intensive Care Units of Hospital Universitário Santa Terezinha (HUST) and Hospital Unimed Meio-Oeste, Joaçaba, Brazil.

Specialist in Intensive Care by the Brazilian Association of Respiratory, Cardiovascular and Critical Care Physiotherapy (ASSOBRAFIR) and the Federal Council of Physiotherapy and Occupational Therapy (COFFITO).

PhD from Fundação Antônio Prudente—AC Camargo Cancer Center

Permanent Professor of the Postgraduate Program in Biosciences and Health, Universidade do Oeste de Santa Catarina, Unoesc, Joaçaba, Brazil.

Daniel Lago Borges Physiotherapist at the Adult Intensive Care Unit of Hospital Universitário of Maranhão Federal University (HUUFMA), São Luis, Maranhão, Brazil

Specialist in Respiratory and Intensive Care Physiotherapy by the Brazilian Association of Respiratory, Cardiovascular and Critical Care Physiotherapy (ASSOBRAFIR) and the Federal Council of Physiotherapy and Occupational Therapy (COFFITO).

PhD from Universidade do Estado do Rio de Janeiro

Luis Felipe da Fonseca Reis Lieutenant Colonel Physiotherapist and Coordinator of the ICU of the Central Hospital of the Military Police of the State of Rio de Janeiro

Intensive Care Physiotherapist at the ICU of the Gafrée Guinle University Hospital of the Federal University of the State of Rio de Janeiro (HUGG-UNIRio)

Specialist in Respiratory and Intensive Care Physiotherapy by the Brazilian Association of Respiratory, Cardiovascular and Critical Care Physiotherapy (ASSOBRAFIR) and the Federal Council of Physiotherapy and Occupational Therapy (COFFITO).

PhD from Federal University of Rio de Janeiro (UFRJ)
Permanent Professor of the Postgraduate Program in Rehabilitation Sciences Augusto Motta University Center (PPGCR-UNISUAM)

Contributors

Antuani Rafael Baptistella Hospital Universitário Santa Terezinha (HUST), Joaçaba, Brazil
Hospital Unimed Meio-Oeste, Joaçaba, Brazil
Universidade do Oeste de Santa Catarina, Unoesc, Joaçaba, Brazil

Shaline Ferla Baptistella Clinical Oncologist, Santa Terezinha University Hospital, Joaçaba, SC, Brazil
Universidade do Oeste de Santa Catarina, Unoesc, Joaçaba, Brazil

Catherine A. Bellissimo Toronto General Hospital Research Institute, University Health Network, Toronto, ON, Canada

Saint-Clair Bernardes Neto Faculdade de Ciências da Saúde (FACISA), Universidade Federal do Rio Grande do Norte (UFRN), Natal, Brazil

Daniel Lago Borges Hospital Universitário of Maranhão Federal University (HUUFMA), São Luis, Maranhão, Brazil
University Hospital of Federal University of Maranhão, São Luís, Maranhão, Brazil

Mayara Gabrielle Barbosa Borges University Hospital of Federal University of Maranhão, São Luís, Maranhão, Brazil

Michele Vaz Pinheiro Canena Federal University of Rio Grande, Rio Grande, Rio Grande do Sul, Brazil

Guilherme Duprat Ceniccola Secretaria de Estado de Saúde do Distrito Federal, Brasília, Brazil

Carmen Chica-Meza International Mechanical Ventilation Group (WeVent), Quillota, Chile
URosario, AMCI, Cartagena, Colombia

André Luiz Lisboa Cordeiro Nobre University Center, University Center of Excellence, Feira de Santana, BA, Brazil
Bahiana School of Medicine and Public Health, Salvador, BA, Brazil

Amanda Pereira Cruz Laboratory of Pulmonary Investigation, Institute of Biophysics Carlos Chagas Filho, Federal University of Rio de Janeiro, Rio de Janeiro, Brazil
Gloria D'Or Hospital, D'Or Institute for Research and Education, Rio de Janeiro, Brazil

Aurio Fajardo-Campoverdi Universidad de la Frontera, Critical Care Unit, Hospital Biprovincial Quillota-Petorca, Quillota, Chile
International Mechanical Ventilation Group (WeVent), Quillota, Chile

Bruno Leonardo da Silva Guimarães Physical Therapy Hospital Niterói D'or, Niterói, RJ, Brazil

Emanuele da Silva Passos Damázio Liga de Medicina Intensiva, UESB, Jequié, Bahia, Brazil

Flávio Maciel de Andrade Pernambuco State Health Department, Recife, Brazil
Regional Council of Physiotherapy and Occupational Therapy of the 1st Region, Recife, Brazil

Diego de Carvalho University of Western Santa Catarina – Unoesc, Joaçaba, Brazil

Leonardo Cordeiro de Souza Physical Therapy School, Universidade Estácio de Sá, Rio de Janeiro, RJ, Brazil

Jonne Doorduin Department of Intensive Care Medicine, Radboud University Medical Center, Nijmegen, The Netherlands

Karoliny dos Santos Isoppo Department of Health Sciences, Federal University of Santa Catarina, Araranguá, Brazil

Nathane Santanna Felix Gloria D'Or Hospital, D'Or Institute for Research and Education, Rio de Janeiro, Brazil

Oellen Stuani Franzosi Nutrition and Dietetic Division, Hospital de Clínicas de Porto Alegre, Universidade Federal do Rio Grande do Sul, Porto Alegre, Brazil

Tim Frenzel Department of Intensive Care Medicine, Radboud University Medical Center, Nijmegen, The Netherlands

Mellina Tamy Fagundes Fujihara Physical Therapy Hospital Niterói D'or, Niterói, RJ, Brazil

Stefany Alves Furtado Health Department of the State of Pernambuco, Garanhuns, Pernambuco, Brazil

Ewan C. Goligher Division of Respirology, Department of Medicine, Toronto General Hospital, University Health Network, Toronto, ON, Canada
Interdepartmental Division of Critical Care Medicine, Department of Physiology, Faculty of Medicine, University of Toronto, Toronto, ON, Canada

Breno Grossi Universidade do Oeste de Santa Catarina, Joaçaba, SC, Brazil
SEDAR – Serviço de Anestesiologia, Hospital Unimed Meio Oeste, Joaçaba, SC, Brazil
SBED – Sociedade Brasileira de Dor, São Paulo, SP, Brazil

Fernando Silva Guimarães Cardiopulmonary and Musculoskeletal Physiotherapy Department, Federal University of Rio de Janeiro, Rio de Janeiro, Brazil

Aline Almeida Gulart Physical Therapy Graduate Program, University of the State of Santa Catarina, Florianópolis, Brazil

Leo M. A. Heunks Department of Intensive Care Medicine, Radboud University Medical Center, Nijmegen, The Netherlands

Marcelo Alcantara Holanda Respiration Laboratory (RespLab/UFC), Internal Medicine Department, Federal University of Ceará (UFC), Fortaleza, CE, Brazil

Sandra R. Justino Federal University of Paraná (UFPR), Curitiba, Brazil

Gabriel Manfro University of Western Santa Catarina – Unoesc, Joaçaba, Santa Catarina, Brazil

Pedro Almir Feitosa Morais Respiration Laboratory (RespLab/UFC), Internal Medicine Department, Federal University of Ceará (UFC), Fortaleza, CE, Brazil

Sergio Nogueira Nemer Niterói Hospital Complex, Rio de Janeiro, Brazil

Darlan Nitz Intensiphysio Fisioterapia Intensiva, Curitiba, Paraná, Brazil

João Rogério Nunes Filho Hospital Universitário Santa Terezinha, UNOESC, Joaçaba, SC, Brazil

Douglas Pellizzaro University of Western Santa Catarina – Unoesc, Joaçaba, Santa Catarina, Brazil
Anesthesiology Department, Hospital Universitário Santa Terezinha, Joaçaba, Santa Catarina, Brazil
Unimed Meio Oeste, Joaçaba, Santa Catarina, Brazil

Gustavo A. Plotnikow Hospital Británico de Buenos Aires, Buenos Aires, Argentina
Facultad de Medicina y Ciencias de la Salud, Universidad Abierta Interamericana, Buenos Aires, Argentina

Wan Cley Rabuske Universidade do Oeste de Santa Catarina, Unoesc, Joaçaba, Brazil

Luis Felipe da Fonseca Reis University Center Augusto Motta, Rio de Janeiro, RJ, Brazil
Intensive Care Unit of the Central Hospital of the Military Police of the State of Rio de Janeiro, Rio de Janeiro, RJ, Brazil
Intensive Care Unit of the Gafrée Guinle University Hospital – Federal University of the State of Rio de Janeiro, Rio de Janeiro, RJ, Brazil
Hospital Universitário Gafree Guinle – HUGG-UNIRio, Rio de Janeiro, Brazil
Hospital Central da Polícia Militar do Estado do Rio de Janeiro, Rio de Janeiro, Brazil
Centro Universitário Augusto Motta (UNISUAM), Rio de Janeiro, Brazil

Ângelo Roncalli Miranda Rocha University of Health Sciences – Alagoas, Maceió, Alagoas, Brazil

Lisanne H. Roesthuis Department of Intensive Care Medicine, Radboud University Medical Center, Nijmegen, The Netherlands

Carina Rossoni Institute of Environmental Health (ISMAB) - Faculty of Medicine, University of Lisbon, Lisbon, Portugal

Isabela Julia Cristiana Santos Silva School of Rehabilitation Science, McMaster University, Hamilton, Canada

Pedro Leme Silva Laboratory of Pulmonary Investigation, Institute of Biophysics Carlos Chagas Filho, Federal University of Rio de Janeiro, Rio de Janeiro, Brazil

Leonardo Pamponet Simões Hospital da Mulher, Salvador, Bahia, Brazil
Aliviare Saúde, Salvador, Bahia, Brazil

Marcelo Taglietti Centro Universitário Fundação Assis Gurgacz (FAG), Cascavel, Brazil

Marcelo Azeredo Terra MTerra Education and Consultancy LTDA, Niterói, Rio de Janeiro, Brazil

Cristina Bueno Terzi Palliative Care Department, State University of Campinas, Campinas, São Paulo, Brazil

Betina Santos Tomaz Respiration Laboratory (RespLab/UFC), Internal Medicine Department, Federal University of Ceará (UFC), Fortaleza, CE, Brazil

Dario S. Villalba Hospital "Santiago Fornos", Chivilcoy, Buenos Aires, Argentina
Santa Catalina Neurorehabilitación Clínica, Buenos Aires, Argentina

Marcia Souza Volpe Department of Sciences of Human Movement, Federal University of São Paulo, São Paulo, Brazil

Chapter 1
Principles of Mechanical Ventilation

Betina Santos Tomaz, Pedro Almir Feitosa Morais, and Marcelo Alcantara Holanda

1.1 History of Mechanical Ventilation

The history of modern mechanical ventilation (MV) began with the polio pandemic of the 1950s. The shortage of iron lungs spurred innovation that led to the treatment of patients with the disease using positive pressure MV via an artificial airway, a cuffed tube inserted into the trachea. The reduction in mortality from acute respiratory failure in polio highlighted the potential of tracheal intubation and mechanical ventilation in medicine and intensive care units (ICUs), born in the 1950s [1–3].

The concept of correcting pulmonary hypoventilation with predefined parameters underscored the need for modern ventilators. Initially, pressure-controlled ventilators, such as the Bird Mark devices, were developed using airway pressure sensors for analysis. Volume-controlled ventilators were then developed by integrating airflow sensors into MV devices. This evolution culminated in the advent of microprocessor-controlled mechanical ventilators as we know them today [1–3].

Despite the significant technological revolution in invasive ventilatory support, new technologies continue to emerge to achieve better outcomes. Substantial efforts are still being made to disseminate knowledge about the management of MV worldwide. This management is based on the synchronization of the patient's neural command and the operator's neural cortex, which monitors and interprets the data and selects the best ventilatory support for each condition. Along with the "invention" of invasive MV, the process of weaning the patient from the ventilator has been identified as one of the most complex. Curiously, the first patient successfully treated by Bjorn Ibsen was submitted to prolonged MV for many years, from 12 to

B. S. Tomaz · P. A. F. Morais · M. A. Holanda (✉)
Respiration Laboratory (RespLab/UFC), Internal Medicine Department, Federal University of Ceará (UFC), Fortaleza, CE, Brazil

A. R. Baptistella et al. (eds.), *Weaning from Mechanical Ventilation*,
https://doi.org/10.1007/978-3-032-01145-9_1

31 years of age. Understanding, preventing, treating, and following patients weaning from MV is the scope of this book. The history of weaning is presented in Chap. 2.

1.2 Principles, Types, and Indications of Mechanical Ventilation

Mechanical ventilation (MV) is used to partially assist or even completely replace the action of the respiratory muscles in maintaining alveolar ventilation of the respiratory system [4]. Alveolar ventilation, in turn, is necessary for gas exchange or pulmonary gas transfer (hematosis) to occur. This process refers to the uptake of inspired oxygen from the alveoli into the arterial blood and the removal of carbon dioxide from the venous circulation into the airways for exhalation [5].

Thus, the term *mechanical pulmonary ventilator*—rather than *mechanical respirator* or *artificial respiration*, as commonly used—more accurately describes the sophisticated devices currently used to support life in patients with respiratory failure (RF). Its primary function is to act as a ventilatory pump, optimizing the physiology of gas exchange as efficiently and safely as possible, ideally allowing for the full recovery of the patient's respiratory autonomy [5, 6].

It is essential to differentiate MV with positive pressure in its form of complete substitution for respiratory muscle activity from what occurs physiologically during the spontaneous breathing cycle, as shown in Fig. 1.1 [7].

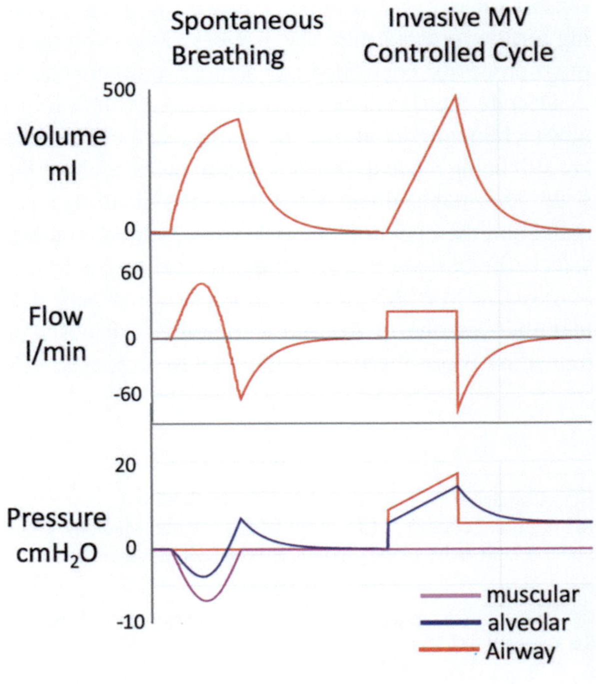

Fig. 1.1 Volume, flow, and airway and alveolar pressures vs. time curves during spontaneous breathing and invasive mechanical ventilation (volume-cycled mode, VCV, a controlled cycle without respiratory muscle effort is shown). The curves are reproduced in the Xlung® Simulator (www.xlung.net)

Note that the airway, alveolar, and muscle pressures, and thus the intrathoracic pressures, are no longer subatmospheric or negative but become positive during total mechanical ventilation. This change has several physiological implications, as we will see below.

1.2.1 Respiratory Cycles and Ventilation Modes

A respiratory cycle consists of a phenomenon that includes four distinct phases: (1) the beginning of inspiration; (2) the phase of lung inflation; (3) the end of inspiration followed by the beginning of expiration; and (4) the expiratory phase, including exhalation and the period until a new respiratory cycle begins. Ventilation mode is defined as the process by which the ventilator determines, in whole or in part, when, how, and with what limitations the mechanical respiratory cycles are delivered to the patient. The mode essentially determines the patient's respiratory pattern during ventilatory support. Thus, a ventilation mode determines how the ventilator controls or influences these four phases of the respiratory cycle [7–9].

Two basic types of respiratory cycles can be defined in MV: controlled and assisted respiratory cycles. In the first, the ventilator "controls" the entire inspiratory phase, i.e., it completely replaces the patient's respiratory muscle effort and neural control. This cycle is referred to here as controlled. In the second type, the ventilator merely aids or assists the active inspiratory musculature, referred to as assisted. Some authors use the term "spontaneous cycle" to define the cycle that occurs during pressure support ventilation (PSV) or inspiratory pressure (IPAP). Instead, the term assisted will be used here to describe this latter type of cycle, maintaining consistency with the above definition and reserving the term spontaneous cycle exclusively for physiological breathing, i.e., the respiratory cycle of an individual not using MV [9–14].

The initiation of respiratory cycles in MV is referred to as triggering. Triggers can be set by the ventilator, initiating cycles at predetermined time intervals, or by the patient using a mechanism sensitive to respiratory muscle effort (setting sensitivity or trigger function). Thus, controlled cycles are triggered by the ventilator, while assisted cycles are triggered by the patient [8, 10–14].

Ventilation mode can be defined as the process by which the ventilator determines how and when mechanical respiratory cycles are delivered to the patient. Thus, the three main modes of invasive mechanical ventilation (IMV) are volume-controlled ventilation (VCV), pressure-controlled ventilation (PCV), and pressure support ventilation (PSV).

VCV and PCV are typically used at the onset of IMV. Their characteristics are shown in Fig. 1.2, along with the differences between controlled cycles (triggered by the ventilator without any respiratory muscle effort) and assisted cycles (initiated by the patient's respiratory muscle effort) based on the ventilator's sensitivity settings.

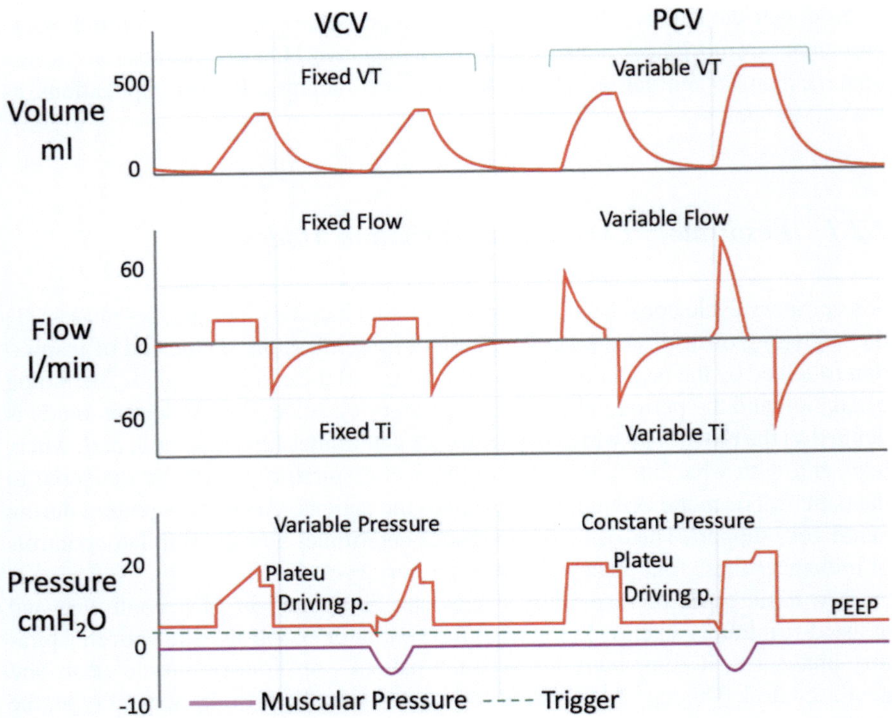

Fig. 1.2 Mechanical ventilation in VCV and PCV modes and their main characteristics in controlled and assisted cycles. In each mode, the first cycle is controlled and the second is assisted. Plateau pressure and driving pressure measurements were obtained with a short pause at the end of inspiration in both modes. The curves are reproduced in the Xlung® Simulator

In PCV mode, the tidal volume (VT) in assisted cycles can vary significantly depending on the patient's respiratory muscle effort and its effect on inspiratory flow. This variability provides greater comfort and improves patient-ventilator interaction in this scenario.

PSV mode differs from PCV in two major ways. First, it does not involve controlled cycles, i.e., it does not deliver time-triggered breaths and therefore requires respiratory drive (neural command). Second, the cycling criterion is not based on a fixed time, but on the deceleration of the inspiratory flow. Cycling occurs when the inspiratory flow reaches a predetermined percentage of peak flow, typically set at 25% on most ventilators. However, this setting can be adjusted to optimize patient-ventilator interaction and prevent asynchrony (Fig. 1.3).

PSV mode is primarily used during the transition period to restore the patient's ventilatory autonomy and gradually wean the patient from IMV.

Table 1.1 summarizes the key features of the basic ventilatory modes.

The basic ventilatory modes have limitations that often result in a lack of patient-ventilator synchronization. However, with a detailed understanding of their functionality, most patients can be ventilated satisfactorily.

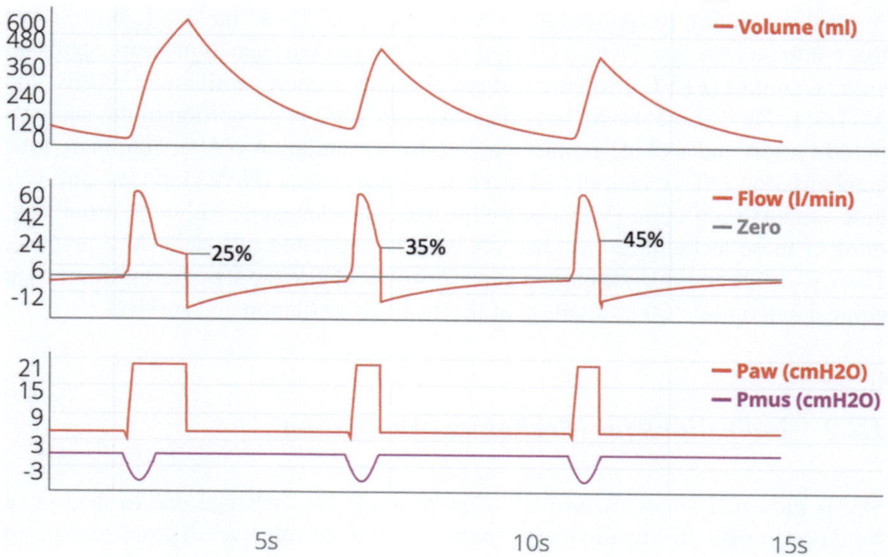

Fig. 1.3 Pressure support ventilation (PSV) cycles with sensitivity to flow of 3 L/min. In this case, the percentage threshold for cycling has been increased from 25% to 35% and then 45%. Observe the effect of this adjustment on Ti, flow curve, and VT. Increasing the threshold reduces Ti and VT, which may benefit patients with COPD and lung hyperinflation. Curves shown in the Xlung® Simulator

Table 1.1 Main characteristics of the basic ventilatory modes

Basic ventilatory modes			
Modes	Volume controlled ventilation (VCV)	Pressure controlled ventilation (PCV)	Pressure support ventilation (PSV)
Principal adjustable variables	Volume tidal (VT) Flow Ti RR	Pressure above PEEP (ΔP) Ti RR	Pressure support % do pico de fluxo para ciclagem
Types of cycles	Assisted and controlled	Assisted and controlled	Assisted
Trigger	Time or patient	Time or patient	Patient
Cycling criterion	Volume	Time	% of peak flow
Main advantage	Control of VT and alveolar pressure Monitoring of respiratory mechanics	Greater synchrony of flow and VT	Greater synchrony of flow, VT, and Ti
Main disadvantage	Lack of synchrony in the assisted cycles	VT and, thus, alveolar pressure not guaranteed	VT and minimum RR not guaranteed
Patient autonomy	Minimum	Moderate	High

New ventilation techniques have been developed. These include hybrid modes that combine features of A/C-VCV and A/C-PCV modes, such as pressure regulated volume control (PRVC), volume assured pressure support ventilation (VAPS), and AUTOFLOW®. Some modes provide airway pressure in proportion to the patient's muscle effort and include proportional assisted ventilation (PAV), automatic tube compensation (ATC), neurally adjusted ventilatory assist (NAVA) modes, and volume support ventilation (VSV) self-adjustment mechanisms. Although promising, most of these techniques have not yet been incorporated into daily MV practice. There is still little evidence of their superiority over basic modes in terms of relevant clinical outcomes such as duration of mechanical ventilation and survival.

1.2.2 Indications for Mechanical Ventilation

MV is indicated when impairment of pulmonary gas exchange due to disease or condition results in impaired oxygenation and/or alveolar ventilation, leading to respiratory failure (RF) and a potential or imminent life-threatening risk.

Main indications for MV:

Oxygenation Failure

Severe hypoxemia: $PaO_2 < 60$ mmHg or $SaO_2 < 90\%$ even with $FIO_2 > 0.6$

Ventilation Failure

Imminent cardiac or respiratory arrest

Severe tachypnea (respiratory rate (RR) > 40 breaths/min) or severe bradypnea (RR < 5 breaths/min)

Hypercapnia with Glasgow Coma Score < 8

Airway obstruction

Neuromuscular disease not improved by noninvasive ventilation

Inability to Protect the Airway

Based on arterial blood gas analysis, respiratory failure can be divided into three main types: hypercapnic, hypoxemic, or mixed [5, 6].

Hypercapnic RF is characterized by an increase in PaCO2 above 45–50 mmHg and resulting acidemia (pH < 7.34). Hypoxemic RF is defined by a PaO2 < 55–60 mmHg in room air or, more critically, despite the use of oxygen therapy. Mixed RF occurs when severe hypoxemia is associated with CO_2 retention and respiratory acidosis [6, 15].

In general, RF is also assessed clinically, with signs such as tachypnea (RR > 30 breaths per minute), excessive sweating (diaphoresis), tachycardia, use of accessory respiratory muscles (sternocleidomastoid and abdominal), supraclavicular, sternal, or intercostal retractions, or even paradoxical respiratory movements suggesting diaphragm dysfunction or fatigue [6, 15].

The goals of MV include:

- Relieve respiratory distress
- Correct respiratory acidosis and hypoxemia
- Reduce respiratory muscle workload
- Reverse respiratory muscle fatigue
- Prevent or reverse atelectasis
- Reduce oxygen consumption by the respiratory muscles

In addition, MV increases oxygen delivery to tissues during circulatory shock, reduces intracranial hypertension in traumatic brain injury, and facilitates surgery requiring general anesthesia and neuromuscular blockade [10, 11].

1.2.3 Initial VM Settings

When initiating MV, it is important to provide adequate oxygenation and alveolar ventilation to rapidly normalize blood gas parameters. Immediately, FIO_2 should be adjusted to achieve an SpO_2 between 92% and 96%, with an initial tidal volume (VT) of 6–8 ml/kg ideal or predicted body weight and a respiratory rate that produces a minute volume (VE, RR x VT) between 5 and 7 l/min, typically achieved at rates between 12 and 18 breaths per minute (bpm). The inspiratory time should be approximately 1 s, while the expiratory time depends on the respiratory rate. For example, at a rate of 15 bpm, the respiratory cycle will have a total duration of 4 s (60 s/15), resulting in an I:E ratio of 1:3, or 1 s of inspiration and 3 s of expiration. The key is to ensure complete expiration of the VT to avoid dynamic hyperinflation and the generation of intrinsic PEEP or auto-PEEP [10–13].

Additionally, PEEP of approximately 5 cmH_2O should be routinely applied to prevent atelectasis caused by the combination of intubation, supine position, and, most importantly, respiratory muscle inactivity. This inactivity increases pleural pressure, especially in the posterior regions of the lung in the supine position, which tend to alveolar collapse [10–13].

After 20 min of initial settings in MV, an arterial blood gas analysis should be performed to record FIO_2, VT, RR, VE, and PEEP for proper interpretation and subsequent parameter adjustment. Respiratory mechanics, including peak airway pressures, inspiratory pause pressure (plateau pressure), and driving pressure, should also be measured at this time [14, 16].

The table provides suggested safe targets for these parameters that are directly affected by mechanical ventilation (Fig. 1.4).

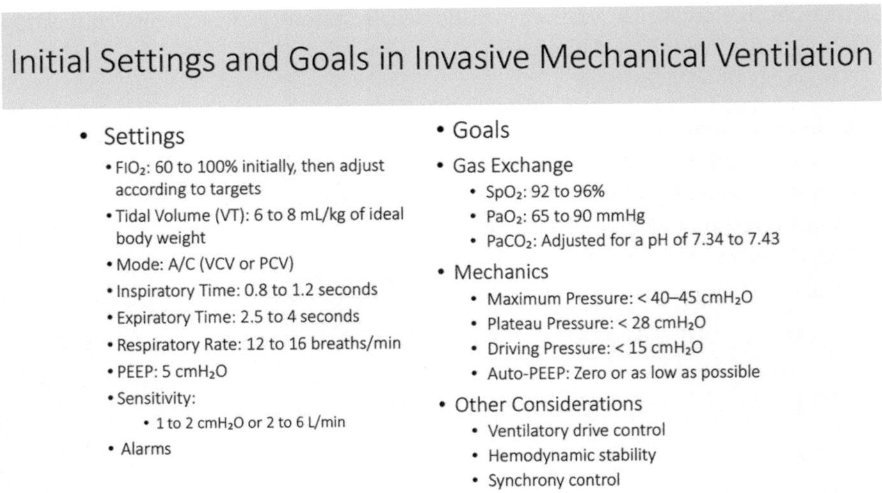

Fig. 1.4 Recommendations for initial settings and goals in invasive mechanical ventilation

1.2.4 Special Care and Complications of Invasive Mechanical Ventilation

As a life support technique, the intubated patient on MV must be cared for in an intensive care environment and by a multidisciplinary team with specific training. Care such as sedation and analgesia, neuromuscular blockade, management of the endotracheal tube and gas circuits, patient positioning, application of inhalation therapy, hemodynamic monitoring, chest imaging analysis, and other procedures are routinely performed in this setting. There is always a risk of complications due to iatrogenic factors or device malfunction. The ventilator should be pre-tested in all patients, and its alarms should be set appropriately on an individual basis. The major complications of MV are listed below:

- Upper airway and tracheal trauma
- Barotrauma (pneumothorax and pneumomediastinum)
- Hemodynamic compromise, hypotension, and shock
- Ventilator-induced lung injury (VILI)
- Ventilator-associated pneumonia
- Multiple organ and system dysfunction (cerebral, renal, digestive, and others)
- Patient-ventilator asynchrony
- Ventilator-induced diaphragm dysfunction (VIDD)

1.3 Prolonged Ventilation: Definition, Risk Factors, Complications, and Outcomes

The number of patients requiring prolonged mechanical ventilation (PMV) is increasing worldwide, placing a significant burden on healthcare systems. Therefore, the study of risk factors, complications, and outcomes is crucial for the proper management of this condition [17, 18].

An American consensus conference first defined PVM as patients requiring 21 days of MV without a 2-day interruption. Prolonged weaning, on the other hand, is specifically related to the gradual discontinuation of MV. It is characterized by patients requiring more than three spontaneous breathing trials (SBTs) or a weaning process lasting longer than 7 days [18, 19]. Thus, while prolonged ventilation focuses on the duration of mechanical ventilation, prolonged weaning emphasizes the complexity and length of the process required to achieve ventilator independence. The following are some risk factors for PMV [18, 21]:

- Systemic comorbidities
  - Chronic respiratory diseases: COPD, bronchiectasis, pulmonary fibrosis
  - Heart failure
  - Cerebrovascular diseases
  - Neuromuscular diseases
  - End-stage renal disease
  - Liver Cirrhosis
  - Malignancy
- Infection: sepsis, multidrug-resistant infection
- Malnutrition
- Reduced respiratory muscle capacity
- Ventilator-induced diaphragm dysfunction
- Critical illness neuromyopathy
- Critical illness encephalopathy
- Hypothyroidism
- Iatrogenic factors
- Psychological factors
- Process of care

Patients who remain on MV for prolonged periods are more susceptible to depression, cognitive decline, and delirium, which can complicate weaning strategies [22]. In addition, several complications may occur, including:

- *Deep Venous Thrombosis (DVT)*: Prolonged immobility increases the risk of thrombosis, highlighting the importance of rehabilitation, mobility enhancement, and pharmacological prophylaxis measures.
- *Orthostatic Hypotension* may be secondary to neurological, hormonal, and humoral changes during extended ventilation. It requires careful management to prevent further complications.

- *Osteoporosis*: Patients may develop bone demineralization due to inactivity and a lack of weight-bearing exercises. Prevention and treatment should include mobilization and calcium and vitamin D supplementation when deficiencies are identified.
- *Pressure Ulcers*: These can occur due to prolonged immobility, necessitating regular mobilization, protection of pressure points, and optimal nutrition to maintain skin integrity.
- *Hyperglycemia*: Elevated blood glucose levels may result from stress, medications, or poor nutritional management, requiring close monitoring and control.
- *Constipation*: Prolonged ventilation may contribute to gastrointestinal motility issues, making constipation a common complication that needs to be addressed with appropriate care and interventions.

PMV is a critical challenge in the management of patients in the ICU. Dependence on ventilatory support for prolonged periods of time often requires tailored weaning strategies that gradually reduce and eventually remove mechanical ventilation support.

Understanding the definitions and classifications of weaning is essential to optimizing care in this patient population. The WIND study provides a comprehensive framework for categorizing weaning based on time to weaning and associated outcomes. These classifications—easy, difficult, and prolonged weaning—not only provide a standardized approach to assessing patient progress but also serve as a predictive tool for prognosis and resource allocation.

Table 1.2 highlights the key definitions of weaning from the WIND study and outlines the associated prognostic implications for each category.

Table 1.2 Main definitions of weaning from the WIND study [20] and the associated prognostic implications for each category

Weaning category	Definition	Prognosis
Simple (short)	Weaning completed in less than 24 h after the first separation attempt (including successful extubation)	*Favorable prognosis*: higher success rate in separation from the ventilator, lower mortality, and shorter ICU and hospital stays Prevalence: 77.98% Mortality: 5.8%
Difficult	Weaning completed between 1 and 7 days after the first separation attempt (with successful extubation)	*Moderate prognosis*: intermediate risk of complications, higher mortality, and hospitalization rates compared to simple weaning but better outcomes than prolonged weaning Prevalence: 15.06% Mortality: 16.5%
Prolonged	More than 7 days without successful weaning after the first separation attempt	*Unfavorable prognosis*: higher mortality rate, longer ICU stays, increased healthcare resource utilization, and greater risk of morbidity Prevalence: 12.96% Mortality: 29.8%

Patients in the prolonged weaning category often experience greater morbidity, require prolonged ventilatory support, and have a higher risk of mortality compared to other categories. Implementation of strategies such as early mobilization, optimization of sedation, and nutritional support can significantly improve outcomes in this vulnerable population [23]. The topic of weaning from mechanical ventilation, including its challenges and key strategies, is discussed in detail in the next chapters.

Finally, it is important to highlight the costs associated with this population. The cost of managing PMV-dependent patients in the United States is substantial, with estimates ranging from $10 billion to $30 billion annually. This makes PMV a significant health care problem, accounting for approximately 12% of total hospitalization expenditures in the country. Similarly, a study conducted in a private intensive care unit in southern Brazil found that 9% of patients required prolonged mechanical ventilation, with an average per capita cost of approximately BRL 300,000. This is significantly higher than the cost of treating non-chronic ICU patients, which averages around BRL 65,000. These figures highlight the financial burden of PMV and underscore the need for effective strategies to manage these patients and reduce associated costs [24, 25].

A significant increase in caregiver burden was observed among PMV caregivers. Home-based PMV resulted in higher levels of physical strain, confinement, work adjustments, and financial stress for caregivers. On the other hand, institutional PMV highlighted emotional adjustments, frustration with changes in the patient, disruptive patient behavior, and a sense of being overwhelmed [26].

1.4 Summary

More than 70 years after its first successful application, MV remains a global challenge for modern medicine. Although only a minority of patients require PMV, they represent a very difficult-to-manage group that undoubtedly requires specific diagnostic and therapeutic approaches. In addition, they have a worse prognosis and represent a significant cost to patients, caregivers, and healthcare systems. This requires a holistic view of each individual and their psychosocial context, with the aim of alleviating their suffering and promoting their happiness with the best possible quality of life.

References

1. Cairo JM. Pilbeam's mechanical ventilation: physiological and clinical applications. Elsevier Health Sciences; 2015.
2. Tobin MJ. Principles and practice of mechanical ventilation. 3rd ed. New York: McGraw Hill; 2006.
3. Slutsky AS, History of Mechanical Ventilation. From Vesalius to ventilator-induced lung injury. Am J Respir Crit Care Med. 2015;191(10):1106–15.

4. Associação de Medicina Intensiva Brasileira. Insuficiência Respiratória Aguda. Em: Fundamentos em Terapia Intensiva. 2ª Ed. REVINTER Ltda. 277 p. 2000.
5. Hughes JMB. Pulmonary gas exchange. Eur Respir Mon. 2005;31:106–26.
6. Ceriana P, Nava S. Hypoxic and hypercapnic respiratory failure. Eur Respir Mon. 2006;36:1–15.
7. Chatburn RL. Classification of ventilator modes: update and proposal for implementation. Respir Care. 2007;52(3):301–23.
8. Bonassa J. Ventilação Mecânica: fundamentos e práticas: princípios do funcionamento dos ventiladores artificiais. Rio de Janeiro: Roca; 2016.
9. Ward J, Noel C. Basic modes of mechanical ventilation. Emerg Med Clin North Am. 2022 Aug;40(3):473–88.
10. Barbas CS, Isola AM, Farias AM, Cavalcanti AB, Gama AM, Duarte AC, et al. Brazilian recommendations of mechanical ventilation 2013. Part I Rev Bras Ter Intensiva. 2014;26(2):89–121.
11. Barbas CS, Ísola AM, Farias AM, Cavalcanti AB, Gama AM, Duarte AC, et al. Brazilian recommendations of mechanical ventilation 2013. Part 2. Rev Bras Ter Intensiva. 2014;26(3):215–239.
12. Carvalho CRR. Ventilação Mecânica. Volume I – Básico. Clínicas Brasileiras de Medicina Intensiva, São Paulo: Ed. Atheneu; 2000.
13. Carvalho CRR. Ventilação Mecânica. Volume II – Avançado. Clínicas Brasileiras de Medicina Intensiva, São Paulo: Ed. Atheneu; 2000.
14. Chatburn RL, Primiano FPJr. A new system for understanding modes of mechanical ventilation. Respir Care. 2001;46(6):604–21.
15. Grippi MA. Respiratory failure: an overview. In: Fishman AP, Elias AJ, Fishman JA, Grippi MA, Senior RM, Pack AL, editors. Fishman's pulmonary diseases and disorders. 4th ed. New York: McGraw Hill; 2008. p. 2509–21.
16. Branson R, Chatburn RL, Hess D. Respiratory care equipment. 2nd ed. Philadelphia: Lippincot; 1998.
17. Damuth E, et al. Long-term survival of critically ill patients treated with prolonged mechanical ventilation: a systematic review and meta-analysis. Lancet Respir Med. 2015;3(7):544–53.
18. Huang SW, Lin HC, Chou YF, Lin TY, Lo CY, Huang HY, et al. The impact of higher protein intake in patients with prolonged mechanical ventilation. Nutrients. 2022;14(20):4395.
19. Boles JM, Bion J, Connors A, Herridge M, Marsh B, Melot C, et al. Weaning from mechanical ventilation. Eur Respir J. 2007;29(5):1033–56.
20. Béduneau G, Pham T, Schortgen F, Piquilloud L, Zogheib E, Jonas M, et al. Epidemiology of weaning outcome according to a new definition. The WIND study. Am J Respir Crit Care Med. 2017;195:772–83.
21. MacIntyre NR, Epstein SK, Carson S, Scheinhorn D, Christopher K, Muldoon S. National Association for medical direction of respiratory care. Management of patients requiring prolonged mechanical ventilation: report of a NAMDRC consensus conference. Chest. 2005;128(6):3937–54.
22. Loss SH. Ventilação Mecânica Prolongada. In: VALIATTI, Jorge Luis dos Santos. Ventilação Mecânica: Fundamentos e prática clínica. Rio de Janeiro: Guanabara Koogan; 2021. p. 778–81.
23. Trudzinski FC, Neetz B, Dahlhoff JC, Wilkens FM, Katzenschlager S, Fähndrich S, et al. A multidimensional approach to the management of patients in prolonged weaning from mechanical ventilation: the concept of treatable traits – a narrative review. Respiration. 2024:1–15. https://doi.org/10.1159/000541965. Epub ahead of print
24. Zanella A, Taboada M, Costa ELV, et al. Cost of prolonged mechanical ventilation in a Brazilian private intensive care unit: a retrospective cohort study. Intensive Care Med. 2023;49(4):568–75. https://doi.org/10.1007/s00134-023-06891-7.
25. Torres A, González-Rivas J, Díaz E, et al. The economic burden of prolonged mechanical ventilation in critically ill patients. J Crit Care. 2022;67:42–8. https://doi.org/10.1016/j.jcrc.2022.03.012.
26. Marcus EL, Jacobs JM, Stessman J. Prolonged mechanical ventilation and caregiver strain: home vs. long-term care facility. Palliat Support Care. 2023;21(3):429–37.

Chapter 2
Principles of Weaning from Invasive Mechanical Ventilation

Antuani Rafael Baptistella, Daniel Lago Borges, and Luis Felipe da Fonseca Reis

2.1 Introduction

During the evolutionary events that formed the current Earth's atmosphere, the increase in O_2 levels that allowed the planet to be surrounded by O_2 probably favored the survival of organisms capable of tolerating its toxicity and safely using the gas to generate energy. The increase in atmospheric oxygen is probably the most significant event in the evolution of human life. To make this process possible, the respiratory system is essential. The lung is the gas exchange organ that provides oxygen and removes carbon dioxide from the blood, and breathing is one of the most primitive functions of the human body. As a basic bodily function, spontaneous breathing is vitally important. The goal of the weaning process is to restore this basic and vital function to the patient [1, 2].

The process of weaning, discontinuing, or withdrawing mechanical ventilation (MV) is an essential and universal issue in the care of critically ill patients, and its

A. R. Baptistella (✉)
Hospital Universitário Santa Terezinha (HUST), Joaçaba, Brazil

Hospital Unimed Meio-Oeste, Joaçaba, Brazil

Universidade do Oeste de Santa Catarina, Unoesc, Joaçaba, Brazil
e-mail: antuani.baptistella@unoesc.edu.br

D. L. Borges
Hospital Universitário of Maranhão Federal University (HUUFMA), São Luis, Maranhão, Brazil

L. F. da Fonseca Reis
Hospital Universitário Gafree Guinle – HUGG-UNIRio, Rio de Janeiro, Brazil

Hospital Central da Polícia Militar do Estado do Rio de Janeiro, Rio de Janeiro, Brazil

Centro Universitário Augusto Motta (UNISUAM), Rio de Janeiro, Brazil

A. R. Baptistella et al. (eds.), *Weaning from Mechanical Ventilation*,
https://doi.org/10.1007/978-3-032-01145-9_2

management can affect the patient's outcome. This process should be initiated as soon as possible, taking into account the control or resolution of the cause that placed the patient on the ventilator [3–5].

The majority of ventilated patients can be weaned without significant problems; however, in approximately 20% of patients, the weaning period is significantly prolonged [6]. In these cases, it has been estimated that the weaning process can take up 42% of the total mechanical ventilation time [7], making it an important focus of critical care research. Many topics related to weaning continue to be widely discussed by the scientific community and experts in the field, such as the criteria for starting weaning, the most appropriate time and method, and failure management, among others, which will be discussed later in this chapter.

2.2 History of Mechanical Ventilation Weaning

Since the first patient was connected to a mechanical ventilator, its operator started to think about how to wean the patient from the ventilator. Therefore, the history of weaning from mechanical ventilation (MV) began with the history of MV.

Although ventilator support was already mentioned in the Bible, Hippocrates' description of tracheal intubation of a human being for artificial ventilation is the first medical report about this process [8]. Nearly 2000 years later, Paracelsus performed many experiments in which a tube was placed in a patient's mouth and air was blown through bellows with the goal of resuscitating the patient. In the 1700s, the discovery of the importance of oxygen for respiration influenced the development of artificial ventilation, leading to the first reported case of mouth-to-mouth resuscitation of a miner rescued from a coal mine by William Tossach in 1774 [9]. A few years later, in 1780, Chaussier presented the first apparatus for noninvasive mechanical ventilation, consisting of a manual bag and mask ventilator [10].

From this point in the history of MV, it is possible to divide the development of MV in a chronological way: negative pressure ventilators, positive pressure noninvasive ventilators (NIV), and positive pressure invasive ventilators with four generations. Some of these types of ventilation coexist during one period [8].

Negative pressure ventilators were the main devices used to artificially ventilate patients in the nineteenth century and the first half of the twentieth century. The description of a full-body ventilator, the "tank ventilator," by John Dalziel in 1838 marked the beginning of the period of negative pressure ventilators [11]. The first working "iron lung," called "spirophore," was developed by the Frenchman Eugene Woillez and presented in 1876 [12], but he was limited by the lack of funding for the project [9]. Subsequently, several models were developed (Eisenmenger in 1901, Sauerbruch in 1904, Hammond in 1905, and Schwake in 1926), but it was not until 1928, with the design of a new iron lung model by Drinker and Shaw [13], that negative pressure ventilation became a clinical reality, playing a fundamental role in the global poliomyelitis epidemics of the next 30 years [14].

After the manual bag and mask ventilator, a much more sophisticated apparatus for noninvasive positive pressure ventilation was developed by Fell in 1887. In 1910, Green and Janeway presented the "rhythmic inflation apparatus," and in 1911, Drager's Pulmotor was introduced, which saved several patients in the following years [8, 10]. However, the most notable ventilators for positive pressure NIV were the Bennett TV and PR and the Bird Mark, both designed in the twentieth century and widely used for life support in the 1960s and 1970s [8].

Invasive positive pressure ventilation was introduced in the 1940s and 1950s and represented a major advance in MV for life support, although it initially provided only volume-controlled ventilation, without patient triggering, monitor, alarms, positive end-expiratory pressure (PEEP), or specific settings. This first generation of ventilators was used until the early 1970s, when the second generation was introduced with some important improvements, as a simple monitor showing tidal volume and respiratory rate, beyond the patient-triggered inspiration and basic alarms. At the end of this generation, the Servo 900C introduced pressure support and pressure control ventilation [15], and in the late 1970s, Hewlett demonstrated the concept of closed-loop ventilation, both of which are still used today. The third generation of ventilators was characterized by microprocessor control, a major event in the development of MV, which allowed any approach to gas delivery and monitoring, flow triggering, that improved the ventilator's response to the patient's needs. These ventilators were the first to display pressure, flow, and volume waveforms beyond the pressure-volume and flow-volume loops [16]. Finally, the fourth generation added a wide variety of ventilation modes, including NIV, high technology aimed at very precise gas delivery, monitoring of multiple parameters, good usability, and user interaction experience, in addition to automated ventilation, which may be the future of MV.

From the eighteenth century until the beginning of modern MV, there was no published knowledge on the pathophysiology of weaning, weaning techniques, predictive tests, or even standardized protocols [17].

The first published study showing results of MV weaning in poliomyelitis patients with respiratory failure was published by Batson and Riley in 1956 [18]. In the early days of intensive care in the United States, a few patients were ventilated for more than 2 days without a tracheostomy. In the first textbook published in the field in 1965, Bendixin and colleagues [19] wrote: "it is our practice to limit endotracheal intubation to approximately forty-eight hours." They also addressed an issue that is still debated today: "to know the proper timing and rate of weaning from the respirator requires considerable judgment and experience. As a rule, weaning should start as soon as possible."

One of the first approaches to weaning a patient from the ventilator was also described by Bendixin and colleagues in the 1960s and was based on taking the patient off the ventilator for 3 or 4 min every half hour and, if tolerated, increasing the time off as rapidly as tolerated [19]. In the 1970s, to be extubated, a patient had to reach a level of recovery, especially from a functional standpoint, that was much higher than what is considered appropriate today. As a list of criteria for extubation,

Egan suggested that the patient should be able to walk short distances consistent with his or her general physical condition. He also listed other criteria: breathing unassisted around the clock, moving a reasonable amount of air without undue effort, satisfactory ventilation, and stable blood gas values [20].

In the 1980s, nearly all weaning attempts were performed using intermittent mandatory ventilation (IMV), which seemed to shorten the weaning period [21], made possible by the development of second-generation ventilators, which made patient-triggered inspiration available in clinical practice. In 1981, pressure support ventilation became available, a novelty introduced by the Servo 900C ventilator [8].

In addition to the advent of patient triggering and pressure support ventilation, several advances have been fundamental milestones in the history of weaning, and the most important are discussed below.

The *predictive tests* used to determine the readiness of patients to be safely weaned from the ventilator marked the beginning of weaning research [17]. The first predictors of successful weaning were minute ventilation <10 l/min and maximal inspiratory pressure > 30 cmH_2O, reported by Sahn and Lakshminarayan in 1973 [22]. In the 1980s, Herrera [23], Sassoon [24], and colleagues reported that a low P0.1 could predict weaning success. The first index integrating different respiratory characteristics was the CROP index, composed of lung compliance, respiratory rate, oxygenation, and maximal inspiratory pressure, proposed by Yang and Tobin in 1991 [25], based on the Milic-Emili proposal published in 1986 [26]. In the same study [25], Yang and Tobin presented the rapid shallow breathing index (RSBI) or f/VT as the most accurate test to predict weaning/extubation outcome. For the first time, a predictor was tested in an experimental design with a validation data set, and the results were presented with important values such as sensitivity, specificity, positive predictive value, negative predictive value, and receiver operating characteristic (ROC) curves. Although many predictive tests have been published since then, this study was a major milestone in the history of weaning, being the most used predictive test to date [27].

Until the 1970s, no significant findings were published on the *pathophysiology of weaning*. It was not until 1977 when Henning and colleagues [28] made detailed measurements of the work of breathing using an esophageal balloon catheter and showed that ventilator-dependent patients had higher work values. In 1982, Cohen and colleagues used electromyography to show that weaning failure was related not only to lung status but also to the respiratory muscle pump [29], and Tobin and colleagues suggested that respiratory center depression, respiratory muscle fatigue, and ventilation-perfusion abnormalities were the mechanisms involved in weaning failure [30].

Until the 1980s, it was thought that a patient connected to a ventilator reduced muscle work to near zero. However, in 1985, Marini and colleagues demonstrated that patients receiving assist-control ventilation performed half the work of the ventilator [31]. In two studies by Brochard and colleagues [32, 33] measuring transdiaphragmatic pressure, electromyography, and work of breathing, they determined the level of pressure support that avoided fatigue but still maintained diaphragmatic activity.

The use of inert gas techniques allowed Torres and colleagues to link acute hypercapnia and ventilation-perfusion maldistribution to rapid shallow breathing [34]. In the early 1990s, Bates and colleagues used the rapid airway occlusion technique to characterize respiratory mechanics and reported the contribution of the chest wall to mechanical disturbances, a process involved in weaning failure [35, 36].

The spontaneous breathing trial (SBT) only became a common practice in intensive care units around the world in the 1990s. Prior to this, Downs and colleagues proposed the concept of the T-piece applied to the IMV for weaning, based on the T-piece introduced by Ayre in 1937 as a valveless anesthesia system for children [37]. In 1989, Tomlinson and colleagues [38] published a randomized controlled trial (RTC) comparing weaning with IMV and T-piece, and in 1994, Brochard and colleagues [32] showed in an RTC that at 21 days, ventilator dependence was less with pressure support than with IMV or T-piece. This study was in contrast to the RTC published by Esteban and colleagues in 1995, where the T-piece proved to be better than pressure support [39]. The best method of SBT is still unclear at this time [40], but the need to perform SBT before extubating a patient is unanimous in the critical care scientific community.

The introduction of the IMV as a mode of ventilation to aid in weaning opened the discussion of *sedation management* as an important step in the weaning process. In 1985, Willatts wrote that the introduction of the IMV could reduce the need for sedation and facilitate weaning [41]. In 1986, the use of ketamine to sedate ICU patients was described [42], and in 1987, the use of propofol was described [43]. Two years later, Aitkenhead and colleagues showed that weaning from mechanical ventilation was significantly faster with propofol than with midazolam [44]. At that time, the use of pressure support ventilation was correlated with less need for sedation [45]. In 1998, Kollef and colleagues showed that the use of continuous intravenous sedation may be associated with prolongation of mechanical ventilation [46]. In 2000, Kress and his colleagues demonstrated for the first time that daily interruption of sedative drug infusions decreased the duration of mechanical ventilation and the length of stay in the intensive care unit [47]. This practice is still used today.

In 1977, Egan suggested that the patient should already be walking short distances consistently to be weaned from MV. Despite the fact that the work of the physiotherapist in the ICU has been discussed for decades since the inception of these units and the concept of mobilization of critically ill patients, *early mobilization* became a common practice only after the 2000s. In 2005, Martin and colleagues demonstrated that weaning outcome improved in chronically ventilated patients after aggressive whole-body and respiratory muscle training [48], and in 2008, Morris and colleagues proposed a mobility protocol that was associated with reduced ICU and hospital length of stay [49]. In the 2010s, the ABCDE bundles proposed early mobility and exercise (E) as one of the essential strategies to "liberate and animate" ventilated ICU patients [50]. Since then, early mobilization has become a common practice for patients under MV.

The use of *noninvasive ventilation after extubation* as an effective method to facilitate weaning was introduced in the 2000s. Nava and colleagues in 2005 and

Ferrer and colleagues in 2006 showed that NIV prevents respiratory failure after extubation in high-risk patients [51, 52]. Three years later, the same group [53] showed that NIV is a good weaning strategy for hypercapnic patients with chronic respiratory diseases, and in 2011, Khilnani and colleagues confirmed these results specifically for patients with chronic obstructive pulmonary disease (COPD) [54]. After these first evidences, NIV after extubation was considered as a good weaning method by different guidelines [3, 5] and meta-analyses [55].

All these milestones, together with other knowledge built up over the last 80 years, allow us to have a broader understanding of weaning and, more importantly, to look forward to what remains to be discovered to improve the outcomes of patients with MV.

2.3 Definition of Weaning

The term "weaning" means to detach from a source of dependence, suggesting a gradual process, and is universally used to describe the process of MV discontinuation or withdrawal. Weaning encompasses the entire process of liberating the patient from MV support and from the endotracheal tube [3].

Weaning should begin when the cause of the patient's need for MV is controlled or resolved, but there is no consensus on the objective point at which the care team should begin weaning. The S2k guideline published by the German Respiratory Society [6] established that the weaning process begins with SBT, while more recently the International Working Group on Mechanical Ventilation (WeVent) [56] proposed that weaning begins with the transition from controlled assisted mode to partial support mode (pressure support ventilation-PSV (pressure support ventilation) or continuous positive airway pressure-CPAP/PEEP).

It is well known that before weaning begins and after weaning is completed, patients go through several stages that require intensive care. Before weaning begins, the cause of respiratory failure must be treated, the patient's sedation must be managed, and intermittent screening for weaning is indicated. Once weaning is complete, the patient must be closely monitored for early management of potential extubation failure.

A six-step weaning process for an intubated patient is proposed here (Fig. 2.1):

First step: Transition from a controlled assisted mode to a partial support mode
Second step: When the ventilator support is gradually reduced—e.g., inspiratory support pressure, PEEP, and FiO_2
Third step: Assessment of spontaneous breathing readiness using the SBT
Fourth step: Extubation outcome prediction tests to assess the risk of failure due to airway-related causes (airway patency/protection tests) and non-airway-related failure.
Fifth step: Extubation.
Sixth step: Post-extubation monitoring/weaning consolidation.

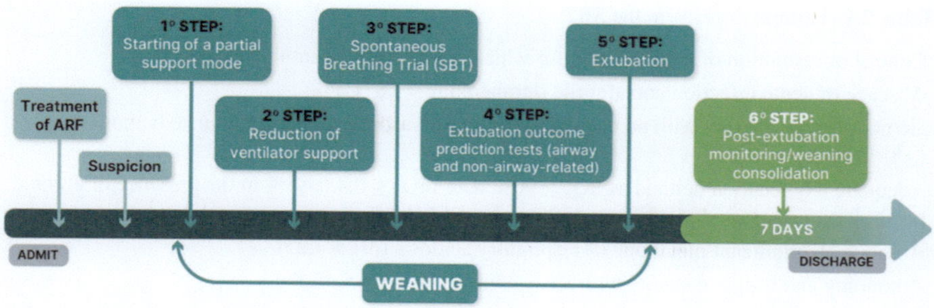

Fig. 2.1 Schematic representation of the six steps of weaning from mechanical ventilation. *ARF* acute respiratory failure, *Suspicion* suspicion that weaning may be possible, *SBT* spontaneous breathing trial. (Adapted from Boles et al. [3])

An international task force provided a definition of weaning success and failure in 2007 [3]. Weaning success was defined as an extubated patient not requiring ventilatory support for at least 48 h after extubation, whereas weaning failure was defined as an unsuccessful SBT or reintubation/recannulation with resumption of MV or death within 48 h of extubation. More recently, the WEAN SAFE trial and the Practical Guidelines on Mechanical Ventilation of the Brazilian Association of Intensive Care Medicine (AMIB) and the Brazilian Society of Pulmonology and Phthisiology (SBPT) defined weaning success as extubation without death or reintubation within the next 7 days [57, 58].

Based on the 2007 Task Force definition, a patient who is successfully ventilated with NIV after extubation or decannulation is not actually weaned and has been placed in an intermediate category known as "weaning in progress" [3]. The S2k guideline defines patients undergoing prolonged weaning as successfully weaned if after completion of the weaning process (extubation or decannulation) they remain dependent on NIV in an outpatient setting or even tracheostomized, MV is no longer required [6].

2.3.1 *When Is the Right Time to Start Weaning?*

Although MV is a life-saving procedure, it is also associated with complications. For this reason, it is indicated to liberate patients from MV as soon as the cause that led the patient to MV has been controlled or resolved, and the patient is able to maintain spontaneous breathing and adequate gas exchange [5].

Unnecessary delays in this weaning process increase the rate of mechanical ventilation complications (e.g., pneumonia, airway trauma), worsen prognosis, and increase hospital length of stay and costs. On the other hand, premature removal of the ventilator can lead to the need for reintubation, difficulty in reestablishing the artificial airway, impaired gas exchange, increased risk of nosocomial pneumonia, and prolonged ICU stay. In fact, both scenarios are associated with a significantly

Table 2.1 Criteria to perform the SBT

Control or resolution of the condition for which the patient was intubated
Absence of acute infection and afebrile (temperature < 38 °C)
Hemodynamic stability with no or minimal need for vasopressors and adequate hemoglobin (≥8–10 g/dL)
Adequate oxygenation defined as $SO_2 \geq 90\%$ with $FiO_2 \leq 0.4$ (>85% in the presence of chronic respiratory failure), or $PaO_2/FiO_2 > 150$ mm hg, PEEP ≤10
Absence of significant metabolic or respiratory acidosis (pH > 7.25)
Autonomy and trigger capacity with RR ≤35/min and VT >5 mL/kg
Absence of sedation or adequate function under sedation (RASS 0/−1)

increased risk of mortality [6]. Accidental self-extubation does not lead to reintubation in nearly 50% of cases, demonstrating that extubation is often delayed [59].

With the goal of initiating weaning at the right time, researchers have proposed objective and subjective criteria over the past three decades to guide the initiation of weaning.

2.3.2 *Weaning Criteria*

Weaning must be initiated as soon as possible, but in order to reduce the duration of mechanical ventilation and increase the likelihood of successful weaning, several prerequisites must be met. Readiness for weaning is based on a number of parameters involving different organs and systems and is not predictive of weaning or extubation. The goal is to indicate which patient is ready to initiate MV weaning.

The first SBT can be planned if the patient meets the following criteria, which are presented in Table 2.1 [3, 4, 6, 56, 57]:

2.4 Classification of Weaning

Weaning can account for 40%–55% of ventilator time [3, 60]. The International Consensus Conference (ICC) classification of weaning is referred to as easy (successful at the first spontaneous breathing trial—SBT), difficult (successful up to the third SBT in the first 7 days), or prolonged if weaning takes longer than 7 days [3, 57]. Recently, a new classification (WIND classification) has been proposed, which defines the initiation of weaning as any type of separation attempt (without taking into account a previous reduction in ventilatory support), calculates the duration of this process and its prognosis, and proposes the following definitions [60]:

For Intubated Patients

Attempted weaning from mechanical ventilation:

SBT with or without extubation, or direct extubation without identified SBT (planned or unplanned extubation, regardless of type).

Successful weaning or separation: Either extubation without death or reintubation within the next 7 days, or discharge from the ICU without invasive ventilation within 7 days, regardless of whether noninvasive ventilation (NIV) was used after extubation. First successful weaning dates were counted retrospectively to the actual extubation date after the patient had gone 7 days without reintubation (or was discharged earlier without reintubation).

For Tracheostomized Patients

Attempted weaning from mechanical ventilation: Spontaneous ventilation via tracheostomy without mechanical ventilation for 24 h or more.

Successful weaning or weaning separation: Spontaneous ventilation via tracheostomy without mechanical ventilation for seven consecutive days or discharge with spontaneous breathing, whichever came first.

Thus, four mutually exclusive groups were proposed based on the duration of the weaning process (i.e., the delay between the first attempt to wean from mechanical ventilation and the completion of weaning), as shown in Table 2.2, including the differences between the ICC and WIND classifications:

The longer the duration of MV, the higher the morbidity [ventilator-associated pneumonia (VAP), ventilator-associated tracheobronchitis (VAT), airway trauma, and mortality] [60, 61]. The incidence of weaning failure varies from 14% to 32% (average 21%). According to Boles and colleagues [3], patients with weaning failure and subsequent prolonged ventilation, although representing only 7% of all ventilated patients, consume 37% of ICU resources. Thus, weaning failure is not only detrimental to the patient but also to the institution and the burden of healthcare in general.

Table 2.2 Classification of ventilator weaning

Classification	ICC	WIND
Group 1	Simple weaning: successful extubation after one SBT	Short weaning: successful separation from MV or death within 24 h
Group 2	Difficult weaning: successful extubation after up to three SBTs in less than 7 days	Difficult weaning: successful separation from MV or death in 1–7 days
Group 3	Prolonged weaning: successful extubation after more than three SBTs or more than 7 days	Prolonged weaning: unsuccessful separation 7 days after the first attempt Subgroup A: eventually separated from MV; B: not separated from MV
Group “no weaning”	–	No separation attempt from MV

ICC international consensus conference (Boules et al. 2007), *WIND* weaning outcome according to a new definition (Béduneau et al. [60]), *MV* mechanical ventilation

2.5 What Modes of Ventilation Should Be Used for Weaning?

Many different modes or methods are used to assess the adequacy of ventilation during weaning. According to the literature, no mode or technique is superior to others in terms of early extubation, reintubation rate, or increase in ventilator-free days.

Initial success with the use of PSV is associated with a shorter weaning period, but it may underestimate the work of breathing that may be required after extubation. It has been suggested that it may be associated with a higher risk of extubation failure. Sklar et al. suggested that PSV may compensate for the additional work imposed by the endotracheal tube, thereby reducing external work of breathing and oxygen consumption by the respiratory muscles during SBT [62]. Daily SBTs led to early extubation in a study by Esteban et al. compared to gradual PSV or SIMV, otherwise known as synchronized intermittent mechanical ventilation, weaning [39]. Brochard et al. compared three methods of gradual weaning from ventilatory support and concluded that gradual PSV weaning had a shorter weaning duration and higher weaning success, including extubation, compared with daily T-piece SBT or SIMV weaning. SIMV and CPAP are no longer used routinely [32].

Closed-loop weaning systems, an automated system that uses physiologic feedback to adjust the weaning process, can facilitate systematic and early identification of spontaneous breathing capacity and the potential for weaning through continuous monitoring and real-time intervention. The concept of closed-loop weaning systems is not new; however, with advanced technology from academia and industry, SmartCare is the first commercial closed-loop system with intelligent modes in clinical use, and adaptive support ventilation, neurally adjusted ventilatory assist, and proportional assisted ventilation (PAV) have been further developed in recent decades. In current studies, closed-loop weaning systems show clinical benefit in terms of reduced weaning time, mechanical ventilation, and ICU length of stay [63, 64].

PAV was first introduced by Younes in 1992 and adjusted the inspiratory pressure proportional to the flow and volume generated by the patient. New software (PAV+) has been developed based on PAV to adapt to clinical needs through semi-continuous measurements and deliver pressure proportional to instantaneous inspiratory flow and volume [63, 65]. PAV is a spontaneous ventilation modality that uses the equation of motion to provide inspiratory pressure (Pvent) proportional to patient effort (Pmus). As the patient's effort is reduced, ventilator assistance is also reduced [66, 67]. PAV+ estimates the work of breathing (WOB) of the patient and the ventilator using the equation of motion and calculates compliance and resistance by applying 300 ms inspiratory micropauses every four to ten ventilator cycles. The main operational advantage of the PAV+ is its automatic synchronization with the patient's inspiratory flow and its adaptability to changes in ventilatory demand. In a meta-analysis, PAV+ showed advantages in reducing the rate of weaning failure and the duration of mechanical ventilation compared to pressure support ventilation. Another meta-analysis found that PAV increased the rate of successful weaning and decreased the proportion of patients requiring reintubation and the length of ICU stay, but did not reduce mortality compared with pressure support ventilation [63, 67].

Other closed-loop ventilation modes have been used in clinical practice, such as adaptive ventilation modes, such as adaptive support ventilation (ASV), a closed-loop controlled ventilator mode used to optimize the patient's work of breathing. A maximum plateau pressure and desired minute ventilation are set, and the ventilatory pattern is automatically selected according to the settings and respiratory mechanics. Neurally adjusted ventilatory assist (NAVA) is a mode of partial ventilatory support in which the proportion of ventilatory support (timing and intensity) is determined by respiratory drive. Respiratory drive is measured by the electrical activity of the diaphragm. Dongelmans et al. showed ASV to be a safer and more useful mode, while extubation time was similar to other modes [68]. Another author tried ASV in chronic respiratory patients and found it to be a cost-saving option in terms of the need for ICU-trained staff and respiratory therapists, and showed that ASV can be used as a weaning mode in severe COPD patients with the benefit of a shorter weaning time [69]. A recent meta-analysis by Yuan et al. concluded that compared with PSV, NAVA was associated with a higher chance of successful weaning, more ventilator-free days, shorter MV duration, and lower hospital mortality [70].

Thus, although a recent systematic review showed promising results with the use of PAV mode, this, as well as other closed-loop ventilation modes such as NAVA and ASV, is not widely available for large-scale use. Perhaps for this reason, the standardized recommendations of weaning guidelines advocate the use of PSV to the detriment of closed-loop ventilation modalities. Therefore, advanced closed-loop mechanical ventilation modes such as PAV, NAVA, ASV, and SmartCare should be restricted to the expertise of services and during individualization of care.

2.6 Spontaneous Breathing Trial (SBT)

The spontaneous breathing trial (SBT) is the final step in the weaning process and is considered a formal assessment of readiness for extubation. It is performed with minimal or no ventilatory support to assess the patient's ability to breathe spontaneously. The SBT can be performed in several ways, including the use of a T-piece, PSV, CPAP, and automatic tube compensation (ATC) [71, 72].

Fig. 2.2 Patient undergoing SBT with T-piece. (Sources: Image by the authors)

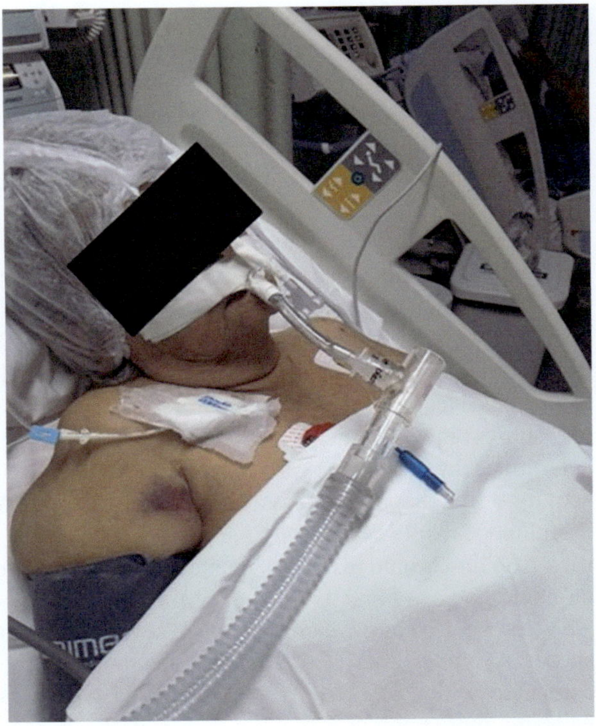

2.6.1 Types of SBT [73]

- T-piece: In this format, supplemental oxygen is delivered through a T-piece connected directly to the endotracheal tube (Fig. 2.2).
- CPAP: Only a low pressure (PEEP) is used.
- PSV (<8 cmH_2O): A low or zero level of support pressure is maintained, with or without PEEP.
- ATC: An option available on some ventilators that compensates for the drop in resistive pressure due to the presence of the endotracheal tube.

2.6.2 Duration of the SBT

A collective task force in 2001 recommended that the SBT should take between 30 and 120 min. In other words, it is necessary to wait at least 30 min to assess tolerance to the test, but one should not wait more than 120 min if tolerance to the test is not clear [4, 74].

The first few minutes of the SBT should be monitored closely to determine whether to continue or interrupt the test. Increased diaphragmatic activity, reflecting

Table 2.3 Criteria for considering discontinuation of SBT

Gas exchange	Hemodynamic	Ventilatory pattern
Objective measures		
$SpO_2 < 85\%–90\%$ $PaO_2 < 50–60$ mmHg pH < 7.32 Increase in $PaCO_2 > 10$ mmHg	HR > 120–140 bpm HR variation >20% Systolic BP > 180–200 mmHg or < 90 mmHg BP variation >20% No need for vasopressors	RR > 30–35 bpm RR variation >50%
Subjective measures		
Change in mental status (e.g., drowsiness, coma, agitation, anxiety) Onset or worsening of respiratory discomfort Sweating Signs of increased respiratory effort (use of accessory respiratory muscles, paradoxical breathing)		

BP blood pressure, *HR* heart rate, $PaCO_2$ arterial partial pressure of carbon dioxide, *PaO_2* arterial partial pressure of oxygen, *RR* respiratory rate, *SpO_2* peripheral oxygen saturation

increased respiratory effort, during the first few minutes of the SBT is likely to be associated with weaning failure [74, 75].

Some studies have compared shorter SBTs (20 or 30 min) with longer SBTs (120 min) and found no significant differences in extubation success and reintubation rates [76–78].

2.6.3 *Signs of Intolerance to SBT*

SBT can be interrupted for a variety of reasons that can be assessed objectively or subjectively (Table 2.3). These criteria should be interpreted in the clinical context, taking into account variations in baseline values, rather than as rigid limits [74].

In case of SBT intolerance (weaning failure), the patient should be returned to ventilatory support, providing comfort and adequate gas exchange for 24 h before repeating the test, with identification of the cause of failure [40, 79].

2.6.4 *What Is the Best Way to Perform the SBT?*

There is no definitive evidence that one approach is superior to another in terms of clinical outcomes.

A large observational study showed that initial SBT was more often performed with PSV with PEEP (49.1%) or T-piece (25.4%), and less often with CPAP (10.8%) or PSV without PEEP (9.5%) [80].

In 2014, a Cochrane review concluded that there was no difference between T-piece and PSV testing with respect to extubation failure and mortality, with low-quality evidence. When considering only patients who successfully completed SBT with simple weaning, the PSV test was considered superior to the T-piece, with moderate-quality evidence [81].

A physiological systematic review showed that patients' respiratory efforts, as assessed by physiological measures, are significantly affected by different types of SBT. Among the types, PSV reduces respiratory effort compared to T-piece testing, and both PSV0/PEEP0 and T-piece appear to more accurately reflect post-extubation physiological conditions [62].

A meta-analysis comparing different SBT techniques found that although there was no prediction of success, patients undergoing SBT in PSV with or without PEEP had an approximately 6% greater chance of remaining extubated compared to T-piece [72]. Therefore, the American Thoracic Society (ATS) and American College of Chest Physicians (ACCP) guidelines issued a conditional recommendation to perform initial SBT in PSV (PS 5–8 cmH_2O) in acutely hospitalized patients ventilated for more than 24 h [82].

Comparing a 30-min SBT with PS of 8 cmH_2O without PEEP (less demanding technique) with a 2-h SBT with T-piece (more demanding technique) in patients intubated for at least 24 h, PSV was found to increase the extubation success rate (defined here as maintenance of spontaneous ventilation for 72 h after the first SBT) by 8.2% without increasing the reintubation rate [78].

In patients intubated for more than 24 h and considered at "high risk" for reintubation (elderly or with any chronic cardiac or pulmonary disease), no difference in ventilation-free days and extubation and reintubation rates was observed when PSV and T-piece SBTs were compared [40].

After successful SBT, whether performed with PSV, CPAP, or T-piece, 1 h of rest on the ventilator with pre-test parameters may reduce reintubation rates within 48 h of extubation in patients intubated for at least 12 h [83].

To date, it remains uncertain which technique or method of performing the SBT is best. It is also unclear which patient profiles may benefit from specific SBT techniques. Therefore, the idea of proper screening for the initiation of SBT is worth considering. More importantly, continuous monitoring during the process to detect early signs of intolerance and avoid prolongation of the test and possible clinical deterioration of the patient is also crucial.

2.7 Extubation

After a successful SBT, it is critical to perform a thorough assessment to determine suitability for extubation. This assessment includes a detailed analysis of factors that may contribute to extubation failure (Table 2.4).

Other factors associated with extubation failure, with their respective likelihood ratios and risk ratios, are presented in Table 2.5 [84]:

Table 2.4 Risk factors for extubation failure [73]

Failure of two or more consecutive spontaneous breathing trials
Chronic heart failure
$PaCO_2 > 45$ mmHg after extubation
More than one coexisting condition other than heart failure
Upper airway stridor on extubation
Age > 65 years
APACHE II score > 12 on the day of extubation
Pneumonia as a cause of respiratory failure

Table 2.5 Variables associated with extubation failure

Variable	Likelihood ratio	Risk ratio (95% CI)
Cough peak flow ≤60 L/min	2.2	4.8 (1.4–16.2)
Secretions ≥2.5 mL/h	1.9	3.0 (1.01–8.8)
Unable to perform all four tasks (open eyes, follow with eyes, grasp hand, and stick out tongue)	4.5	4.3 (1.8–10.4)
Any two of the above risks	3.8	6.7 (2.3–19.3)

Although a few studies have examined how extubation decisions are made, they should be patient-centered and consider [85]:

(1) A dynamic assessment of each patient's extubation readiness and the risks and consequences of failure
(2) A plan for extubation failure
(3) Reducing the risk of extubation failure with strategic interventions before or after extubation

Extubation failure is characterized by the need for reintubation within 48 h of extubation, although more recent publications have considered a period of 7 days [57, 58]. Reintubation is directly associated with prolonged ICU and hospital stay and increased incidence of tracheostomy [86].

The reintubation rate, which is calculated by dividing the number of reintubated patients by the total number of extubated patients, is widely used as an indicator of the effectiveness of the weaning process in the ICU. An excessively high rate indicates that weaning is being performed prematurely, while an excessively low rate indicates the use of unnecessary conservative practices. A reintubation rate between 5% and 20% is generally considered acceptable [74].

Post-extubation management should be planned before the procedure to ensure clarity of action in the event of clinical deterioration of the patient. Patients who show signs of respiratory failure after extubation should be immediately reintubated [85].

2.7.1 *Cuff Leak Test (CLT)*

Post-extubation stridor due to airway edema potentially increases the risk of reintubation. The CLT can identify airway edema and guide steroid therapy to increase extubation success rates [87].

The ATS/ACCP recommends that CLT be performed in adult mechanically ventilated patients who meet extubation criteria and have risk factors for post-extubation stridor, including traumatic intubation, intubation for more than 6 days, large endotracheal tube, female sex, and reintubation after unplanned extubation (conditional recommendation, very low certainty of evidence) [82].

For adults who have a positive CLT (presence of edema) but are ready for extubation, the ATS/ACCP suggests systemic steroid administration at least 4 h before extubation (conditional recommendation, moderate certainty of evidence), with no need to repeat the CLT before extubation [82].

Table 2.6 describes how to perform the cuff leak test in mechanically ventilated patients [79, 88].

Although CLT can help identify laryngeal edema prior to extubation and reduce the risk of post-extubation stridor, it can also delay extubation due to false-positive results [82].

Some predictors of extubation failure have been described in the literature, as shown in Table 2.7.

Table 2.6 How to perform the cuff leak test in mechanically ventilated patients

1. Before performing the cuff leak test, aspirate tracheal and oral secretions and set the ventilator to assist control mode in volume-controlled ventilation (VCV)
2. With the cuff inflated, record the inspiratory and expiratory tidal volumes and ensure they are similar
3. Deflate the cuff
4. Record the expiratory tidal volume (VTe) over six respiratory cycles, noting that VTe will plateau after a few cycles
5. If VTe is less than 10% of the inspiratory tidal volume (set) or the difference is greater than 110 ml, the test is considered negative (for edema)

Table 2.7 Predictors of extubation failure [89]

Airway failure	Non-airway failure
Female gender Baseline pathology with coma as the reason for intubation Acute respiratory failure as the reason for intubation Duration of mechanical ventilation >8 days Copious secretions at the time of extubation Absence of strong cough before extubation	Nonobese status Baseline pathology with coma as the reason for intubation Acute respiratory failure as the reason for intubation Absence of strong cough before extubation Sequential organ failure assessment (SOFA) score ≥ 8

References

1. Bailey DM. Oxygen, evolution and redox signalling in the human brain; quantum in the quotidian. J Physiol. 2019;597:15–28.
2. Carvalho O, Maina JN. Respiratory system. Em: Brüne M, Schiefenhövel W, organizadores. Oxf Handb Evol Med [Internet]. Oxford University Press; 2019 [citado 8 de outubro de 2024]. p. 485–530. Recuperado de: https://academic.oup.com/edited-volume/27973/chapter/211624992.
3. Boles J-M, Bion J, Connors A, Herridge M, Marsh B, Melot C, et al. Weaning from mechanical ventilation. Eur Respir J. 2007;29:1033–56.
4. MacIntyre NR, Cook DJ, Ely EW, Epstein SK, Fink JB, Heffner JE, et al. Evidence-based guidelines for weaning and discontinuing ventilatory support: a collective task force facilitated by the American College of Chest Physicians; the American Association for Respiratory Care; and the American College of Critical Care Medicine. Chest. 2001;120:375S–95S.
5. Ouellette DR, Patel S, Girard TD, Morris PE, Schmidt GA, Truwit JD, et al. Liberation from mechanical ventilation in critically ill adults: an official American College of Chest Physicians/American Thoracic Society clinical practice guideline. Chest. 2017;151:166–80.
6. Schönhofer B, Geiseler J, Dellweg D, Fuchs H, Moerer O, Weber-Carstens S, et al. Prolonged weaning: S2k guideline published by the German respiratory society. Respiration. 2020;99:982–1084.
7. Esteban A, Alía I, Ibañez J, Benito S, Tobin MJ. Modes of mechanical ventilation and weaning. A national survey of Spanish hospitals. The Spanish Lung Failure Collaborative Group. Chest. 1994;106:1188–93.
8. Kacmarek RM. The mechanical ventilator: past, present, and future. Respir Care. 2011;56:1170–80.
9. Hidalgo J, Hyzy RC, Mohamed Reda Taha A, Tolba YYA. Personalized mechanical ventilation: improving quality of care. Cham: Springer; 2023.
10. Mushin WW, Rendell-Baker L, Thompson PW. Automatic ventilation of the lungs. 3rd ed. Oxford: Blackwell Scientific Publications; 1980.
11. Baker AB. Artificial respiration, the history of an IDEA. Med Hist. 1971;15:336–51.
12. Emerson CJ. The evolution of iron lungs. Cambridge; 1978.
13. Drinker P, Shaw LA. An apparatus for the prolonged administration of artificial respiration. J Clin Invest. 1929;7:229–47.
14. Hodes H. Treatment of respiratory difficulty in poliomyelitis. Polio Pap Discuss Present Third Int Poliomyeliytis Conf. 1955.
15. McPherson S, Spearman C. Respiratory therapy equipment. 2nd ed. Mosby; 1981.
16. Hewlett AM, Platt AS, Terry VG. Mandatory minute volume: a new concept in weaning from mechanical ventilation. Anaesthesia. 1977;32:163–9.
17. Tobin MJ. Remembrance of weaning past: the seminal papers. Intensive Care Med. 2006;32:1485–93.
18. Batson R, Riley HD. Respiratory failure in poliomyelitis: results in weaning from respiratory aids. J Tenn State Med Assoc Tenn State Med Assoc. 1956;49:341–5.
19. Bendixen H, Egbert L, Hedley-Whyte J, Laver M, Pontoppidan H. Respiratory care. 149th ed. 1965. p. 148.
20. Egan D. Fundamentals of respiratory therapy. 3rd ed. St Louis: Mosby; 1977.
21. Venus B, Smith RA, Mathru M. National survey of methods and criteria used for weaning from mechanical ventilation. Crit Care Med. 1987;15:530–3.
22. Sahn SA, Lakshminarayan S. Bedside criteria for discontinuation of mechanical ventilation. Chest. 1973;63:1002–5.
23. Herrera M, Blasco J, Venegas J, Barba R, Doblas A, Marquez E. Mouth occlusion pressure (P0.1) in acute respiratory failure. Intensive Care Med. 1985;11:134–9.

24. Sassoon CS, Te TT, Mahutte CK, Light RW. Airway occlusion pressure. An important indicator for successful weaning in patients with chronic obstructive pulmonary disease. Am Rev Respir Dis. 1987;135:107–13.
25. Yang KL, Tobin MJ. A prospective study of indexes predicting the outcome of trials of weaning from mechanical ventilation. N Engl J Med. 1991;324:1445–50.
26. Milic-Emili J. Is weaning an art or a science? Am Rev Respir Dis. 1986;134:1107–8.
27. Baptistella AR, Sarmento FJ, da Silva KR, Baptistella SF, Taglietti M, Zuquello RÁ, et al. Predictive factors of weaning from mechanical ventilation and extubation outcome: a systematic review. J Crit Care. 2018;48:56–62.
28. Henning RJ, Shubin H, Weil MH. The measurement of the work of breathing for the clinical assessment of ventilator dependence. Crit Care Med. 1977;5:264–8.
29. Cohen CA, Zagelbaum G, Gross D, Roussos C, Macklem PT. Clinical manifestations of inspiratory muscle fatigue. Am J Med. 1982;73:308–16.
30. Tobin M, Perez W, Guenther S, Semmes B, Mador M, Allen S, et al. The pattern of breathing during successful and unsuccessful trials of weaning from mechanical ventilation. Am Rev Respir Dis. 1986;134:1111–8.
31. Marini JJ, Capps JS, Culver BH. The inspiratory work of breathing during assisted mechanical ventilation. Chest. 1985;87:612–8.
32. Brochard L, Rauss A, Benito S, Conti G, Mancebo J, Rekik N, et al. Comparison of three methods of gradual withdrawal from ventilatory support during weaning from mechanical ventilation. Am J Respir Crit Care Med. 1994;150:896–903.
33. Brochard L, Pluskwa F, Lemaire F. Improved efficacy of spontaneous breathing with inspiratory pressure support. Am Rev Respir Dis. 1987;136:411–5.
34. Torres A, Reyes A, Roca J, Wagner PD, Rodriguez-Roisin R. Ventilation-perfusion mismatching in chronic obstructive pulmonary disease during ventilator weaning. Am Rev Respir Dis. 1989;140:1246–50.
35. Bates JH, Baconnier P, Milic-Emili J. A theoretical analysis of interrupter technique for measuring respiratory mechanics. J Appl Physiol. 1988;64:2204–14.
36. Polese G, Rossi A, Appendini L, Brandi G, Bates JH, Brandolese R. Partitioning of respiratory mechanics in mechanically ventilated patients. J Appl Physiol. 1991;71:2425–33.
37. Downs JB, Klein EF, Desautels D, Modell JH, Kirby RR. Intermittent mandatory ventilation: a new approach to weaning patients from mechanical ventilators. Chest. 1973;64:331–5.
38. Tomlinson JR, Miller KS, Lorch DG, Smith L, Reines HD, Sahn SA. A prospective comparison of IMV and T-piece weaning from mechanical ventilation. Chest. 1989;96:348–52.
39. Esteban A, Frutos F, Tobin MJ, Alía I, Solsona JF, Valverdu V, et al. A comparison of four methods of weaning patients from mechanical ventilation. N Engl J Med. 1995;332:345–50.
40. Thille AW, Gacouin A, Coudroy R, Ehrmann S, Quenot J-P, Nay M-A, et al. Spontaneous-breathing trials with pressure-support ventilation or a T-piece. N Engl J Med. 2022;387:1843–54.
41. Willatts SM. Alternative modes of ventilation. Part I. Disadvantages of controlled mechanical ventilation: intermittent mandatory ventilation. Intensive Care Med. 1985;11:51–5.
42. Brown DL. Use of ketamine to wean a patient with sleep apnea. Crit Care Med. 1986;14:167–8.
43. Grounds RM, Lalor JM, Lumley J, Royston D, Morgan M. Propofol infusion for sedation in the intensive care unit: preliminary report. BMJ. 1987;294:397–400.
44. AlanR A, SheilaM W, Park Gilbert R, Collins Charles H, Mca LI, Pepperman Michael L, et al. Comparison of PROPOFOL and midazolam for sedation in critically ill patients. Lancet. 1989;334:704–9.
45. Stewart KG. Clinical evaluation of pressure support ventilation. Br J Anaesth. 1989;63:362–4.
46. Kollef MH, Levy NT, Ahrens TS, Schaiff R, Prentice D, Sherman G. The use of continuous IV sedation is associated with prolongation of mechanical ventilation. Chest. 1998;114:541–8.
47. Kress JP, Pohlman AS, O'Connor MF, Hall JB. Daily interruption of sedative infusions in critically ill patients undergoing mechanical ventilation. N Engl J Med. 2000;342:1471–7.
48. Martin UJ, Hincapie L, Nimchuk M, Gaughan J, Criner GJ. Impact of whole-body rehabilitation in patients receiving chronic mechanical ventilation. Crit Care Med. 2005;33:2259–65.

49. Morris PE, Goad A, Thompson C, Taylor K, Harry B, Passmore L, et al. Early intensive care unit mobility therapy in the treatment of acute respiratory failure*. Crit Care Med. 2008;36:2238–43.
50. Pandharipande P, Banerjee A, McGrane S, Ely EW. Liberation and animation for ventilated ICU patients: the ABCDE bundle for the back-end of critical care. Crit Care. 2010;14:157.
51. Ferrer M, Valencia M, Nicolas JM, Bernadich O, Badia JR, Torres A. Early noninvasive ventilation averts extubation failure in patients at risk: a randomized trial. Am J Respir Crit Care Med. 2006;173:164–70.
52. Nava S, Gregoretti C, Fanfulla F, Squadrone E, Grassi M, Carlucci A, et al. Noninvasive ventilation to prevent respiratory failure after extubation in high-risk patients*. Crit Care Med. 2005;33:2465–70.
53. Ferrer M, Sellarés J, Valencia M, Carrillo A, Gonzalez G, Badia JR, et al. Non-invasive ventilation after extubation in hypercapnic patients with chronic respiratory disorders: randomised controlled trial. Lancet. 2009;374:1082–8.
54. Khilnani GC, Galle AD, Hadda V, Sharma SK. Non-invasive ventilation after extubation in patients with chronic obstructive airways disease: a randomised controlled trial. Anaesth Intensive Care. 2011;39:217–23.
55. Boscolo A, Pettenuzzo T, Sella N, Zatta M, Salvagno M, Tassone M, et al. Noninvasive respiratory support after extubation: a systematic review and network meta-analysis. Eur Respir Rev. 2023;32:220196.
56. Fajardo-Campoverdi A, González-Castro A, Adasme-Jeria R, Roncalli-Rocha A, Ibarra M, Chica-Meza C, et al. Mechanical ventilator liberation protocol. Recommendation based on review of the evidence. J Mech Vent. 2023;4:31–41.
57. AMIB, SBPT. Orientações práticas em Ventilação Mecânica AMIB SBPT. 2024.
58. Pham T, Heunks L, Bellani G, Madotto F, Aragao I, Beduneau G, et al. Weaning from mechanical ventilation in intensive care units across 50 countries (WEAN SAFE): a multicentre, prospective, observational cohort study. Lancet Respir Med. 2023;11:465–76.
59. Epstein SK, Nevins ML, Chung J. Effect of unplanned extubation on outcome of mechanical ventilation. Am J Respir Crit Care Med. 2000;161:1912–6.
60. Béduneau G, Pham T, Schortgen F, Piquilloud L, Zogheib E, Jonas M, et al. Epidemiology of weaning outcome according to a new definition. The WIND study. Am J Respir Crit Care Med. 2017;195:772–83.
61. Ely EW, Baker AM, Dunagan DP, Burke HL, Smith AC, Kelly PT, et al. Effect on the duration of mechanical ventilation of identifying patients capable of breathing spontaneously. N Engl J Med. 1996;335:1864–9.
62. Sklar MC, Burns K, Rittayamai N, Lanys A, Rauseo M, Chen L, et al. Effort to breathe with various spontaneous breathing trial techniques. A physiologic meta-analysis. Am J Respir Crit Care Med. 2017;195:1477–85.
63. Delgado M, Zavala E, Tomás R, Fernandez R. Clinical factors associated with success of proportional assist ventilation in the acute phase of critical illness: pilot study. Med Intensiva Engl Ed. 2014;38:65–72.
64. Ou-Yang L-J, Chen P-H, Jhou H-J, Su VY-F, Lee C-H. Proportional assist ventilation versus pressure support ventilation for weaning from mechanical ventilation in adults: a meta-analysis and trial sequential analysis. Crit Care. 2020;24:556.
65. Kataoka J, Kuriyama A, Norisue Y, Fujitani S. Proportional modes versus pressure support ventilation: a systematic review and meta-analysis. Ann Intensive Care. 2018;8:123.
66. Kacmarek RM. Proportional assist ventilation and neurally adjusted ventilatory assist. Respir Care. 2011;56:140–52.
67. Lellouche F, Brochard L. Advanced closed loops during mechanical ventilation (PAV, NAVA, ASV, SmartCare). Best Pract Res Clin Anaesthesiol. 2009;23:81–93.
68. Dongelmans DA, Veelo DP, Paulus F, De Mol BAJM, Korevaar JC, Kudoga A, et al. Weaning automation with adaptive support ventilation: a randomized controlled trial in cardiothoracic surgery patients. Anesth Analg. 2009;108:565–71.

69. Kirakli C, Ozdemir I, Ucar ZZ, Cimen P, Kepil S, Ozkan SA. Adaptive support ventilation for faster weaning in COPD: a randomised controlled trial. Eur Respir J. 2011;38:774–80.
70. Yuan X, Lu X, Chao Y, Beck J, Sinderby C, Xie J, et al. Neurally adjusted ventilatory assist as a weaning mode for adults with invasive mechanical ventilation: a systematic review and meta-analysis. Crit Care. 2021;25:222.
71. Burns KEA, Raptis S, Nisenbaum R, Rizvi L, Jones A, Bakshi J, et al. International practice variation in weaning critically ill adults from invasive mechanical ventilation. Ann Am Thorac Soc. 2018;15:494–502.
72. Burns KEA, Soliman I, Adhikari NKJ, Zwein A, Wong JTY, Gomez-Builes C, et al. Trials directly comparing alternative spontaneous breathing trial techniques: a systematic review and meta-analysis. Crit Care. 2017;21:127.
73. Zein H, Baratloo A, Negida A, Safari S. Ventilator weaning and spontaneous breathing trials; an educational review. Emerg Tehran Iran. 2016;4:65–71.
74. MacIntyre NR. The ventilator discontinuation process: an expanding evidence base discussion. Respir Care. 2013;58:1074–86.
75. Liu L, Liu H, Yang Y, Huang Y, Liu S, Beck J, et al. Neuroventilatory efficiency and extubation readiness in critically ill patients. Crit Care. 2012;16:R143.
76. Esteban A, Alía I, Tobin MJ, Gil A, Gordo F, Vallverdú I, et al. Effect of spontaneous breathing trial duration on outcome of attempts to discontinue mechanical ventilation. Am J Respir Crit Care Med. 1999;159:512–8.
77. Perren A, Domenighetti G, Mauri S, Genini F, Vizzardi N. Protocol-directed weaning from mechanical ventilation: clinical outcome in patients randomized for a 30-min or 120-min trial with pressure support ventilation. Intensive Care Med. 2002;28:1058–63.
78. Subirà C, Hernández G, Vázquez A, Rodríguez-García R, González-Castro A, García C, et al. Effect of pressure support vs T-piece ventilation strategies during spontaneous breathing trials on successful Extubation among patients receiving mechanical ventilation: a randomized clinical trial. JAMA. 2019;321:2175.
79. Barbas CSV, Ísola AM, Farias AMDC, Cavalcanti AB, Gama AMC, Duarte ACM, et al. Brazilian recommendations of mechanical ventilation 2013. Part I Rev Bras Ter Intensiva [Internet]. 2014; [citado 16 de outubro de 2024];26. Recuperado de: https://criticalcarescience.org/article/brazilian-recommendations-of-mechanical-ventilation-2013-part-i/
80. Burns KEA, Rizvi L, Cook DJ, Lebovic G, Dodek P, Villar J, et al. Ventilator weaning and discontinuation practices for critically ill patients. JAMA. 2021;325:1173.
81. Ladeira MT, Ribeiro Vital FM, Andriolo RB, Andriolo BN, Atallah ÁN, Peccin MS. Pressure support versus T-tube for weaning from mechanical ventilation in adults. Cochrane Emergency and Critical Care Group, organizador. Cochrane Database Syst Rev [Internet]. 2014; [citado 13 de outubro de 2024]; 2018. Recuperado de. http://doi.wiley.com/10.1002/14651858.CD006056.pub2
82. Schmidt GA, Girard TD, Kress JP, Morris PE, Ouellette DR, Alhazzani W, et al. Official executive summary of an American Thoracic Society/American College of Chest Physicians Clinical Practice Guideline: liberation from mechanical ventilation in critically ill adults. Am J Respir Crit Care Med. 2017;195:115–9.
83. Fernandez MM, González-Castro A, Magret M, Bouza MT, Ibañez M, García C, et al. Reconnection to mechanical ventilation for 1 h after a successful spontaneous breathing trial reduces reintubation in critically ill patients: a multicenter randomized controlled trial. Intensive Care Med. 2017;43:1660–7.
84. Salam A, Tilluckdharry L, Amoateng-Adjepong Y, Manthous CA. Neurologic status, cough, secretions and extubation outcomes. Intensive Care Med. 2004;30:1334–9.
85. Burns KEA, Rochwerg B, Seely AJE. Ventilator weaning and extubation. Crit Care Clin. 2024;40:391–408.
86. Thille AW, Harrois A, Schortgen F, Brun-Buisson C, Brochard L. Outcomes of extubation failure in medical intensive care unit patients*. Crit Care Med. 2011;39:2612–8.

87. Fan E, Zakhary B, Amaral A, McCannon J, Girard TD, Morris PE, et al. Liberation from mechanical ventilation in critically ill adults. An official ATS/ACCP clinical practice guideline. Ann Am Thorac Soc. 2017;14:441–3.
88. Miller RL, Cole RP. Association between reduced cuff leak volume and postextubation stridor. Chest. 1996;110:1035–40.
89. Jaber S, Quintard H, Cinotti R, Asehnoune K, Arnal J-M, Guitton C, et al. Risk factors and outcomes for airway failure versus non-airway failure in the intensive care unit: a multicenter observational study of 1514 extubation procedures. Crit Care. 2018;22:236.

Chapter 3
The Epidemiology of Weaning from Mechanical Ventilation

Lisanne H. Roesthuis, Tim Frenzel, Jonne Doorduin, and Leo M. A. Heunks

Weaning from mechanical ventilation is a crucial step in recovering from severe respiratory failure and can take up to 40% of total ventilation time [1]. Weaning is the process of transitioning a patient from ventilator support to spontaneous (unassisted) breathing. The epidemiology of weaning encompasses the study of factors affecting the weaning process, including weaning methods, outcomes, patient demographics, clinical conditions, and comorbidities. Understanding these factors is essential for improving weaning practices, patient outcomes, and health-care resource use.

3.1 Definition of Weaning

Historically, the weaning process was not clearly defined, leading to wide variations in weaning definitions and practices. This lack of standardization made it challenging to compare, conduct, and interpret epidemiological studies. As a result, the impact of weaning difficulties on patient outcome was poorly understood [2]. In 2007, recommendations regarding the weaning process were proposed [3]. However, these recommendations had limitations: they only considered patients who could be weaned and assumed that a spontaneous breathing trial (SBT) was a universal practice in every patient [3].

Recently, two large multicenter multinational observational studies, namely the WIND [2] and WEAN SAFE [4] studies, have described the weaning process in more detail. Consequently, the following definitions are derived from these studies. The first attempt to separate the patient from the ventilator marks the start of the

L. H. Roesthuis · T. Frenzel · J. Doorduin · L. M. A. Heunks (✉)
Department of Intensive Care Medicine, Radboud University Medical Center, Nijmegen, The Netherlands
e-mail: Leo.Heunks@radboudumc.nl

A. R. Baptistella et al. (eds.), *Weaning from Mechanical Ventilation*, https://doi.org/10.1007/978-3-032-01145-9_3

weaning process. In intubated patients, this separation attempt can be an SBT, that is, a short period with minimal or no ventilator support as a test to predict extubation success, or a direct extubation without SBT. In tracheotomized patients, this involves a short period of spontaneous ventilation through tracheostomy with minimal or no ventilator support, with or without oxygen supply. Minimal support is defined as continuous positive airway pressure ≤ 5 cmH_2O, or pressure support (PS) with positive end-expiratory pressure (PEEP) ≤ 5 cmH_2O and PS ≤ 7 cmH_2O). Weaning success in intubated patients is defined as extubation without death or reintubation within the next 7 days, or discharge from the intensive care unit (ICU) without invasive ventilation within 7 days. For tracheotomized patients, this includes ventilation through tracheostomy without ventilator support during seven consecutive days or discharge from the ICU without ventilator support. From these definitions, weaning duration can be defined as the number of days from the first separation attempt to the point of weaning success [2, 4].

According to the WEAN SAFE study [4], which included patients receiving invasive ventilation for at least 2 days, patients can be classified into weaning groups based on weaning duration (Table 3.1). Group 1 includes patients who never have a separation attempt. These patients die or are transferred to another hospital before entering the weaning phase. Patients who can be extubated within one day after the first separation attempt belong to the short wean group (group 2). If weaning takes longer than one day but less than one week after the first separation attempt, patients belong to the intermediate wean group (group 3). Prolonged weaning (group 4) is defined when patients need at least 7 days after the first separation attempt before they can be extubated. Finally, the group of patients that undergo at least one

Table 3.1 Weaning groups and outcomes

Group	Definition	Population (%)	Median ventilation time (# days (IQR))	Reintubations (%)	Tracheostomy (%)	Hospital mortality (%)
1: No SA	No SA, no extubation	1346 (22.9)	6 (4–11)	–	–	82.4
2: Short	Extubation <1 day after 1st SA	2927 (49.9)	5 (3–8)	1.6	10.8	10.1
3: Intermediate	Extubation >1 day and < 7 days after 1st SA	457 (7.8)	10 (8–15)	23.6	31.5	13.6
4: Prolonged	Extubation >7 days after 1st SA	433 (7,4)	20 (15–28)	44.6	63.3	17.9
5: Failure	Failed SA, no extubation	706 (12.0)	11 (7–18)	21.2	33.1	78.3

Data are given as numbers (percentage) of the whole study population (WEAN SAFE study), as number of days, or as percentage of the weaning group
SA separation attempt, *IQR* interquartile range

separation attempt but cannot be extubated (group 5), because they die or are transferred to another hospital (Table 3.1). This last group was added by the WEAN SAFE investigators [4] as a modification of the WIND classification [2].

3.2 Weaning Readiness

A number of key events occur after intubation and before entering the weaning process (Fig. 3.1). After tracheal intubation, in more than half of the patients, it takes more than one day for diaphragm activity to resume, with a median of 22 h [5]. Most patients show signs of spontaneous breathing activity within 3 days after tracheal intubation [4]. Besides controlled ventilation, an important reason for this delay is the use of sedatives, especially propofol and fentanyl. The higher the cumulative dose of sedative infusions in the first 24 h on mechanical ventilation, the longer the delay for the resumption of diaphragm activity [5]. Therefore, sedation should be titrated to the lowest effective level that allows spontaneous breathing, ensuring safe ventilation for both the lungs and respiratory muscles [6].

Once the patient has recovered from the acute phase of respiratory failure, weaning from mechanical ventilation should be considered [6]. In general, screening criteria for SBT readiness are based on improving PaO_2/FiO_2, low FiO_2, and minimal level of PS and/or PEEP. Currently used screening criteria are mainly based on expert opinion. Screening criteria using higher support/oxygenation

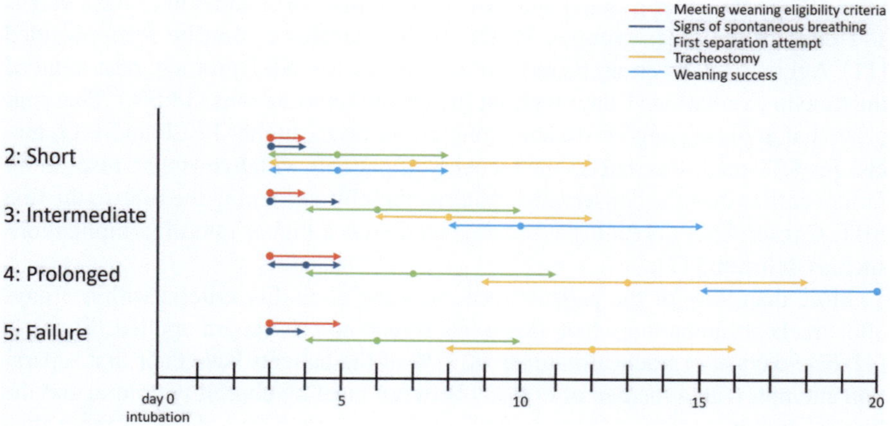

Fig. 3.1 Graph showing the weaning groups (y-axis) with key events during the weaning process: starting from intubation (day 0 on x-axis), signs of spontaneous breathing (dark blue), meeting weaning eligibility criteria (red), first separation attempt (green), and tracheostomy (yellow) until weaning success (light blue) (i.e., missing in the failure group). Results are shown from the WEAN SAFE study. A large variation can be seen for the different events between the different groups, particularly in days from intubation (x-axis) until first separation attempt, tracheostomy, and weaning success (i.e., per definition). Of note, group 1 is not depicted in this figure because this group never enters the weaning phase

levels will lead to earlier initiation of SBTs and a higher percentage of patients succeeding the first SBT [7], making these criteria less suitable as a screening test. Lower support levels may delay weaning and prolong the duration of mechanical ventilation. Additionally, subjective global clinical assessment and non-respiratory factors may play a role, such as patient comfort or hemodynamic stability, leading to a wide variation in practices. Until recently, optimal ventilator settings during SBTs were unknown. SBTs using higher support levels are easier to pass but will underestimate the work of breathing after extubation, with the opposite being true for SBTs using lower support levels [7–9]. In contrast, a recent multicenter randomized controlled trial in patients with high risk of extubation failure showed no difference between SBT using inspiratory pressure support or T-piece with oxygen supply with respect to ventilator-free days at day 28 [10]. To clarify the apparent conflicting results from these studies, a recent multicenter randomized trial compared the effectiveness of paired combinations of aggressive versus conservative screening and SBT strategies [11]. Aggressive screening criteria included higher support levels (PEEP ≤10 cmH_2O and $FiO_2 \leq 50\%$; comparable to WEAN SAFE study [4]), whereas conservative screening criteria included lower support levels (PEEP ≤8 cmH_2O and $FiO_2 \leq 40\%$). The aggressive SBT protocol consisted of PS 8 cmH_2O with PEEP 5 cmH_2O, whereas the conservative SBT protocol consisted of PS 5 cmH_2O with PEEP 0 cmH_2O. Aggressive screening paired with an aggressive SBT protocol increased the number of reintubations (20% versus 13%–16% in the other groups). On the other hand, conservative screening with a conservative SBT protocol had a lower number of reintubations but was at the cost of a lower percentage of simple weaning (45.7% versus more than 71% in the other groups) and extended the time to extubation (3 days versus 1–2 days in the other groups). Hence, both strategies cannot be recommended [11]. Aggressive screening paired with a conservative SBT protocol best reduced the time to extubation (1 day) without increasing reintubations (14.6%). This suggests that applying aggressive screening criteria (i.e., higher PEEP and FiO_2 levels) for SBT readiness detects the recovery of patients with hypoxemic respiratory failure earlier than the conservative criteria, thereby shortening the time to the first SBT. Conservative screening was associated with a higher rate of complications such as delirium [11].

More than 90% of the patients meet weaning eligibility criteria within 3 days after tracheal intubation when aggressive screening criteria are applied (Fig. 3.1) [4]. Five days after tracheal intubation, 77% of the patients have their first separation attempt, with a median of one day between meeting eligibility criteria and the first separation attempt. However, 22% of the patients have a delay of more than 5 days. Factors associated with weaning delays include frailty, trauma, and non-traumatic neurological events. Additionally, potentially modifiable factors, such as use of continuous neuromuscular blocking agents and moderate to deep sedation levels, also contribute to weaning delays [4]. Therefore, to reduce weaning delays, it is important to evaluate whether it is safe and tolerable to reduce or stop neuromuscular blocking agents and sedation.

3.3 Weaning Outcome According to Weaning Classification

Table 3.1 describes the most important weaning outcomes according to the different weaning groups from the WEAN SAFE study [4]. Almost half of the patients belong to the short wean group, having the shortest duration of invasive ventilation. Patients belonging to the prolonged wean group had the longest duration of invasive ventilation, twice as long as the intermediate wean group. Not unexpected, this group had the most reintubations and tracheostomies. Sixty-five percent of all patients were successfully weaned after 90 days. Not surprisingly, the group of patients who never entered the weaning phase had the highest mortality, shortly followed by the failure group (Table 3.1) [4].

3.4 Risk Factors Weaning Failure

Now that the weaning process and classification of wean groups are defined, demographics and clinical conditions associated with weaning failure can be described. As explained before, sedation is an important independent risk factor for delayed initiation of weaning. Both delayed weaning and high sedation levels are potentially modifiable factors associated with weaning failure. Patients that are older, immunocompromised, and more frail have a higher risk of weaning failure [4]. In contrast, younger patients generally exhibit better weaning outcomes owing to fewer comorbidities and greater physiological reserve [3]. Primary reasons for ICU admission associated with weaning failure are cardiac arrest, non-traumatic neurological event, non-neurological SOFA score, and pre-existing limitations of care [4]. Respiratory variables, such as higher respiratory rate, PEEP, and driving pressure at the beginning of the weaning process, are also associated with increased risk of weaning failure. These higher support levels may indicate either that patients have not recovered from respiratory failure or that SBTs are initiated earlier [4].

3.5 Conclusions

It is important to have a clear definition of the weaning process, to be able to compare, conduct, and interpret (epidemiological) studies. Sedation plays a critical role during invasive ventilation: it delays the resumption of diaphragm activity and increases weaning delays. Therefore, it is important to titrate sedation regularly to the lowest possible level, taking into account patient comfort and lung- and diaphragm-protective ventilation. Defining the weaning process helps to identify patients ready for weaning and classifying patients into specific wean groups with known outcomes. Applying aggressive screening criteria for weaning eligibility leads to an earlier SBT; combined with a conservative SBT protocol, this strategy best reduces the time to extubation without increasing the rate of reintubations.

References

1. Esteban A, Alia I, Ibanez J, Benito S, Tobin MJ. Modes of mechanical ventilation and weaning. A national survey of Spanish hospitals. The Spanish Lung Failure Collaborative Group. Chest. 1994;106(4):1188–93.
2. Beduneau G, Pham T, Schortgen F, Piquilloud L, Zogheib E, Jonas M, Grelon F, Runge I, Nicolas T, Grange S, Barberet G, Guitard PG, Frat JP, Constan A, Chretien JM, Mancebo J, Mercat A, Richard JM, Brochard L, Group WS, the RNdd. Epidemiology of weaning outcome according to a new definition. The WIND study. Am J Respir Crit Care Med. 2017;195(6):772–83.
3. Boles JM, Bion J, Connors A, Herridge M, Marsh B, Melot C, Pearl R, Silverman H, Stanchina M, Vieillard-Baron A, Welte T. Weaning from mechanical ventilation. Eur Respir J. 2007;29(5):1033–56.
4. Pham T, Heunks L, Bellani G, Madotto F, Aragao I, Beduneau G, Goligher EC, Grasselli G, Laake JH, Mancebo J, Penuelas O, Piquilloud L, Pesenti A, Wunsch H, van Haren F, Brochard L, Laffey JG, Investigators WS. Weaning from mechanical ventilation in intensive care units across 50 countries (WEAN SAFE): a multicentre, prospective, observational cohort study. Lancet Respir Med. 2023;11(5):465–76.
5. Sklar MC, Madotto F, Jonkman A, Rauseo M, Soliman I, Damiani LF, Telias I, Dubo S, Chen L, Rittayamai N, Chen GQ, Goligher EC, Dres M, Coudroy R, Pham T, Artigas RM, Friedrich JO, Sinderby C, Heunks L, Brochard L. Duration of diaphragmatic inactivity after endotracheal intubation of critically ill patients. Crit Care. 2021;25(1):26.
6. Goligher EC, Jonkman AH, Dianti J, Vaporidi K, Beitler JR, Patel BK, Yoshida T, Jaber S, Dres M, Mauri T, Bellani G, Demoule A, Brochard L, Heunks L. Clinical strategies for implementing lung and diaphragm-protective ventilation: avoiding insufficient and excessive effort. Intensive Care Med. 2020;46(12):2314–26.
7. Subira C, Hernandez G, Vazquez A, Rodriguez-Garcia R, Gonzalez-Castro A, Garcia C, Rubio O, Ventura L, Lopez A, de la Torre MC, Keough E, Arauzo V, Hermosa C, Sanchez C, Tizon A, Tenza E, Laborda C, Cabanes S, Lacueva V, Del Mar FM, Arnau A, Fernandez R. Effect of pressure support vs T-piece ventilation strategies during spontaneous breathing trials on successful Extubation among patients receiving mechanical ventilation: a randomized clinical trial. JAMA. 2019;321(22):2175–82.
8. Burns KEA, Soliman I, Adhikari NKJ, Zwein A, Wong JTY, Gomez-Builes C, Pellegrini JA, Chen L, Rittayamai N, Sklar M, Brochard LJ, Friedrich JO. Trials directly comparing alternative spontaneous breathing trial techniques: a systematic review and meta-analysis. Crit Care. 2017;21(1):127.
9. Sklar MC, Burns K, Rittayamai N, Lanys A, Rauseo M, Chen L, Dres M, Chen GQ, Goligher EC, Adhikari NKJ, Brochard L, Friedrich JO. Effort to breathe with various spontaneous breathing trial techniques. A physiologic meta-analysis. Am J Respir Crit Care Med. 2017;195(11):1477–85.
10. Thille AW, Gacouin A, Coudroy R, Ehrmann S, Quenot JP, Nay MA, Guitton C, Contou D, Labro G, Reignier J, Pradel G, Beduneau G, Dangers L, Saccheri C, Prat G, Lacave G, Sedillot N, Terzi N, La Combe B, Mira JP, Romen A, Azais MA, Rouze A, Devaquet J, Delbove A, Dres M, Bourenne J, Lautrette A, de Keizer J, Ragot S, Frat JP, Network RR. Spontaneous-breathing trials with pressure-support ventilation or a T-piece. N Engl J Med. 2022;387(20):1843–54.
11. Hernandez Martinez G, Rodriguez P, Soto J, Caritg O, Castellvi-Font A, Mariblanca B, Garcia AM, Colinas L, Anon JM, Parrilla-Gomez FJ, Silva-Obregon JA, Masclans JR, Propin A, Cuadra A, Dalorzo MG, Rialp G, Suarez-Sipmann F, Roca O. Effect of aggressive vs conservative screening and confirmatory test on time to extubation among patients at low or intermediate risk: a randomized clinical trial. Intensive Care Med. 2024;50(2):258–67.

Chapter 4
Sedation and Weaning

João Rogério Nunes Filho and Breno Grossi

4.1 Introduction

Sedation and analgesia are essential practices in the intensive care unit (ICU), providing comfort, pain relief, and anxiety reduction for critically ill patients. The appropriate administration of sedatives and analgesics is critical to improving clinical outcomes, minimizing complications, and reducing costs associated with ICU care. It is commonly used in patients undergoing mechanical ventilation (MV), where it helps achieve patient-ventilator synchrony and improves tolerance to the ventilator. However, withdrawal of sedation is an essential step in initiating the weaning process from MV, allowing assessment of the patient's readiness for extubation and reducing the risks associated with prolonged ventilation [1–4].

This chapter reviews the principles, pharmacologic agents, and management strategies for sedoanalgesia during weaning of ICU patients from mechanical ventilation.

J. R. Nunes Filho (✉)
Hospital Universitário Santa Terezinha, UNOESC, Joaçaba, SC, Brazil

B. Grossi
Universidade do Oeste de Santa Catarina, Joaçaba, SC, Brazil

SEDAR – Serviço de Anestesiologia, Hospital Unimed Meio Oeste, Joaçaba, SC, Brazil

SBED – Sociedade Brasileira de Dor, São Paulo, SP, Brazil

A. R. Baptistella et al. (eds.), *Weaning from Mechanical Ventilation*,
https://doi.org/10.1007/978-3-032-01145-9_4

4.2 Daily Patient Assessment

Several strategies have been proposed to improve the management of mechanically ventilated patients, aiming for early awakening, optimization of ventilation time, and reduction of complications.

The ABCDEF bundle integrates interventions in a structured manner to assess and address various factors that may interfere with the success of this process and is currently recommended for daily use at the bedside to optimize performance and outcomes. The bundle recommends the following interventions [5]:

- **A**: Assess, prevent, and manage pain
- **B**: Both spontaneous awakening trials (SATs) and spontaneous breathing trials (SBTs)
- **C**: Choice of analgesia and sedation
- **D**: Delirium: Assess, prevent, and manage
- **E:** Early mobility and exercise
- **F**: Family engagement and empowerment

Pain assessment and management, arousal protocols, spontaneous breathing tests, and the indications and contraindications for the major analgesics and sedatives are the scope of this chapter and will be discussed in more detail below.

4.3 Principles of Sedoanalgesia

The main goals of sedoanalgesia in the intensive care unit include:

- Relief of pain and anxiety
- Facilitating invasive procedures
- Promoting sleep and rest
- Preventing delirium and agitation

4.4 Assessment of Pain

Pain, characterized as an unpleasant sensory and emotional experience associated with, or similar to, actual or potential tissue injury, is a common symptom in mechanically ventilated patients and should be routinely assessed and managed.

Accurate assessment, grading, and treatment of pain are essential for the proper titration or withdrawal of sedatives, facilitating the weaning process from mechanical ventilation.

The most common symptoms associated with pain are tachycardia, sweating, hypertension, mydriasis, and ventilator resistance. However, these symptoms are nonspecific and may be associated with other conditions, such as the underlying pathologies that brought the patient to the ICU [3, 5, 6].

If inadequately controlled, pain can lead to several complications, including delirium, anxiety, increased inflammatory response, insomnia, and even impaired recovery, making the weaning process from mechanical ventilation more challenging. Its accurate assessment is essential to implement effective analgesic interventions, improve patient comfort, and optimize clinical outcomes. Therefore, the use of standardized pain scales is recommended to aid in the diagnosis, management, and monitoring of pain control interventions [3, 6, 7].

4.5 Pain Assessment Methods

4.5.1 Subjective Assessment

Subjective pain assessment involves patient self-report. In patients who are conscious and able to communicate, self-report is the gold standard for measuring pain. The most commonly used pain scales include:

- *Numerical Pain Scale (NPS)*: Patients rate their pain on a scale of 0–10, where 0 represents no pain and 10 represents the worst pain imaginable.
- *Visual Analog Scale (VAS)*: Consists of a 10 cm straight line on which the patient marks the intensity of pain, ranging from "no pain" to "most pain possible" (Fig. 4.1).
- *Wong-Baker Faces Pain Scale*: Often used with pediatric patients or those with communication difficulties, it presents drawings of faces ranging from happy (no pain) to sad (severe pain).

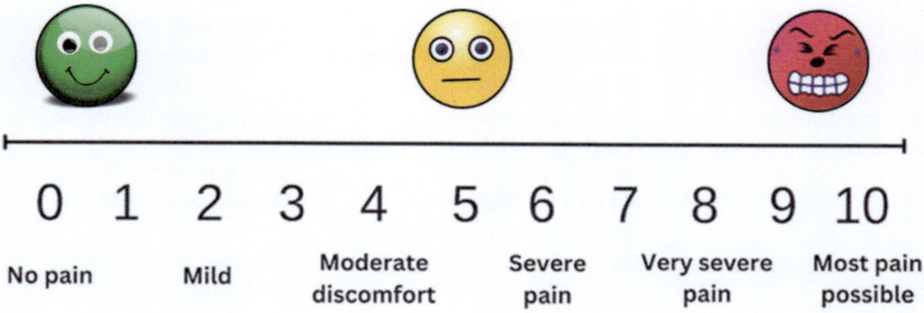

Fig. 4.1 Visual analog scale. (Adapted from Hayes and Patterson [8]. Image created with clip arts from opencliart.org)

4.5.2 Behavioral Assessment

For patients who are unable to communicate verbally, pain assessment should be based on behavioral and physiologic signs. Some of the tools used are:

- *Behavioral Pain Scale (BPS)*: Assesses facial expressions, upper limb movements, and compliance with mechanical ventilation on a scale of 1–12.
- *Critical-Care Pain Observation Tool (CPOT)*: Assesses facial expressions, body movements, muscle tension, and compliance with mechanical ventilation on a scale of 0–8 (Table 4.1).

4.5.3 Physiological Assessment

Physiological indicators can complement behavioral and subjective assessments but should not be used in isolation due to their non-specificity. Common indicators include:

- Heart rate
- Blood pressure
- Respiratory rate
- Sweating

Table 4.1 Comparison between BPS and CPOT pain scales

Component	Behavioral pain scale (BPS)	Critical-care pain observation tool (CPOT)
1. Facial expression	Relaxed +1 Partially tightened +2 Fully tightened +3 Grimacing +4	Relaxed, neutral = 0 Tense +1 Grimacing +2
2. Upper limbs	No movement +1 Partially bent +2 Fully bent with finger flexion +3 Permanently retracted +4	Relaxed = 0 Tense, rigid +1 Very tense or rigid +2
3. Compliance with mechanical ventilation	Tolerating movement +1 Coughing but tolerating ventilation for most of the time + 2 Fighting ventilator +3 Unable to control ventilation +4	Tolerating ventilator or movement = 0 Coughing but tolerating +1 Fighting ventilator +2
4. Body movements	NA	Absence of movements = 0 Protection +1 Restlessness +2

BPS: Scores range from 3 (no pain) to 12 (maximum pain)
CPOT: Scores vary from 0 (no pain) to 8 (maximum pain)

4.6 Sedatives

After adequate recognition of pain and the establishment of an effective strategy to control it, the use of one or more sedatives may or may not be necessary.

A small group of mechanically ventilated patients, such as those with intracranial hypertension, severe hemodynamic instability, and severe acute respiratory distress syndrome (ARDS), may currently have indications for deep sedation and even the use of neuromuscular blocking agents. For other patients, sedation goals should be more superficial, or even involve no sedation at all.

The Richmond Agitation-Sedation Scale (RASS) has been widely used with the goal of keeping patients conscious on mechanical ventilation while preventing discomfort or agitation. For patients with a target of light sedation, the aim is a RASS score between 0 and −2, with the patient being calm, alert, and cooperative [9–12].

When sedation is indicated, the most commonly used agents are dexmedetomidine, propofol, and benzodiazepines. Table 4.2 lists the drugs, initial doses, main side effects, and primary actions of the most commonly used sedatives.

Benzodiazepines

Benzodiazepines are sedatives that act centrally on the GABA system, enhancing the action of inhibitory neurotransmitters. They have anxiolytic effects at low doses and cause sedation and retrograde amnesia at higher doses. They do not have intrinsic analgesic effects.

Table 4.2 Main medications and their doses in the use of sedoanalgesia in intensive care

Drug	Initial dose	Main side effects	Main action
Midazolam	0.01–0.05 mg/kg/h	Respiratory depression, hypotension, delirium	Sedation, anxiolytic, amnesic
Propofol	5–50 mcg/kg/min	Hypotension, respiratory depression, hyperlipidemia	Rapid sedation, antiemetic effect
Fentanyl	0.7–10 mcg/kg/h	Respiratory depression, bradycardia, muscle rigidity	Powerful analgesia, rapid onset
Dexmedetomidine	0.2–1.5 mcg/kg/h	Hypotension, bradycardia, dry mouth	Mild to moderate sedation, analgesic
Ketamine	1–2 mg/kg bolus, 0.1–2 mg/kg/h	Hallucinations, hypertension, tachycardia	Dissociative analgesia, sedation, bronchodilation
Morphine	0.05–0.1 mg/kg	Respiratory depression, nausea, constipation	Powerful analgesia, sedation
Remifentanil	0.05–2 mcg/kg/min	Respiratory depression, bradycardia, hypotension	Fast-acting, short-duration analgesia
Haloperidol	0.5–2 mg	Neuroleptic malignant syndrome, extrapyramidalism	Sedation, delirium control
Lorazepam	0.02–0.06 mg/kg	Respiratory depression, hypotension, amnesia	Prolonged sedation, anxiolytic

Benzodiazepines, such as midazolam and lorazepam, are commonly used for their anxiolytic and amnesic properties. However, major adverse effects include respiratory depression, delirium, hypotension, and the development of dependence.

- Midazolam: It has a rapid onset of action and a short half-life but is metabolized in the liver to an active metabolite that is eliminated renally and may accumulate in patients with hepatic or renal impairment. When infused in large volumes and for prolonged periods, it can have a prolonged residual effect, making arousal unpredictable.
- Diazepam: Generally used as a bolus because of its rapid onset of action and efficient penetration of the blood-brain barrier. Its continuous use is rare in the ICU setting because of its large volume of distribution and active metabolites, which can lead to prolonged sedation, especially in the elderly and in patients with hepatic or renal impairment.
- Lorazepam: Commonly used for continuous sedation in ventilated patients. It has a slower onset of action but has a smaller volume of distribution, no active metabolites, and a lower risk of drug interactions, making it a reasonable choice among benzodiazepines.

Propofol

Propofol is a fast-acting sedative with hypnotic and amnesic properties. It is preferred for short-term sedation due to its rapid onset and offset, making it easier to awaken mechanically ventilated patients. It acts on the GABA system with anxiolytic, anticonvulsant, and muscle relaxant effects, but it does not provide analgesia.

Propofol is presented as a lipid emulsion with 1.1 kcal/ml, which must be considered in the nutritional assessment of patients, and serum triglycerides should be monitored during continuous infusion. Because it contains soybean oil, egg lecithin, and glycerin, it may cause allergic reactions in predisposed individuals. It may also cause irritation at the injection site when used in peripheral access, as well as increase the risk of infection associated with central lines.

The most feared side effect is propofol infusion syndrome, a rare but highly fatal condition associated with high-dose infusions (>4 mg/kg/h) and prolonged use (>48 h). This syndrome is characterized by bradycardia, severe metabolic acidosis, rhabdomyolysis, hyperlipidemia, hypercalcemia, acute kidney injury, hepatomegaly, and cardiovascular collapse.

Dexmedetomidine

Dexmedetomidine is a highly selective agonist of alpha-2 adrenergic receptors with sedative, anxiolytic, and analgesic properties that potentiate the effects of opioids. It provides sedation without causing significant respiratory depression, is useful for mild to moderate sedation, and is also useful in the prevention of delirium. It has a rapid onset and offset of action, allowing for daily reassessment with rapid awakening of the patient. It is usually given as a continuous infusion.

The most common side effects are hypotension and bradycardia. After prolonged use, abrupt discontinuation of dexmedetomidine may cause withdrawal symptoms such as agitation, delirium, tachycardia, and hypertension.

Ketamine
Ketamine is widely used as a sedoanalgesic in intensive care due to its unique pharmacological properties. It acts as an NMDA receptor antagonist, providing both analgesia and sedation without causing significant respiratory depression. Its sympathomimetic effects are particularly beneficial in hemodynamically unstable patients, as it helps maintain blood pressure and cardiac output.

Ketamine can induce a dissociative state, allowing patients to remain responsive while experiencing pain relief. It is important to monitor for psychotomimetic effects, such as hallucinations, which can be minimized with the concomitant use of benzodiazepines.

4.7 Analgesics

Opioids
In addition to providing analgesia, opioids reduce anxiety, which may make it easier to connect the patient to the ventilator. However, they also have the ability to decrease respiratory drive and cause respiratory depression, requiring caution in patients without an established airway.

Major side effects of opioids include hypotension, hallucinations, delirium, histamine release, pruritus, adynamic ileus, vomiting, and urinary retention.

The most commonly used opioids in mechanically ventilated patients are morphine and fentanyl. They are effective in controlling pain but require careful monitoring due to the risk of respiratory depression and dependence.

- Morphine: It has a longer duration of action, with a half-life of 3–5 h and is metabolized in the liver with renal elimination of its metabolites. It is associated with greater histamine release and, because of accumulation, is often given in intermittent doses. Its onset of action is slower, and its duration is longer, making it useful for controlling persistent pain.
- Fentanyl: A synthetic derivative of morphine with 100 times greater potency, fentanyl causes less histamine release and is therefore preferred in patients with bronchospasm. Its onset of action is faster because it crosses the blood-brain barrier quickly. Because of its short half-life (2–3 h), it is generally administered as a continuous infusion, although it may have a prolonged residual effect on adipose tissue after discontinuation. Its rapid onset and short duration make it ideal for fast-track procedures and control of acute pain.
- Remifentanil: With an ultra-short half-life, it allows for rapid dose adjustments and rapid recovery after discontinuation.
- Methadone: A synthetic opioid that is not widely used for pain control in ICU patients because of its long duration of action and difficulty in handling and adjusting the dose. Unlike other opioids, methadone has unique properties, such as the ability to antagonize NMDA receptors, which may be beneficial in the treatment of neuropathic pain. In addition, methadone has high oral bioavailability

and a prolonged half-life, allowing for less frequent dosing and potentially improving treatment adherence. However, its use is associated with several contraindications and precautions. Patients with a history of cardiac arrhythmias should be closely monitored, as methadone can prolong the QT interval, increasing the risk of Torsades de Pointes. In addition, dose adjustment is required in patients with hepatic or renal impairment due to the risk of accumulation and toxicity. Interactions with other drugs, especially those that also affect the QT interval or are metabolized by cytochrome P450, should be carefully evaluated. Methadone can also cause severe respiratory depression, especially at high doses or in combination with other central nervous system depressants, making continuous monitoring of patients' vital signs and respiratory function essential.

Non-opioid Analgesics

Non-opioid analgesics used in the ICU include dipyrone, paracetamol, and neuropathic pain medications such as gabapentin, carbamazepine, and pregabalin. Nonsteroidal anti-inflammatory drugs (NSAIDs) should be used with caution because of their effects on platelet aggregation, renal function, and risk of gastric mucosal damage.

4.8 Daily Awakening from Sedation and Weaning from Mechanical Ventilation

Due to the side effects and potential complications associated with maintaining patients in deep sedation, some strategies aim to keep patients more awake on mechanical ventilation, as long as they remain comfortable and receive adequate analgesia. Deep sedation, regardless of the sedative used, has been associated with longer mechanical ventilation times, extended ICU stays, prolonged hospital stays, and higher mortality rates [2, 3].

Currently, in the absence of clinical contraindications such as intracranial hypertension, hemodynamic instability, or the need for high ventilatory parameters, the goal is to keep patients comfortable with light or no sedation. Strategies such as daily sedation interruption, the use of bolus analgesia and sedation, or nurse-controlled sedation protocols are routinely employed in ICUs to achieve this goal [2, 9–11, 13–15].

Daily sedation interruption, where sedation is halted until the patient is awake and able to follow commands (or until they become agitated or uncomfortable, requiring re-sedation), has been associated with shorter mechanical ventilation times, fewer ICU days, and reduced benzodiazepine use. This approach also allows for more frequent assessment of the patient's neurological status. There does not appear to be a higher incidence of complications such as accidental extubation, post-traumatic stress, ICU-related complications, or coronary ischemia [9, 16].

Combining this strategy with spontaneous breathing protocols appears to result in further reductions in coma duration, hospital length of stay, ICU length of stay, and 1-year mortality compared to standard care [13].

Non-sedation consists of using bolus opioid analgesia to synchronize patients with mechanical ventilation, administering sedatives only to those who remain uncomfortable. When this strategy was compared with light sedation and daily sedation breaks, no differences were found in the number of ventilator-free days, ICU stays, or hospitalizations. Additionally, there appear to be no negative long-term psychological outcomes when non-sedation protocols are implemented [10, 14].

The success of nurse-controlled sedation protocols seems to be directly related to the nurse-to-patient ratio, with better outcomes observed when this ratio is close to 1:1, leading to shorter mechanical ventilation times and a lower incidence of tracheostomies. However, this staffing ratio may not be common in most ICUs, which could overburden the nursing team [11, 15].

Therefore, the adoption of sedation weaning protocols tailored to the local characteristics of intensive care services is essential to optimize this process, leading to shorter ICU and hospital stays without increasing the risk of long-term hospital or inpatient complications.

4.9 Conclusion

Sedoanalgesia is a central practice in managing critically ill patients, particularly those on mechanical ventilation. Balancing effective sedation and analgesia with minimizing complications remains a constant challenge in the ICU. Daily awakening strategies, the rational use of sedatives and analgesics, and the adoption of nurse-controlled sedation protocols are essential measures to optimize patient outcomes, reduce complications, and shorten the length of stay.

The continued development of evidence-based practices, such as the implementation of the ABCDEF bundle, and educating healthcare professionals on best practices for pain management, sedation, and delirium are critical steps in improving ICU care. These efforts ensure a more comprehensive, patient-centered approach that focuses on faster and safer recovery.

References

1. Aragón, et al. Pain, agitation, and delirium in critically ill patients: management and outcomes. Crit Care. 2019;23:130. https://doi.org/10.1186/s13054-019-2394-9.
2. Kollef MH, Levy NT, Ahrens TS, Schaiff R, Prentice D, Sherman G. The use of continuous iv sedation is associated with prolongation of mechanical ventilation. Chest. 1998;114:541–8. https://doi.org/10.1378/chest.114.2.541.

3. Payen JF, Chanques G, Mantz J, et al. Current practices in sedation and analgesia for mechanically ventilated critically ill patients: a prospective multicenter patient-based study. Anesthesiology. 2007;106(4):687–95. https://doi.org/10.1097/01.anes.0000264747.00275.c1.
4. Reade MC, Finfer S. Sedation and delirium in the intensive care unit. N Engl J Med. 2014;370(5):444–54. https://doi.org/10.1056/NEJMra1208705.
5. Barr J, Fraser GL, Puntillo K, et al. Clinical practice guidelines for the management of pain, agitation, and delirium in adult patients in the intensive care unit. Crit Care Med. 2013;41(1):263–306. https://doi.org/10.1097/CCM.0b013e3182783b72.
6. Gélinas C, Fillion L, Puntillo KA, et al. Validation of the critical-care pain observation tool in adult patients. Am J Crit Care. 2006;15(4):420–7. https://doi.org/10.4037/ajcc2006.15.4.420.
7. Devlin JW, Skrobik Y, Gélinas C, et al. Clinical practice guidelines for the prevention and management of pain, agitation/sedation, delirium, immobility, and sleep disruption in adult patients in the ICU. Crit Care Med. 2018;46(9) https://doi.org/10.1097/CCM.0000000000003299.
8. Hayes MHS, Patterson DG. Experimental development of the graphic rating method. Psychol Bull. 1921;18:98–9.
9. Kress JP, et al. Daily interruption of sedative infusions in critically ill patients undergoing mechanical ventilation. N Engl J Med. 2000;342:1471–7. https://doi.org/10.1056/NEJM200005183422002.
10. Olsen HT, et al. Nonsedation or light sedation in critically ill mechanically ventilated patients. N Engl J Med. 2020;382:1103–11. https://doi.org/10.1056/NEJMoa190675.
11. Brook AD, et al. Effect of a nursing-implemented sedation protocol on the duration of mechanical ventilation. Crit Care Med. 1999;27(12):2609–15. https://doi.org/10.1097/00003246-199912000-00001.
12. Sessler CN, Gosnell MS, Grap MJ, et al. The Richmond agitation-sedation scale: validity and reliability in adult intensive care unit patients. Am J Respir Crit Care Med. 2002;166(10):1338–44. https://doi.org/10.1164/rccm.2107138.
13. Girard TD, et al. Efficacy and safety of a paired sedation and ventilator weaning protocol for mechanically ventilated patients in intensive care (Awakening and breathing controlled trial). Lancet. 2008;371 https://doi.org/10.1016/S0140-6736(08)60105-1.
14. Strom T, Martinussen T, Toft P. A protocol of no sedation for critically ill patients receiving mechanical ventilation: a randomised trial. Lancet. 2010;375(9713):475–80. https://doi.org/10.1016/S0140-6736(09)62072-9.
15. Bucknall TK, et al. A randomized trial of protocol-directed sedation management for mechanical ventilation in an Australian intensive care unit. Crit Care Med. 2008;36(5):1444–50. https://doi.org/10.1097/CCM.0b013e318168f82d.
16. Mehta S, Burry L, Cook D, et al. Daily sedation interruption in mechanically ventilated critically ill patients cared for with a sedation protocol: a randomized controlled trial. JAMA. 2012;308(19):1985–92. https://doi.org/10.1001/jama.2012.13872.

Chapter 5
Predictors of Weaning Outcome

Antuani Rafael Baptistella, Diego de Carvalho, and Marcelo Taglietti

5.1 Introduction

- What is the cost of weaning failure?
- When this question is answered, it is likely that professionals and institutions will focus on establishing best practices with standardized protocols to improve the outcome of patients weaning from MV.
- The answer to the above question is: it costs lives, and it costs money.
- Failure to extubate can increase the risk of death by 25%–700% [1, 2] and double the length of hospital stay [1, 3] and therefore cost.

Prediction is the act of anticipating whether an event will occur in the future based on knowledge or experience. In the case of weaning, parameters, scores, or indices that can predict the outcome allow the right patient to be selected to continue weaning and be extubated, as well as identify patients at high risk of extubation failure, thus avoiding reintubation and the consequences of that failure, which is a longer hospital stay and greater risk of death.

The WEAN SAFE study [4], which collected data from 481 ICUs in 50 countries, showed that among 4523 patients who had at least one weaning attempt, the

A. R. Baptistella (✉)
Hospital Universitário Santa Terezinha (HUST), Joaçaba, Brazil

Hospital Unimed Meio-Oeste, Joaçaba, Brazil

Universidade do Oeste de Santa Catarina, Unoesc, Joaçaba, Brazil
e-mail: antuani.baptistella@unoesc.edu.br

D. de Carvalho
University of Western Santa Catarina – Unoesc, Joaçaba, Brazil

M. Taglietti
Centro Universitário Fundação Assis Gurgacz (FAG), Cascavel, Brazil

A. R. Baptistella et al. (eds.), *Weaning from Mechanical Ventilation*,
https://doi.org/10.1007/978-3-032-01145-9_5

weaning failure rate was 15.6% and the extubation failure rate was 13.7%, even though most of these patients had undergone SBT.

SBT is a well-established technique to assess the spontaneous breathing capacity of patients during weaning from MV. In fact, SBT is the most important predictor of weaning outcome, and other weaning or extubation predictors will not replace SBT. The main objective of other weaning and extubation predictors is try to separate the group of patients who tolerate SBT and will be successfully extubated from those who tolerate SBT and will fail extubation, worsening the outcome of these patients. This is the true role of the weaning/extubation predictors (Fig. 5.1).

Extubation failure in patients who tolerated SBT can be divided into airway failure (45%) and non-airway failure (50%) (5% are mixed airway and non-airway failure) [5]. Airway failure includes upper airway obstruction (stridor related to laryngeal edema) and lower airway obstruction (aspiration or excessive respiratory secretions), while non-airway failure is related to many different causes, the most common being respiratory failure, heart failure, brain dysfunction, respiratory muscle weakness or fatigue, and endocrine and metabolic dysfunction [5, 6]. Based on this, the predictors have been divided into non-airway-related and airway-related.

Before presenting the predictors of weaning, it is very important to clarify certain concepts. Weaning is the process of MV discontinuation that starts with the transition from a controlled ventilation mode to a spontaneous ventilation mode [7], goes through SBT, and ends with extubation [8]. In this sense, a predictor of weaning is one where the failure group includes patients who failed SBT and those who failed extubation. In addition, there are predictors of SBT outcome only and predictors of extubation outcome. In this chapter, the predictors have also been divided into weaning, SBT, and extubation outcome predictors.

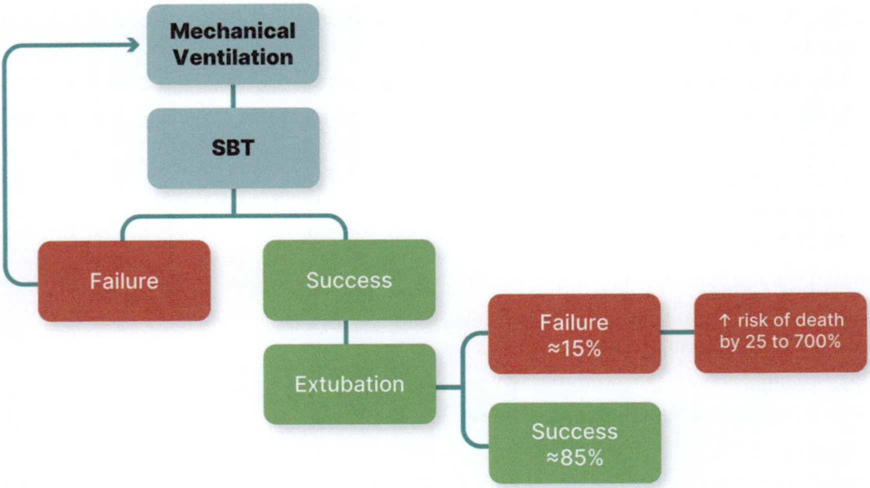

Fig. 5.1 Schematic flowchart of the weaning process

Most of the weaning predictors were tested, including in the failure group with the patients who failed SBT and those who failed extubation. As it has been presented that the pathophysiology of SBT and extubation failure may be different [9], predictors specifically tested to predict the outcome of SBT or those tested to predict only extubation seem to be better options to be used in clinical practice.

Another point is whether it makes sense to predict the outcome of SBT, whether it is possible to perform SBT and have the real result (not just a prediction) in 30 min, without risks or adverse effects to the patient.

Finally, it is important to note that only one clinical trial tested a predictor of weaning, the work published by Tanios and colleagues in 2006 [10], which showed that the use of Rapid Shallow Breathing Index (RSBI) increased the duration of weaning. Keep in mind that it is not possible to support a theory that the use of predictors delays weaning based on only one study that tested an index that does not seem to be the most appropriate for predicting the outcome of weaning. It is extremely important that other predictors be tested in clinical trials.

Presented here is the scientific concept of a predictor applied to health science as well as the parameters that can predict weaning and the predictive scores and indices.

5.2 What Is a Predictor?

The ability to foresee the future is an amazing feature that is explored in many fantasy stories. However, when it comes to real life, this ability relies on solid clues that indicate the probability of an outcome occurring or not. Thus, a good predictor is that cue or set of cues that indicates with a good degree of certainty a possible outcome that, when analyzed retrospectively, has consistently been the correct outcome; in other words, it has a good degree of accuracy.

At this point, it is possible to perceive that a predictor is not infallible because it relies on probability. However, as will be shown in this section, there are characteristics that make either good or bad predictors.

First, a good predictor in health (and in other fields) cannot be more laborious to collect the data than to observe the outcome itself. Sounds almost absurd, but imagine that there is a type of disease that causes severe fatigue in some patients. To predict this fatigue, researchers could develop a complex model requiring extensive genetic testing and psychological assessments. However, a much simpler and more effective predictor might be the presence of specific symptoms, such as frequent sleep disturbances or reduced physical activity. The ease of collecting this symptom data—observed during a routine visit—makes it a more practical predictor than relying on cumbersome tests that could discourage patients from seeking timely care.

In other words, a good predictor should be both meaningful and easy to collect. For example, consider a health predictor such as body mass index (BMI) in relation to obesity. Measuring BMI requires only height and weight, which can be easily obtained during a routine physical examination. In contrast, determining the actual health outcome, such as the onset of obesity-related diseases, typically involves more complex processes, including various tests and assessments. This simplicity of data collection makes BMI a practical and effective predictor, allowing healthcare professionals to quickly assess risk with little effort.

Of course, this is not to dismiss the importance of complex health predictors depending on the outcomes they predict. For example, if genetic mapping predicts the risk of a serious type of cancer, the outcome justifies the complex method of collecting the predictor's data. It is a trade-off between risk and benefit, just like any drug used to treat a disease.

Second, the accuracy of the predictor should be good. How good? Again, it depends on the severity of the predicted outcome. If a disease is rapidly evolving for a severe condition and a marker predicts with 68% accuracy which patient will be badly affected or not, this accuracy might be sufficient if no other predictor exists and there are some treatment options available to avoid the bad outcome.

Remember that accuracy is the ability to correctly predict the outcome. However, in science, there are other metrics that are better than overall accuracy. Sensitivity and specificity, along with receiver operating characteristic (ROC) curves, are commonly used for a predictor in health. And the usual metric for the quality of the predictor is the area under the ROC curve (AUC), where AUCs close to 1 represent better predictors and close to 0.5 represent predictors as good as random choices. As artificial intelligence advances into health, other quality metrics such as precision, recall, and F1 score are used [11].

Third, a good predictor should be most useful when it comes to public health. This means that it should be simple, inexpensive, and easy to collect so that it can be widely used in diverse populations. Predictors that require complex or invasive measurements may limit their use in large-scale health monitoring or in resource-limited settings. Therefore, the more simple and accessible the predictor, the more effective it will be in identifying health risks and guiding public health interventions.

In the field of health, there has been a tremendous increase in publications on predictors. For example, in PubMed from 2013 to 2023, there was a 238% increase in the number of publications when "predictors AND health" was searched. This increase in papers demonstrates the importance of predictors in health and science in general. However, there is often confusion in terms of the definitions of predictors and prognostic factors.

A *predictor* is a variable that can be used to estimate or predict a specific outcome, often in response to a particular intervention or treatment. In healthcare, predictors are used to assess how a patient may respond to a therapeutic intervention, such as medication or surgery. For example, in diabetes management, baseline blood glucose levels can serve as a predictor of how well a patient will respond to a particular treatment regimen. Predictors are typically used in clinical decision making to tailor treatments to individual patients based on their expected responses [12, 13].

In contrast, a *prognostic factor* is any variable that provides information about the likely course or outcome of a disease, regardless of treatment. Prognostic factors help clinicians understand the natural history of a condition and estimate the future course of a disease. For example, in cancer, the stage of the tumor at diagnosis is a key prognostic factor—it provides insight into the likely survival or progression of the disease without necessarily being influenced by treatment options. In contrast to predictors, prognostic factors provide an overall view of the patient's condition over time. In brief, while both predictors and prognostic factors provide valuable information, predictors are specific to treatment response and prognostic factors focus on disease progression. Both play an essential role in personalized medicine, guiding decisions about interventions and long-term management [14].

In summary, predictors play a critical role in modern healthcare by enabling more personalized and effective medical interventions. By using specific variables such as genetic markers, lifestyle factors, or clinical data, healthcare providers can estimate how individuals or populations will respond to treatments, identify at-risk groups, and implement preventive measures. The simplicity and accessibility of these predictors can significantly improve public health outcomes by enabling early intervention and minimizing the burden of disease. In addition, predictors help clinicians make informed decisions that reduce trial and error, improve patient outcomes, and optimize resource use [15].

As the field of data analytics continues to evolve, the future of healthcare will increasingly rely on predictive and *prescriptive analytics*. Predictive analytics, fueled by large-scale data from electronic health records, wearable devices, and genomic data, will provide more accurate and timely insights into patient health trends and risks. This approach will allow for earlier detection of potential health issues, enabling proactive management rather than reactive treatment. For example, machine learning algorithms could predict the likelihood of a heart attack based on subtle changes in patient data over time, prompting early intervention.

Beyond prediction, prescriptive analytics takes data-driven healthcare a step further by providing actionable recommendations based on predictive insights. This approach enables personalized treatment plans that not only forecast patient outcomes but also suggest the most effective interventions tailored to each individual's unique characteristics. Prescriptive analytics could revolutionize healthcare in the future by making treatment decisions more precise, reducing inefficiencies, improving overall patient care, and transforming the way prevention and treatment in public health are approached.

In critical care, particularly in the management of patients requiring mechanical ventilation, predictors are invaluable in guiding treatment decisions and improving patient outcomes. By using data-driven predictions, critical care teams can make more informed decisions about when to initiate or discontinue mechanical ventilation, optimizing patient recovery and resource allocation. As predictive models become more sophisticated, their role in critical care will continue to expand, offering personalized approaches to managing critically ill patients and improving the overall quality of care.

5.3 Predictors of Weaning Outcome

Two systematic reviews have identified a large number of parameters, characteristics, signs, scores, and indexes that predict weaning. Baptistella et al. [16] found 56 parameters associated with weaning and extubation, with the Rapid Shallow Breathing Index (RSBI) being the most common predictor in most studies, followed by age and maximal inspiratory pressure. The second review proposed by Torrini et al. [17] identified a total of 26 factors significantly associated with extubation failure, with 12 factors being more relevant according to the meta-analysis. These factors include: age, history of cardiac disease, history of respiratory disease, Simplified Acute Physiologic Score II, pneumonia, duration of mechanical ventilation, heart rate, Rapid Shallow Breathing Index, negative inspiratory force, lower PaO_2/FiO_2 ratio, lower hemoglobin level, and lower Glasgow Coma Scale before extubation, with the last factor having the strongest association with extubation outcome.

The most important predictors, including individual parameters, clinical or demographic characteristics, signs, scores, and indices, are presented here, divided into predictors of weaning outcome (those included in the failure group, patients who failed SBT and those who failed extubation), predictors of SBT outcome, and predictors of extubation outcome (Fig. 5.2).

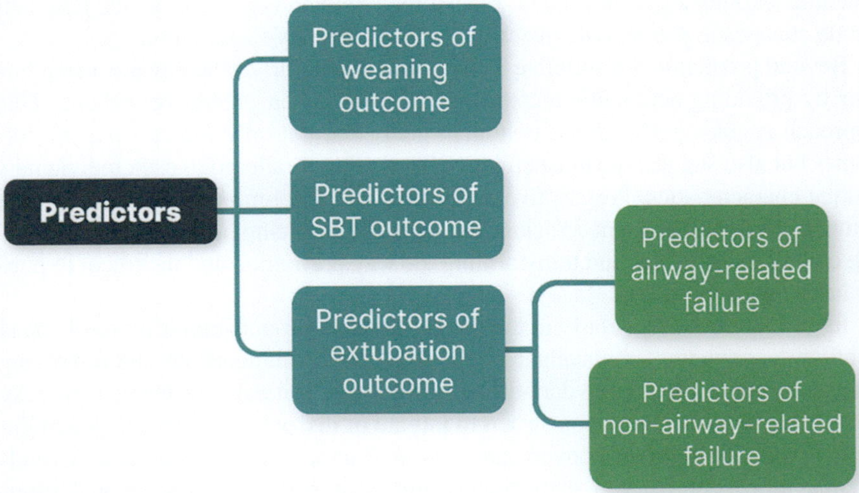

Fig. 5.2 Schematic flowchart of weaning outcome predictors

5.3.1 *Weaning Predictors*

Age

The conventional parameters used for weaning may not always be applicable for deciding when to discontinue mechanical ventilation (MV) in older adults [18]. Research has highlighted significant differences in the ages of patients who are successfully weaned (SW) compared to those who are not (Failed Weaning [FW]). Studies report that the age of SW patients typically ranges from 43.2 to 56 years, whereas FW patients are generally older, ranging from 59.6 to 73 years [19–22]. These differences have been attributed to the physiological changes that occur with aging. Another study found a small but statistically significant age difference between the groups (SW at 68.2 ± 0.9 years and FW at 71.4 ± 0.9 years), despite the small biological difference between 68 and 71 years [23].

Further research dividing age into quartiles (≤42, 43–54, 55–62, and 63+ years) showed a decrease in successful weaning rates with increasing age, with percentages of 91%, 91%, 87%, and 84%, respectively [24]. Based on these findings, many researchers suggest that age over 65 or 70 years serves as a negative predictor of successful weaning and extubation [22, 23, 25]. In addition, in patients 80 years of age or older, age combined with the number of days on mechanical ventilation exceeding 100 may indicate a poorer prognosis [26].

Duration of IMV in Days

Several studies have found that the longer the duration of invasive mechanical ventilation (IMV), the lower the likelihood of successful weaning and extubation, and that a duration of ≥21 days may be a predictor of weaning failure [20, 25, 27].

Respiratory Muscle Assessments

Mechanical ventilation is known to cause rapid weakening of the diaphragm, which is critical for generating the necessary tidal volume to meet the physiological needs of the body [28]. Several bedside assessments are used to evaluate respiratory muscle function and predict weaning outcomes in ICU patients. These include maximal inspiratory pressure (PImax), maximal expiratory pressure, diaphragm thickening fraction (DTF), diaphragm excursion (DE), end-expiratory and end-inspiratory diaphragm thickness (Tdiee and Tdiei), airway closing pressure (P0.1), and both voluntary and involuntary assessments of transdiaphragmatic and airway opening pressures [29].

Maximum inspiratory pressure (MIP) is a valuable parameter for assessing respiratory muscle strength and is often used as a predictor of successful weaning from mechanical ventilation. Previous research has shown that MIP values below −30 cmH_2O are associated with a greater likelihood of weaning success, whereas values above −20 cmH_2O are associated with a greater likelihood of weaning failure [30]. However, some researchers point out the variability of normal MIP values, which can be influenced by the level of voluntary effort. This variability makes it difficult to use in uncooperative patients. In addition, MIP is more representative of diaphragmatic contractile force during deep breathing than during normal quiet breathing [31], which limits its predictive value due to high sensitivity but relatively low specificity [32].

Efforts to improve the predictive power of MIP for weaning outcomes have led to the identification of the occlusion pressure (P0.1)/MIP ratio as a superior indicator of extubation success compared to traditional weaning indices [19]. In addition, other research has shown that sustained maximal inspiratory pressures (SMIP) have better sensitivity and specificity than MIP in predicting weaning outcomes [32]. As the diaphragm plays a central role in spontaneous breathing, assessment of its function should theoretically provide insight into extubation outcomes [33].

Several studies have shown that ultrasound (US) assessment of diaphragm function can serve as an important marker influencing weaning and extubation decisions [33–35] (*read more about US and weaning in* Chap. 11). The percentage change in diaphragm thickness (Tdi) between end-expiration and end-inspiration (ΔTdi%), particularly in the apposition zone, has been associated with extubation success, with a sensitivity of 88% and a specificity of 71% when the change is ≥30% [34]. Another study found that a Δtdi% greater than 20 was a reliable predictor of successful extubation within 48 h of ultrasound evaluation [36]. More recently, a threshold of Δtdi% greater than 34.2 was identified as a key marker of extubation success [35].

A systematic review and meta-analysis of the accuracy of respiratory muscle assessments found that PImax had a sensitivity of 63%, DE had a sensitivity of 75%, DTF had a sensitivity of 77%, P0.1 had a sensitivity of 74%, Tdi_{ei} had a sensitivity of 69%, and Tdi_{ee} had a sensitivity of 37% for predicting weaning success at a fixed specificity of 80%. DE and DTF were significantly more accurate than PImax in predicting weaning success. In addition, DTF was significantly more accurate than DE in predicting weaning success [29].

Arterial Blood Gas (ABG)

ABG analysis is widely used to monitor arterial pH, gas levels, and bicarbonate concentrations in patients and plays an important role in ventilator settings. Parameters such as $PaCO_2$ [37–39], PaO_2 [22, 39], PaO_2/FiO_2 ratio [21, 22, 27], pH [21, 39], HCO_3 [37], and oxygen saturation [40] have been identified as valuable indicators for predicting weaning and extubation outcomes.

Renal Function

Renal function is another important factor to consider, as studies have shown that indicators such as blood urea nitrogen (BUN) [23, 27], creatinine levels (> 1.3 mg%; ≥1.5 mg/dL) [27, 41, 42], and the need for hemodialysis [43] are also predictive of weaning and extubation outcomes.

Fluid Balance

Fluid balance, which is often adjusted in the management of critical illness, may influence the success of extubation. One study showed that a positive fluid balance in the 24 h prior to extubation may be a predictor of extubation failure [37]. In addition, another study suggested that a positive fluid balance observed not only in the last 24 h but also over 48 and 72 h, or accumulated since the patient's admission to the hospital, significantly increases the risk of weaning failure [44].

Nutrition

Nutritional status also plays a role in weaning success. Malnutrition can lead to increased fatigue, decreased inspiratory and expiratory muscle strength, decreased endurance, and decreased diaphragm muscle mass, all of which affect respiratory function [45]. The relationship between nutrition and weaning has been demonstrated by various measures, such as total protein [46], creatinine level index [46], hypophosphatemia [47–49], and albumin levels [27], which correlate with weaning outcomes.

Anemia, as indicated by hemoglobin levels, has been shown to be a predictor of weaning success [37, 46]. Patients with hemoglobin levels below 10 g/dL are more than five times more likely to have an unsuccessful extubation than those with levels above 10 g/dL [50]. The mechanism by which low hemoglobin levels increase the risk of extubation failure is not fully understood, but anemia may exacerbate global oxygen delivery insufficiency and myocardial ischemia, conditions commonly observed in patients who fail weaning [51, 52].

Furthermore, hypophosphatemia is associated with respiratory muscle weakness, as reflected by a decrease in spontaneous tidal volume, decreased static lung compliance and impaired lung function, increased length of stay in the ICU, and time on mechanical ventilation, leading to weaning failure [49]. Hypophosphatemia significantly affected weaning from MV in acute exacerbations of chronic obstructive pulmonary disease (AECOPD) patients (with a threshold of 0.87 mmol/l) [49], also in the general ICU population [47, 48], and in COVID-19 patients (with a threshold of 0.80 mmol/l) [48].

Following the identification of many individual parameters related to weaning outcome, some researchers have proposed scores that consider multiple parameters systematically combined with the aim of improving the ability to predict weaning.

Here, scores and indices are presented for predicting weaning, SBT, and extubation outcomes.

Morganroth Scoring System

The first score to predict weaning outcome was developed by Morganroth and colleagues and published in 1984 [53] with the goal of creating a scoring system as a criterion for weaning patients from prolonged MV. At that time, the SBT was not well established and standardized. Progression of weaning was determined by increasing the time the patient remained off the ventilator. Weaning success was determined when the patient was able to tolerate 24 consecutive hours without mechanical ventilation without signs of fatigue. The authors do not mention whether patients were extubated. This score consists of two tables: the first table evaluates ventilator parameters (Ventilator Score) with a total of 27 points, while the second table evaluates adverse factors (Adverse Factor Score) with a total of 48 points. Evaluating the sum of the two scores as a test of weaning ability, using all determinations for all patients, gives a sensitivity of 93% and a specificity of 86%.

Rapid Shallow Breathing Index

In 1991, Yang and Tobin [54] published the comparison of two new indices (f/VT and CROP, or compliance, rate, oxygenation, and pressure) with some parameters used to predict weaning outcome, such as minute ventilation and maximal inspiratory pressure (Pimax). The f/VT or RSBI is quantified as the respiratory frequency divided by the tidal volume (VT) in liters. This measurement was taken with the patient breathing spontaneously for 1 min while connected to a spirometer.

The primary outcome was the ability to maintain spontaneous breathing for more than 24 h after extubation. Weaning failure was considered to be those patients who had mechanical ventilation reinitiated at the end of the weaning trial or who required reintubation within 24 h. RSBI was the most accurate predictor of success with an AUC of 0.89. The authors also suggested a threshold of ≤105 breaths/min/L.

In the following years, the RSBI became the most studied index to predict weaning or extubation outcome and has been used in different situations and patient groups, measured with ventilometers as well as in the mechanical ventilator, at different moments of the SBT [16].

Despite the cutoff established by Yang and Tobin, other studies have shown that other values are better predictors. Upadya and colleagues [44] showed that patients who were successfully extubated had an RSBI around 50 breaths/min/L, while those who failed SBT or extubation had an RSBI around 80 breaths/min/L. Chatila and colleagues [55] showed that RSBI measured at the beginning of SBT did not correlate with outcome, but RSBI measured at 30–60 min of SBT was more predictive of weaning outcome (92.2 ± 24.7 and 132.0 ± 57.4 for weaning success and failure groups, respectively). A similar result was observed by Kuo and colleagues [56], where there were no differences in RSBI between success and failure groups at 1 min SBT, but RSBI at 120 min was significantly higher in extubation failure (95.9 ± 20.6) and trial failure (98.0 ± 50.0) patients than in weaning success (64.6 ± 26.3) patients.

In a different approach, Segal and colleagues [57] measured RSBI every 30 min during 2 h of SBT. Initial RSBI was similar in the extubation success and failure groups (77.0 ± 4.8 and 77.0 ± 4.8, respectively). However, RSBI remained unchanged or decreased in the extubation success group and increased in the extubation failure group. Wysocki and colleagues [58] showed that the RSBI in the first minute of SBT was statistically lower in the success group (60 [30–161]) than in the failure group (116 [68–277]).

On the other hand, Savi and colleagues [22] showed in a study of 500 patients that RSBI at both 1 min and 30 min of SBT was statistically higher in the extubation failure group.

However, subsequent predictive statistical analyses showed that changes in RSBI during SBT, or RSBI at either 1 min or 30 min of SBT, did not predict extubation outcome.

In the only randomized controlled trials (RCTs) published to date to evaluate scores or indices predictive of weaning, Tanios and colleagues [10] compared a group of 151 patients in whom RSBI was measured but not used in the weaning decision with 153 patients in whom RSBI was used (threshold of 105 breaths/min). Patients who passed the 2-h SBT were eligible for extubation. Median weaning time was significantly shorter in the group not using the weaning predictor, with no difference in extubation failure rate, in-hospital mortality, tracheostomy, or unplanned extubation. The authors concluded that the RSBI should not be used routinely to guide weaning decisions.

In a recent meta-analysis that included 48 studies with 10,946 patients, Trivedi and colleagues [59] showed that the sensitivity for RSBI of <105 in predicting extubation success was moderate (0.83) and the specificity was poor (0.58), with a diagnostic OR (DOR) of 5.91. Similar sensitivity, specificity, and DOR were obtained for thresholds of <80 or 80–105. These results were consistent across multiple subgroup analyses.

CROP

In the same study in which Yang and Tobin [54] published the RSBI, they also proposed the CROP index. Once again, CROP is an acronym for Compliance, Rate, Oxygenation, and Pressure:

$$\text{CROP} = \left(C_{dyn} \times P_{Imax} \times \left[PaO_2 / P_AO_2\right]\right) / \text{rate}$$

In the original study, CROP had an AUC of 0.78, and the authors suggested a threshold of ≥13 ml/breath/min for CROP as a predictor of weaning success.

Gluck and Corgian Scoring System

In 1996, Gluck and Corgian proposed the Gluck and Corgian scoring system [60] to predict eventual weaning success or failure in patients receiving long-term MV. It is composed of five respiratory parameters (RSBI, VD/VT [dead space to tidal volume ratio], static lung compliance, resistance, $PaCO_2$), scored from 0 to 2, with a lower score more indicative of weaning success, and was used at the time of admission to a long-term ventilator facility in adult patients ventilated for an average of 3 weeks. Patients were considered weaned if they could tolerate 48 consecutive hours without pressure or flow support from a mechanical ventilator. The sensitivity of the scoring system was 100%, while the specificity was 77%, using a threshold of 3. A score less than 3 was associated with weaning success, while a score greater than 3 predicted failure, with sensitivity and specificity of 100% and 91%, respectively, with a score of 3 being nondiscriminatory. Thus, the positive predictive value of a score less than 3 was 83% and the negative predictive value of a score greater than 3 was 100%.

Integrative Weaning Index (IWI)

The Integrative Weaning Index (IWI), proposed by Nemer and colleagues in 2009 [61], is composed of the static compliance of the respiratory system (Cst,rs), arterial oxygen saturation (SaO_2), and the f/VT (or RSBI):

$$\text{IWI} = \text{Cst,rs} \times SaO_2 / \left(f / V_T\right)$$

In a prospective validation cohort, 183 patients were evaluated, and the primary outcome was successful weaning, considered if the patient maintained spontaneous breathing for more than 48 h after extubation. Weaning failure was defined if the patient failed SBT, was reintubated, or died within 48 h of extubation. The threshold for distinguishing between successful and unsuccessful weaning was 25 ml/cmH_2O

breaths/minute/liter or greater. IWI showed an area under the ROC curve of 0.96, significantly higher than RSBI (0.85), with a higher probability of successful weaning when the test was positive (0.99) and a lower probability when the test was negative (0.14). The authors suggested that the measurement of Cst,rs during the weaning process may be considered one of the limitations of the method.

TIE Index

The timed inspiratory effort (TIE) index was developed by Souza and colleagues and published in 2015 [62], with the premise that patients with poorer neuromuscular efficiency require more time to develop maximal effort during the occlusion maneuver. Measurement of maximal inspiratory pressure (MIP) involves the imposition of a respiratory discomfort that challenges autonomic and voluntary control of breathing. After a period of time, the MIP is reached due to the progressive increase in respiratory drive. The TIE index is calculated as the ratio between the MIP and the corresponding time to reach it during 60 s of observation (Fig. 5.3).

The primary outcome of the study was weaning failure, defined as patients showing signs of intolerance during the SBT or within 48 h after weaning from mechanical ventilation. Using a cutoff of 1 cmH_2O/sec, the AUC of TIE was 0.90, with a sensitivity of 0.78 and specificity of 0.86, demonstrating that it was a better predictor of weaning than RSBI (AUC = 0.80 with a cutoff of 90).

In 2023, Godoy and colleagues [63], from the same research group, showed in a randomized, controlled, non-inferiority trial that the TIE index was not inferior to the T-piece trial as a decision tool for extubation, which could allow a reduction in decision time.

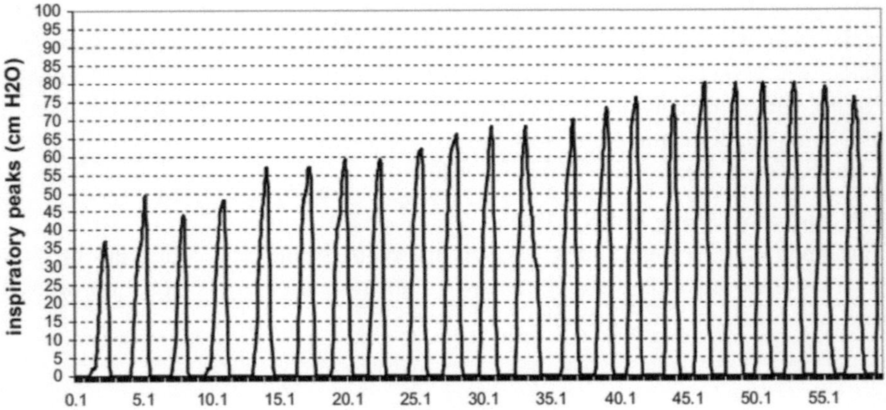

Fig. 5.3 Graph showing inspiratory peaks during 60 s of observation. Maximum inspiratory pressure was reached at 46.5 s. In this case, the TIE index was 1.72 cmH_2O/sec. (Figure from Souza et al. 2015, doi: 10.1177/0885066613483265)

D-RSBI

The Diaphragmatic Rapid Shallow Breathing Index (D-RSBI) was developed by Spadaro and colleagues and published in 2016 [64]. They replaced VT with ultrasound assessment of diaphragmatic displacement (DD) to predict weaning failure:

$$\text{D}-\text{RSBI} = \text{respiratory rate}\left(\text{RR}\right) / \text{diaphragmatic displacement}\left(\text{DD}\right)$$

The authors hypothesized that although the diaphragm generates VT in healthy subjects, when diaphragmatic efficiency is impaired, the accessory inspiratory muscles may contribute to ventilation, but these muscles can sustain this process for a limited period of time because they are less efficient and more fatigable than the diaphragm, resulting in weaning failure in the following hours. By replacing VT with DD, the authors reasoned that this new index could evaluate diaphragmatic capacity without the interference of accessory muscles.

In this study, all patients underwent SBT with a T-tube for 2 h, and 30 min after the start of SBT, diaphragmatic displacement was evaluated by ultrasound. The outcomes evaluated were weaning success (extubation and spontaneous breathing for more than 48 h) or weaning failure (SBT failure, reintubation, or NIV within 48 h of extubation). D-RSBI greater than 1.3 predicted weaning failure with an AUC of 0.89, sensitivity of 94.1%, and specificity of 64.7%, whereas the AUC of RSBI greater than 62 was 0.72 (sensitivity of 52.9% and specificity of 97.1%). These results demonstrated that the D-RSBI (RR/DD) is more accurate than the traditional RSBI (RR/VT) in predicting weaning outcome.

BICYCLE Score

In 2023, Schreiber and colleagues [65] published the BICYCLE score, a prediction model for weaning success in patients with traumatic spinal cord injuries (tSCI). The primary outcome was weaning success from MV at ICU discharge, and a parsimonious model was developed and validated by Bootstrap.

Of the 459 patients analyzed, 72% were weaned and discharged alive from the ICU. Factors associated with weaning success were blunt injury, Injury Severity Score (ISS), complete syndrome, age, and cervical lesion. Linear combination of the regression coefficients of these five predictors generated the BICYCLE score:

31 – 109 [if injury of Blunt type] + 2 * (ISS)
+ 64 [if Complete Syndrome present]
+ 2*age [Years]
+ 51 [if Cervical Lesion present]
*(where a + 31 intercept was added to provide as score range starting from 0)

The BICYCLE score showed a larger area under the curve than the ISS (0.689 vs. 0.537). Factors predicting weaning success also predicted time to liberation and showed good discriminative ability after internal validation.

The authors suggested that external validation in an independent cohort of patients with tSCI could ensure the generalizability of the model, and in the absence of new evidence, this score could provide valuable information, in addition to individual patient history, disease course, and clinical examination, to predict weaning outcome in patients with tSCI.

5.3.2 SBT Predictors

Weaning Index (WI)—(Jabour, 1991) In 1991, Jabour and colleagues published the Weaning Index (WI) [66], which integrates ventilatory endurance and gas exchange efficiency using the formula:

$$WI = PTI \times \left(V_{E40} / V_{Tsb}\right)$$

PTI is the pressure-time index and reflects the strength and duration of inspiratory muscle contraction, calculated using the formula PTI = (Pbreath/NIP) × (Tr/Ttot), where NIP is the negative inspiratory pressure, Tr is the inspiratory time, and Ttot is the total breathing cycle time. Pbreath is calculated using the formula Pbreath = (Ppeak − PEEP) × (VTsb/VTmv), where VTsb is the patient's spontaneous tidal volume and VTmv is the tidal volume during mechanical ventilation.

VE40 is calculated using the formula VE40 = (f × [VTmv/BW]) × ($PaCO_2$mv/40), where f is the respiratory rate during mechanical ventilation, BW is the body weight, and $PaCO_2$mv is the arterial pressure of CO_2 during mechanical ventilation.

The primary outcome was weaning failure, defined as intolerance to the weaning trial (not described if it was an SBT). All 24 trials in which the WI was >4 min^{-1} failed, whereas 18 of 19 trials in which the WI was <4 min^{-1} succeeded. The authors also proposed a simplified WI (SWI) without PTI measurement.

Despite the great complexity in assessing this index, the authors concluded that WI successfully predicts the outcome of weaning trials and also provides valuable insight into the mechanisms responsible for weaning failure.

CORE Index
In 2011, Delisle and colleagues [67] described the CORE index, the first tool to predict the success or failure of SBT. The authors did not test the impact of CORE on extubation outcome. The CORE index added P0.1 to the CROP index:

$$CORE = \left[C_{dyn} \times \left(P_{Imax} / P_{0.1}\right) \times \left(P_aO_2 / P_AO_2\right)\right] / f$$

They compared the ability of CORE, CROP, P0.1, and RSBI to predict SBT success/failure and found AUC of 1.00, 0.91, 0.81, and 0.77, respectively, demonstrating that the CORE index is a more accurate predictor of weaning outcome than the CROP index and RSBI.

COBRE-US Trial
The COBRE-US trial published by Varón-Vega and colleagues in 2023 [68] proposed a predictive model for SBT outcome (for both 30-min T-piece or pressure support ventilation) and a model for extubation success (see Extubation Predictors—Sect. 5.3.3).

Based on a multivariate logistic regression analysis, only cough and diaphragmatic contraction velocity (DCV) were associated with SBT success, which is the basis for the following equation:

$$(0.56 \times \text{cough}) - (0.13 \times \text{DCV}) + 0.25$$

In this model, DCV is a continuous variable, and cough ranges from 0 to 3:

0 = No presence of cough.
1 = Audible movement of air through the orotracheal tube, but no audible cough.
2 = Strong cough with mobilization of secretions within the orotracheal tube.
3 = Strong cough with mobilization of secretions outside the orotracheal tube (expectoration). The cutoff point was ≥0.83, with sensitivity of 91.5% and specificity of 22.1%, with an overall accuracy of 76.2%.

5.3.3 Predictors of Extubation Outcome

5.3.3.1 Predictors of Non-Airway-Related Failure

Lung Compliance

Lung compliance, which reflects the pressure required to produce the appropriate volume for the body's physiological needs, has been identified as a predictor of extubation outcome [25, 58].

ICU-Acquired Weakness

ICU-acquired weakness, which includes polyneuropathy, myopathy, and muscle atrophy [69–71], is clinically recognized as limb paresis but can also affect all respiratory muscles, resulting in decreased inspiratory and expiratory strength, as well as pharyngeal muscles. This condition can ultimately lead to generalized respiratory muscle weakness [72, 73] and dysphagia [74].

Limb muscle strength is assessed using the Medical Research Council (MRC) score for the three muscle groups of each limb, with an overall score ranging from 0 (total paralysis) to 60 (normal muscle strength); ICU-acquired weakness was defined as an MRC sum score of less than 48, and severe weakness as a sum score of less than 36 [75]. The lower the MRC sum score, the greater the difficulty of weaning and delayed extubation in mechanically ventilated patients [72, 74–77] and its association with extubation failure [36, 78].

Burns Wean Assessment Program (BWAP) and Modified BWAP (M-BWAP)

The Burns Wean Assessment Program (BWAP) was proposed by Burns and colleagues in 2010 [24]. The BWAP is a 26-factor weaning assessment worksheet and scoring tool consisting of 12 general assessment questions and 14 respiratory assessment questions. Responses are yes, no, or not rated based on the previous 24 h. A yes response indicates that the factor meets the established threshold definition. The BWAP score is calculated by dividing the total number of yes responses by 26 (resulting in a percentage of yes responses). Results showed that patients with BWAP scores >50 were significantly more likely to be successfully extubated than patients with lower scores. Since the primary outcome was defined as reintubation and/or reinstitution of mechanical ventilation within 24 h of extubation, BWAP can be considered the first score specifically tested to predict extubation outcome.

In 2014, Jiang and colleagues [25] published the modified BWAP (m-BWAP), adding age, cardiac function, level of consciousness, lung compliance, airway resistance, and minute ventilation to the original version. The results showed that the m-BWAP score was higher in patients with successful extubation compared to those who failed. Using a cutoff of 60, the sensitivity and specificity of the m-BWAP for predicting successful extubation were 81.4% and 82.1%, respectively. m-BWAP showed similar results when tested as a predictor of SBT.

Weaning Index (WI)—(Huaringa, 2013)

Huaringa and colleagues published the Weaning Index (WI) in 2013 [51]. This index, which integrates three indices (RSBI × EI × VDI), was compared to RSBI alone.

$$\mathrm{WI} = \mathrm{RSBI} \times \mathrm{EI} \times \mathrm{VDI}$$

The elastance index (EI) was expressed as the ratio of peak pressure (at a VT of 8 mL/kg ideal body weight) to the strength of the inspiratory muscles measured by negative inspiratory force (NIF), also called maximal inspiratory pressure (PImax). EI is peak pressure/NIF.

The ventilatory demand index (VDI) was determined by obtaining the minute ventilation with the patient at complete rest and fully supported by assist/control ventilation (A/C). The minute ventilation was then divided by 10.

In this study of 59 patients, the AUC of the WI was 95.9, and when the authors evaluated the accuracy of a WI ≤100 to predict extubation outcome, the sensitivity was 97%, specificity 89%, positive predictive value (PPV) 95%, and negative predictive value (NPV) 94%. The authors concluded that the WI is a simple, easily obtained, and reproducible value that integrates breathing pattern, compliance, inspiratory muscle strength, and ventilatory demand, with a high sensitivity and specificity.

Integrative Index

In 2017, Wu and colleagues proposed an integrative index that combines three parameters: albumin, hemoglobin, and Glasgow Coma Scale (GCS) to predict extubation outcome [79]. Authors showed that an integrative index considering lower serum albumin (<2.6 g/dL), lower hemoglobin (<10.0 g/dL) and lower GCS (≤ 8) predicted extubation failure with an area under the receiver operating characteristic curve of 0.84 (the AUC for RSBI in this study was 0.61), and sensitivity and specificity of 78.6% and 75.9%, respectively.

The authors concluded that although this index is easy to use, further studies should include parameters such as airway secretions, cardiac function, and cough strength, and should be tested in a larger population.

ExPreS: Extubation Predictive Score

This score was developed, validated, and published by Baptistella and colleagues in 2021 [3]. Based on the hypothesis that extubation failure is multifactorial and often involves changes in various organs and systems of the critically ill patient, the authors developed a statistical model that used logistic regression to group patient clinical characteristics associated with extubation outcome. The best model was composed of eight characteristics (RSBI, lung compliance, days of MV, estimated Glasgow Coma Scale (eGCS), muscle strength, hematocrit, creatinine, and neurological comorbidity) and resulted in an AUC of 0.87 in the derivation cohort and 0.97 in the validation cohort (AUC of RSBI alone in the derivation cohort was 0.77) (Fig. 5.4).

The Youden index from the ROC analysis was used to determine the cutoff values of ExPreS for predicting extubation success. The OR for extubation success was 23.07 ($p = 0.004$) for patients with ExPreS ≥59 points and 0.82 ($p = 0.004$) for patients with ExPreS ≤44 points (Fig. 5.5).

In the validation cohort, where patients were extubated based on ExPreS values, the extubation failure rate was 2.4%. Before the use of ExPreS, the extubation failure rate in the derivation cohort was 8.2%. Additionally, in the validation cohort, no patients with ExPreS ≥59 failed extubation.

The ExPreS, a multi-parameter score developed by incorporating several respiratory and non-respiratory parameters associated with extubation outcome, is a reliable predictor of extubation outcome in patients receiving IMV in the ICU. It is a simple method that can be easily applied at the bedside, and an app is available for free for Android and iOS (Fig. 5.6).

COBRE-US Trial

In addition to the model for predicting SBT success (see SBT Predictors), Varón-Vega and colleagues also published a model for predicting extubation success in the same study [68].

Based on a multivariate logistic regression analysis and SBT score, cough and diaphragm contraction velocity (DCV) were associated with extubation success. The prediction model is based on the following equation:

$$(5.7 \times \text{SBT}) + (0.75 \times \text{Cough}) - (0.25 \times \text{DCV}) - 4.5$$

Fig. 5.4 ExPreS—Extubation Predictive Score Tool

EXTUBATION PREDICTIVE SCORE – ExPreS

PARAMETER	VALUE	SCORE
RSBI in SBT (breaths/min/L)	≤42	25
	43–54	20
	55–76	10
	77–90	5
	≥91	0
Dynamic Lung Compliance (ml/cmH2O)	≥63	15
	51–62	10
	43–50	7
	32–42	3
	< 32	0
Days of Mechanical Ventilation	1–3	10
	4–5	7
	6–8	4
	9–10	1
	≥11	0
Estimated Glasgow Coma Scale	≥13.5	10
	11.7–13.4	6
	8.9–11.6	3
	< 8.9	0
Muscle Strength (MRC)	49–60	10
	37–48	7
	25–36	4
	13–24	1
	0–12	0
Hematocrit (%)	≥37	10
	32–36	7
	26–31	3
	22–25	1
	< 22	0
Creatinine (mg/dL)	≤0.99	10
	1.0–1.2	7
	1.3–1.5	4
	1.6–2.9	1
	≥3	0
Neurological Comorbidity	No	10
	Yes	0
Total		=

In this equation, SBT is a dichotomous variable (1 = successful SBT, 0 = unsuccessful SBT), cough was scored from 0 to 3 (see COBRE-US study for SBT predictors), and DCV was scored as a continuous variable.

Extubation success was defined as the absence of death or need for reintubation within 48 h of extubation. Using a cutoff of ≥1.25, the sensitivity was 96.8%, the specificity was 78.4%, and the overall accuracy was 91.5%.

ExPreS	Sensitivity	Specificity	Success rate (%)	Success probability
ExPreS ≤ **44 points**	0.960	0.333	57.1	Low
ExPreS from **45 to 58 points**	0.950 - 0.667	0.333 - 0.772	88.3	Intermediate
ExPreS ≥ **59 points**	0.889	0.752	98.7	High

Fig. 5.5 Cutoff points of the ExPreS—Extubation Predictive Score—and the sensitivity, specificity, success rate, and probability of success for each point

Fig. 5.6 QR code to download the ExPreS app

Artificial Intelligence Predicting Extubation Outcome

In the last decade, several studies have been published that present the potential use of artificial intelligence (AI) to predict extubation outcomes.

In 2015, Kuo and colleagues [80] presented an artificial neural network (ANN) with eight variables: age, reasons for intubation, duration of mechanical ventilation, APACHE II score, mean inspiratory and expiratory times, mean respiratory frequency, and mean expiratory tidal volume in a 30-min SBT (pressure support ventilation of 5 cmH_2O and PEEP of 5 cmH_2O). The area under the receiver operating characteristic curve of the ANN model was 0.83, demonstrating better than RSBI and maximum inspiratory pressure (MIP) to predict extubation outcome at 48 h.

In 2018, Hsieh and colleagues [81] published another ANN with the following parameters: age, APACHE II score, Therapeutic Intervention Scoring System (TISS), GCS, chronic hemodialysis, diabetes, active cancer, duration of ventilator use, RSBI, MIP, maximum expiratory pressure (MEP), and pre-extubation assessment of pulse rate, PaO_2/FiO_2, hemoglobin, hematocrit, and blood urea nitrogen (BUN). The AUC of this model was 0.85, and the authors concluded that it performed well in predicting extubation failure.

In 2023, Menguy and colleagues [82] showed that a model composed of body mass index (BMI), P0.1, and heart rate analysis parameters (low frequency/high frequency [LF/HF]), both measured before SBT, and heart rate during SBT, had an accuracy of 83% in predicting extubation success at 72 h.

5.3.3.2 Predictors of Airway-Related Failure

Cuff Leak Test

The cuff leak test ensures that there is adequate airflow around the endotracheal tube after cuff deflation to confirm that the airway is free of significant laryngeal edema. An absolute volume of <110 ml has been used most consistently in the literature, measured during assisted control ventilation within 24 h of extubation, and has been associated with a higher risk of post-extubation stridor [83].

The cuff leak test has a low diagnostic accuracy, with a sensitivity of 27%–46%, a specificity of 70%–88%, a very low positive predictive value of 14%–19%, and a negative predictive value of 92%–93% [84]. Therefore, cuff leak testing has limited diagnostic power and may unnecessarily prolong the duration of mechanical ventilation.

Neurological Status, Cough, and Endotracheal Secretions

Airway parameters such as cough strength and the presence of endotracheal secretions are critical in predicting a patient's ability to generate an effective cough, expel secretions, and maintain a clear airway—all of which are associated with successful weaning and extubation [50, 85].

Several methods have been used to assess the relationship between cough strength and weaning/extubation outcomes. One study of 150 patients measured involuntary peak inspiratory flow (CPFi) elicited by 2 mL of normal saline at the end of inspiration and found that the cough reflex could predict successful extubation in patients who passed a spontaneous breathing trial (SBT) [86]. These results correlated moderately with a cough strength scale and the amount of endotracheal secretions, which have been shown to be important predictors of extubation outcome [50]. However, there is no standardized scale that categorizes the type and amount of secretions into a reproducible score. Two other studies [85, 87] demonstrated that peak cough expiratory flow may be a useful parameter for predicting weaning and extubation outcomes.

In addition to the cough reflex and the volume of endotracheal secretions, the patient's level of consciousness is another critical factor in determining the ability to protect the airway and facilitate safe extubation. Consciousness is assessed using the Glasgow Coma Scale (GCS) [25] and the modified GCS [27]. Lower scores on these scales are associated with unsuccessful weaning and extubation outcomes [25, 27, 88].

In patients with severe brain injury submitted to mechanical ventilation, the success in the SBT is not sufficient to predict the extubation success, due to the neurological status that may complicate the airway protection ability. Here, the scores are presented, focused on evaluating the risk of extubation failure in relation to airway.

Airway Care Score (Coplin Score)

Coplin and colleagues in 2000 [89], in a prospective observational cohort study of patients with acute brain injury in the ICU, developed the airway care score (ACS), a semiquantitative score divided into six parts to assess airway function. The higher the ACS, the worse the airway function that was associated with a delay in extubation. Patients with an ACS score ≥ 10 were classified as having poor airway function. The six components of the ACS (spontaneous cough, gag, sputum quantity, sputum viscosity, sputum character, and suction frequency) are scored from 0 to 3 (Table 5.1).

In 2017, in a prospective cohort study of patients with stroke or intracerebral hemorrhage, Steidl and colleagues [90] proposed a modified ACS in which sputum viscosity (watery: 0, frothy: 1, thick: 2) and character (clear: 0, tan/yellow: 1) were shortened. Extubation failure was associated with a worse modified ACS.

Table 5.1 Semiquantitative Airway Care Score (ACS) [89]

Score	Spontaneous cough	Gag	Sputum quantity	Sputum viscosity	Sputum character	Suction frequency
0	Vigorous	Vigorous	None	Watery	Clear	> 3 h
1	Moderate	Moderate	1 pass	Frothy	Tan	q 2–3 h
2	Weak	Weak	2 passes	Thick	Yellow	q 1–2 h
3	None	None	≥ 3 passes	Tenacious	Green	≤ 1 h

Table 5.2 VISAGE Score Calculation Worksheet

Clinical features	Assigned points according to items
Age < 40 year old (yes/no)	1/0
Visual pursuit (yes/no)	1/0
Swallowing attempts (yes/no)	1/0
Glasgow Coma Scale score > 10 (yes/no)	1/0

VISAGE Score

In 2017, Asehnoune and colleagues [91] developed and published the VISAGE score (visual pursuit, swallowing, age, and Glasgow for extubation) to predict successful extubation specifically for patients with brain injury. These four clinical features were associated with successful extubation: age less than 40 years, visual pursuit, swallowing attempts, and a Glasgow Coma Scale greater than 10 (Table 5.2).

Each of these items counted as one. A score of 3 or greater was associated with 90% extubation success. The area under the receiver operator curve was 0.75, and after internal validation, the AUC was 0.73.

ENIO Score

In 2022, Cinotti and colleagues [92] proposed the ENIO score in an international multicenter observational study conducted in 73 ICUs with a training and validation cohort. In this study, they evaluated neurocritical care patients with a baseline GCS score ≤ 12 who were under MV for at least 24 h. Extubation failure was defined as reintubation in the first 5 days after extubation. Although the score was composed of 20 variables independently associated with extubation outcome, the authors proposed a simplified, user-friendly model with seven predictors: traumatic brain injury diagnosis, vigorous cough, gag reflex, swallowing attempts, endotracheal suctioning frequency ≤ 2 q h, GCS motor score = 6, and body temperature. The area under the curve of this optimal model was 0.65 (95% CI 0.53–0.76) in the validation cohort.

The Future

Future predictive scores should combine predictive factors for airway and non-airway failure in the same score, since different causes of failure need to be predicted by different factors. This will increase the predictive power of the scores.

Furthermore, more important than creating new scores is the testing of existing scores in randomized and multicenter controlled trials.

References

1. Epstein SK, Ciubotaru RL, Wong JB. Effect of failed Extubation on the outcome of mechanical ventilation. Chest. 1997;112:186–92.
2. Thille AW, Richard J-CM, Brochard L. The decision to Extubate in the intensive care unit. Am J Respir Crit Care Med. 2013;187:1294–302.
3. Baptistella AR, Mantelli LM, Matte L, da Rosa Ulanoski Carvalho ME, Fortunatti JA, Costa IZ, et al. Prediction of extubation outcome in mechanically ventilated patients: development and validation of the Extubation predictive score (ExPreS) (Pasin L, editor). PLos One. 2021;16:e0248868.
4. Pham T, Heunks L, Bellani G, Madotto F, Aragao I, Beduneau G, et al. Weaning from mechanical ventilation in intensive care units across 50 countries (WEAN SAFE): a multicentre, prospective, observational cohort study. Lancet Respir Med. 2023;11:465–76.
5. Jaber S, Quintard H, Cinotti R, Asehnoune K, Arnal J-M, Guitton C, et al. Risk factors and outcomes for airway failure versus non-airway failure in the intensive care unit: a multicenter observational study of 1514 extubation procedures. Crit Care. 2018;22:236.
6. Heunks LM, Van Der Hoeven JG. Clinical review: the ABC of weaning failure – a structured approach. Crit Care. 2010;14:245.
7. Fajardo-Campoverdi A, González-Castro A, Adasme-Jeria R, Roncalli-Rocha A, Ibarra M, Chica-Meza C, et al. Mechanical ventilator liberation protocol. Recommendation based on review of the evidence. J Mech Vent. 2023;4:31–41.
8. Schönhofer B, Geiseler J, Dellweg D, Fuchs H, Moerer O, Weber-Carstens S, et al. Prolonged weaning: S2k guideline published by the German respiratory society. Respiration. 2020;99:982–1084.
9. MacIntyre NR. Evidence-based guidelines for weaning and discontinuing ventilatory support. Chest. 2001;120:375S–95S.
10. Tanios MA, Nevins ML, Hendra KP, Cardinal P, Allan JE, Naumova EN, et al. A randomized, controlled trial of the role of weaning predictors in clinical decision making*. Crit Care Med. 2006;34:2530–5.
11. Agarwal R. Predictive analysis in health care system using AI. In: Garg L, Basterrech S, Banerjee C, Sharma TK, editors. Artif Intell Healthc [internet]. Singapore: Springer; 2022. p. 117–31. Available from: https://link.springer.com/10.1007/978-981-16-6265-2_8. [cited 2024 Oct 22].
12. Hayes DF. Prognostic and predictive factors revisited. Breast. 2005;14:493–9.
13. Italiano A. Prognostic or predictive? It's time to get Back to definitions! J Clin Oncol. 2011;29:4718.
14. Sechidis K, Papangelou K, Metcalfe PD, Svensson D, Weatherall J, Brown G. Distinguishing prognostic and predictive biomarkers: an information theoretic approach. Bioinformatics 2018;34:4139.
15. Kent P, Cancelliere C, Boyle E, Cassidy JD, Kongsted A. A conceptual framework for prognostic research. BMC Med Res Methodol. 2020;20:172.

16. Baptistella AR, Sarmento FJ, Da Silva KR, Baptistella SF, Taglietti M, Zuquello RÁ, et al. Predictive factors of weaning from mechanical ventilation and extubation outcome: a systematic review. J Crit Care. 2018;48:56–62.
17. Torrini F, Gendreau S, Morel J, Carteaux G, Thille AW, Antonelli M, et al. Prediction of extubation outcome in critically ill patients: a systematic review and meta-analysis. Crit Care. 2021;25:391.
18. Krieger BP, Ershowsky PF, Becker DA, Gazeroglu HB. Evaluation of conventional criteria for predicting successful weaning from mechanical ventilatory support in elderly patients. Crit Care Med. 1989;17:858–61.
19. Capdevïla XJ, Perrigault PF, Perey PJ, Roust An JPA, d'Athis F. Occlusion pressure and its ratio to maximum inspiratory pressure are useful predictors for successful Extubation following T-piece weaning trial. Chest. 1995;108:482–9.
20. Montgomery AB, Holle RHO, Neagley SR, Pierson DJ, Schoene RB. Prediction of successful ventilator weaning using airway occlusion pressure and Hypercapnic challenge. Chest. 1987;91:496–9.
21. Papanikolaou J, Makris D, Saranteas T, Karakitsos D, Zintzaras E, Karabinis A, et al. New insights into weaning from mechanical ventilation: left ventricular diastolic dysfunction is a key player. Intensive Care Med. 2011;37:1976–85.
22. Savi A, Teixeira C, Silva JM, Borges LG, Pereira PA, Pinto KB, et al. Weaning predictors do not predict extubation failure in simple-to-wean patients. J Crit Care. 2012;27:221.e1–8.
23. Scheinhorn DJ, Hassenpflug M, Artinian BM, LaBree L, Catlin JL. Predictors of weaning after 6 weeks of mechanical ventilation. Chest. 1995;107:500–5.
24. Burns SM, Fisher C, Tribble SSE, Lewis R, Merrel P, Conaway MR, et al. Multifactor clinical score and outcome of mechanical ventilation weaning trials: Burns wean assessment program. Am J Crit Care. 2010;19:431–9.
25. Jiang J, Yen S, Chien J, Liu H, Wu Y, Chen C. Predicting weaning and extubation outcomes in long-term mechanically ventilated patients using the modified Burns Wean Assessment Program scores. Respirology. 2014;19:576–82.
26. Cohen IL, Lambrinos J, Fein IA. Mechanical ventilation for the elderly patient in intensive care. Incremental changes and benefits. JAMA. 1993;269:1025–9.
27. Wu Y-K, Kao K-C, Hsu K-H, Hsieh M-J, Tsai Y-H. Predictors of successful weaning from prolonged mechanical ventilation in Taiwan. Respir Med. 2009;103:1189–95.
28. Levine S, Nguyen T, Taylor N, Friscia ME, Budak MT, Rothenberg P, et al. Rapid disuse atrophy of diaphragm fibers in mechanically ventilated humans. N Engl J Med. 2008;358:1327–35.
29. Poddighe D, Van Hollebeke M, Choudhary YQ, Campos DR, Schaeffer MR, Verbakel JY, et al. Accuracy of respiratory muscle assessments to predict weaning outcomes: a systematic review and comparative meta-analysis. Crit Care. 2024;28:70.
30. Bien UDS, Souza GF, Campos ES, Farah De Carvalho E, Fernandes MG, Santoro I, et al. Maximum inspiratory pressure and rapid shallow breathing index as predictors of successful ventilator weaning. J Phys Ther Sci. 2015;27:3723–7.
31. Jiang H, Li T. Inhibition of Bleomycin-induced pulmonary fibrosis by Okam extract J201. Chest. 2004;126:889S.
32. Bruton A. A pilot study to investigate any relationship between sustained maximal inspiratory pressure and extubation outcome. Heart Lung. 2002;31:141–9.
33. Blumhof S, Wheeler D, Thomas K, McCool FD, Mora J. Change in diaphragmatic thickness during the respiratory cycle predicts Extubation success at various levels of pressure support ventilation. Lung. 2016;194:519–25.
34. DiNino E, Gartman EJ, Sethi JM, McCool FD. Diaphragm ultrasound as a predictor of successful extubation from mechanical ventilation. Thorax. 2014;69:431–5.
35. Farghaly S, Hasan AA. Diaphragm ultrasound as a new method to predict extubation outcome in mechanically ventilated patients. Aust Crit Care. 2017;30:37–43.
36. Jeong B, Nam J, Ko MG, Chung CR, Suh GY, Jeon K. Impact of limb weakness on extubation failure after planned extubation in medical patients. Respirology. 2018;23:842–50.

37. Boniatti VM, Boniatti MM, Andrade CF, Zigiotto CC, Kaminski P, Gomes SP, et al. The modified integrative weaning index as a predictor of Extubation failure. Respir Care. 2014;59:1042–7.
38. Farghaly S, Galal M, Hasan AA, Nafady A. Brain natriuretic peptide as a predictor of weaning from mechanical ventilation in patients with respiratory illness. Aust Crit Care. 2015;28:116–21.
39. Mabrouk AA, Mansour OF, El-Aziz AAA, Elhabashy MM, Alasdoudy AA. Evaluation of some predictors for successful weaning from mechanical ventilation. Egypt J Chest Dis Tuberc. 2015;64:703–7.
40. El-Gazzar AG, El-Salahy MM, Essway TS, Mohammed SN, Elnaggar ME. Effect of acute kidney injury on weaning from mechanical ventilation in chronic obstructive pulmonary diseases patients with respiratory failure. Egypt J Bronchol. 2020;14:13.
41. Datta D, Foley RJ, Wu R, Grady J, Scalise P. Renal function, weaning, and survival in patients with ventilator-dependent respiratory failure. J Intensive Care Med. 2019;34:212–7.
42. Vieira JM, Castro I, Curvello-Neto A, Demarzo S, Caruso P, Pastore L, et al. Effect of acute kidney injury on weaning from mechanical ventilation in critically ill patients*. Crit Care Med. 2007;35:184–91.
43. Muzaffar SN, Gurjar M, Baronia AK, Azim A, Mishra P, Poddar B, et al. Predictors and pattern of weaning and long-term outcome of patients with prolonged mechanical ventilation at an acute intensive care unit in North India. Rev Bras Ter Intensiva [Internet]. 2017;29. Available from: https://criticalcarescience.org/article/predictors-and-pattern-of-weaning-and-long-term-outcome-of-patients-with-prolonged-mechanical-ventilation-at-an-acute-intensive-care-unit-in-north-india/. [cited 2024 Oct 13]
44. Upadya A, Tilluckdharry L, Muralidharan V, Amoateng-Adjepong Y, Manthous CA. Fluid balance and weaning outcomes. Intensive Care Med. 2005;31:1643–7.
45. Doley J, Mallampalli A, Sandberg M. Nutrition Management for the Patient Requiring Prolonged Mechanical Ventilation. Nutr Clin Pract. 2011;26:232–41.
46. Datta D, Foley R, Wu R, Grady J, Scalise P. Can creatinine height index predict weaning and survival outcomes in patients on prolonged mechanical ventilation after critical illness? J Intensive Care Med. 2018;33:104–10.
47. Alsumrain MH, Jawad SA, Imran NB, Riar S, DeBari VA, Adelman M. Association of hypophosphatemia with failure-to-wean from mechanical ventilation. Ann Clin Lab Sci. 2010;40:144–8.
48. Wozniak H, Dos Santos RA, Beckmann TS, Larpin C, Buetti N, Quintard H, et al. Hypophosphatemia on ICU admission is associated with an increased length of stay in the ICU and time under mechanical ventilation. J Clin Med. 2022;11:581.
49. Zhao Y, Li Z, Shi Y, Cao G, Meng F, Zhu W, et al. Effect of hypophosphatemia on the withdrawal of mechanical ventilation in patients with acute exacerbations of chronic obstructive pulmonary disease. Biomed Rep. 2016;4:413–6.
50. Khamiees M, Raju P, DeGirolamo A, Amoateng-Adjepong Y, Manthous CA. Predictors of Extubation outcome in patients who have successfully completed a spontaneous breathing trial. Chest. 2001;120:1262–70.
51. Huaringa AJ, Wang A, Haro MH, Leyva FJ. The weaning index as predictor of weaning success. J Intensive Care Med. 2013;28:369–74.
52. Jubran A, Mathru M, Dries D, Tobin MJ. Continuous recordings of mixed venous oxygen saturation during weaning from mechanical ventilation and the ramifications thereof. Am J Respir Crit Care Med. 1998;158:1763–9.
53. Morganroth ML. Criteria for weaning from prolonged mechanical ventilation. Arch Intern Med. 1984;144:1012.
54. Yang KL, Tobin MJ. A prospective study of indexes predicting the outcome of trials of weaning from mechanical ventilation. N Engl J Med. 1991;324:1445–50.
55. Chatila W, Jacob B, Guaglionone D, Manthous CA. The unassisted respiratory rate-tidal volume ratio accurately predicts weaning outcome. Am J Med. 1996;101:61–7.

56. Kuo P-H, Kuo S-H, Yang P-C, Wu H-D, Lu B-Y, Chen M-T. Predictive value of rapid shallow breathing index measured at initiation and termination of a 2-hour spontaneous breathing trial for weaning outcome in ICU patients. J Formos Med Assoc. 2006;105:390–8.
57. Segal LN, Oei E, Oppenheimer BW, Goldring RM, Bustami RT, Ruggiero S, et al. Evolution of pattern of breathing during a spontaneous breathing trial predicts successful extubation. Intensive Care Med. 2010;36:487–95.
58. Wysocki M, Cracco C, Teixeira A, Mercat A, Diehl J-L, Lefort Y, et al. Reduced breathing variability as a predictor of unsuccessful patient separation from mechanical ventilation*. Crit Care Med. 2006;34:2076–83.
59. Trivedi V, Chaudhuri D, Jinah R, Piticaru J, Agarwal A, Liu K, et al. The usefulness of the rapid shallow breathing index in predicting successful Extubation. Chest. 2022;161:97–111.
60. Gluck EH, Corgian L. Predicting eventual success or failure to wean in patients receiving long-term mechanical ventilation. Chest. 1996;110:1018–24.
61. Nemer SN, Barbas CS, Caldeira JB, Cárias TC, Santos RG, Almeida LC, et al. A new integrative weaning index of discontinuation from mechanical ventilation. Crit Care. 2009;13:R152.
62. De Souza LC, Guimarães FS, Lugon JR. Evaluation of a new index of mechanical ventilation weaning: the timed inspiratory effort. J Intensive Care Med. 2015;30:37–43.
63. Godoy MDP, Souza LCD, Silva Neto AED, Lugon JR. Comparison of the timed inspiratory effort index with the T-piece trial as a decision-making tool for extubation: a randomized controlled non-inferiority trial. Braz J Med Biol Res. 2023;56:e12824.
64. Spadaro S, Grasso S, Mauri T, Dalla Corte F, Alvisi V, Ragazzi R, et al. Can diaphragmatic ultrasonography performed during the T-tube trial predict weaning failure? The role of diaphragmatic rapid shallow breathing index. Crit Care. 2016;20:305.
65. Schreiber AF, Garlasco J, Urner M, McFarlan A, Baker A, Rigamonti A, et al. Mechanical ventilation after traumatic spinal cord injury—a multicentric cohort study-based prediction model for weaning success: the BICYCLE score. Ann Am Thorac Soc. 2023;20:1156–65.
66. Jabour ER, Rabil DM, Truwit JD, Rochester DF. Evaluation of a new weaning index based on ventilatory endurance and the efficiency of gas exchange. Am Rev Respir Dis. 1991;144:531–7.
67. Delisle S, Francoeur M, Albert M, Ouellet P, Bellemare P, Arsenault P. Preliminary evaluation of a new index to predict the outcome of a spontaneous breathing trial. Respir Care. 2011;56:1500–5.
68. Varón-Vega F, Giraldo-Cadavid LF, Uribe AM, Rincón A, Palacios J, Crevoisier S, et al. Utilization of spontaneous breathing trial, objective cough test, and diaphragmatic ultrasound results to predict extubation success: COBRE-US trial. Crit Care. 2023;27:414.
69. Hermans G, Van Den Berghe G. Clinical review: intensive care unit acquired weakness. Crit Care. 2015;19:274.
70. Latronico N, Bolton CF. Critical illness polyneuropathy and myopathy: a major cause of muscle weakness and paralysis. Lancet Neurol. 2011;10:931–41.
71. Piva S, Fagoni N, Latronico N. Intensive care unit–acquired weakness: unanswered questions and targets for future research. F1000Res. 2019;8:508.
72. De Jonghe B, Bastuji-Garin S, Durand M-C, Malissin I, Rodrigues P, Cerf C, et al. Respiratory weakness is associated with limb weakness and delayed weaning in critical illness*. Crit Care Med. 2007;35:2007–15.
73. Jung B, Moury PH, Mahul M, De Jong A, Galia F, Prades A, et al. Diaphragmatic dysfunction in patients with ICU-acquired weakness and its impact on extubation failure. Intensive Care Med. 2016;42:853–61.
74. Mirzakhani H, Williams J-N, Mello J, Joseph S, Meyer MJ, Waak K, et al. Muscle weakness predicts pharyngeal dysfunction and symptomatic aspiration in long-term ventilated patients. Anesthesiology. 2013;119:389–97.
75. De Jonghe B. Paresis acquired in the intensive care UnitA prospective multicenter study. JAMA. 2002;288:2859.

76. Dres M, Jung B, Molinari N, Manna F, Dubé B-P, Chanques G, et al. Respective contribution of intensive care unit-acquired limb muscle and severe diaphragm weakness on weaning outcome and mortality: a post hoc analysis of two cohorts. Crit Care. 2019;23:370.
77. Dres M, Dubé B-P, Mayaux J, Delemazure J, Reuter D, Brochard L, et al. Coexistence and impact of limb muscle and diaphragm weakness at time of liberation from mechanical ventilation in medical intensive care unit patients. Am J Respir Crit Care Med. 2017;195:57–66.
78. Garnacho-Montero J, Amaya-Villar R, García-Garmendía JL, Madrazo-Osuna J, Ortiz-Leyba C. Effect of critical illness polyneuropathy on the withdrawal from mechanical ventilation and the length of stay in septic patients*. Crit Care Med. 2005;33:349–54.
79. Wu T-J, Shiao JS-C, Yu H-L, Lai R-S. An integrative index for predicting Extubation outcomes after successful completion of a spontaneous breathing trial in an adult medical intensive care unit. J Intensive Care Med. 2019;34:640–5.
80. Kuo H-J, Chiu H-W, Lee C-N, Chen T-T, Chang C-C, Bien M-Y. Improvement in the prediction of ventilator weaning outcomes by an artificial neural network in a medical ICU. Respir Care. 2015;60:1560–9.
81. Hsieh M-H, Hsieh M-J, Chen C-M, Hsieh C-C, Chao C-M, Lai C-C. An artificial neural network model for predicting successful Extubation in intensive care units. J Clin Med. 2018;7:240.
82. Menguy J, De Longeaux K, Bodenes L, Hourmant B, L'Her E. Defining predictors for successful mechanical ventilation weaning, using a data-mining process and artificial intelligence. Sci Rep. 2023;13:20483.
83. Pluijms WA, Van Mook WN, Wittekamp BH, Bergmans DC. Postextubation laryngeal edema and stridor resulting in respiratory failure in critically ill adult patients: updated review. Crit Care. 2015;19:295.
84. Darmon J-Y, Rauss A, Dreyfuss D, Bleichner G, Elkharrat D, Schlemmer B, et al. Evaluation of risk factors for laryngeal edema after tracheal Extubation in adults and its prevention by dexamethasone a placebo-controlled, double-blind. Multicent Stud Anesthesiol. 1992;77:245–51.
85. Smina M, Salam A, Khamiees M, Gada P, Amoateng-Adjepong Y, Manthous CA. Cough peak flows and Extubation outcomes. Chest. 2003;124:262–8.
86. Su W-L, Chen Y-H, Chen C-W, Yang S-H, Su C-L, Perng W-C, et al. Involuntary cough strength and Extubation outcomes for patients in an ICU. Chest. 2010;137:777–82.
87. Beuret P, Roux C, Auclair A, Nourdine K, Kaaki M, Carton M-J. Interest of an objective evaluation of cough during weaning from mechanical ventilation. Intensive Care Med. 2009;35:1090–3.
88. Salam A, Tilluckdharry L, Amoateng-Adjepong Y, Manthous CA. Neurologic status, cough, secretions and extubation outcomes. Intensive Care Med. 2004;30:1334–9.
89. Coplin WM, Pierson DJ, Cooley KD, Newell DW, Rubenfeld GD. Implications of Extubation delay in brain-injured patients meeting standard weaning criteria. Am J Respir Crit Care Med. 2000;161:1530–6.
90. Steidl C, Boesel J, Suntrup-Krueger S, Schoenenberger S, Al-Suwaidan F, Warnecke T, et al. Tracheostomy, Extubation, reintubation: airway management decisions in intubated stroke patients. Cerebrovasc Dis. 2017;44:1–9.
91. Asehnoune K, Seguin P, Lasocki S, Roquilly A, Delater A, Gros A, et al. Extubation success prediction in a multicentric cohort of patients with severe brain injury. Anesthesiology. 2017;127:338–46.
92. Cinotti R, Mijangos JC, Pelosi P, Haenggi M, Gurjar M, Schultz MJ, et al. Extubation in neurocritical care patients: the ENIO international prospective study. Intensive Care Med. 2022;48:1539–50.

Chapter 6
Weaning in Patients with Chronic Obstructive Pulmonary Disease (COPD)

Ângelo Roncalli Miranda Rocha

6.1 Introduction

Chronic obstructive pulmonary disease (COPD) is a prevalent condition that contributes significantly to overall morbidity and mortality and often requires invasive mechanical ventilation (IMV) during acute exacerbations. The incidence of IMV in patients with acute exacerbations of COPD has been reported in studies showing a general downward trend over time. In a study analyzing data from the OUTCOMEREA database, the proportion of COPD patients treated with IMV decreased from 51% between 1997 and 2002 to 35% between 2013 and 2018 [1]. Another study examining trends in the United States from 2001 to 2011 reported a decrease in initial IMV use from 8.7% to 5.9% [2]. Similarly, data from Spain showed a decrease in IMV use from 1.39% in 2001–2003 to 0.67% in 2013–2015 [3].

This downward trend in the use of IMV may be due to the increasing use of non-invasive ventilation (NIV) as a first-line treatment for COPD exacerbations, which has been shown to have favorable outcomes, such as lower intubation rates and lower mortality [4]. The decline in the use of IMV reflects an evolution in clinical practice that favors less invasive methods when appropriate due to the risks and complications associated with invasive ventilation.

It should be considered that some patients with COPD exacerbation will inevitably progress to IMV and are particularly challenging. Studies show significant in-hospital mortality rates, ranging from 28% to 39.9%, depending on the presence of comorbidities and the duration of mechanical ventilation [5, 6]. Factors such as a higher severity score and the presence of malignancy are associated with increased mortality. The need for prolonged ventilation (>72 h) has also been associated with higher mortality [5]. This justifies the need for professionals managing mechanical ventilation to develop strategies that allow earlier weaning from IMV.

Â. R. M. Rocha (✉)
University of Health Sciences – Alagoas, Maceió, Alagoas, Brazil

A. R. Baptistella et al. (eds.), *Weaning from Mechanical Ventilation*,
https://doi.org/10.1007/978-3-032-01145-9_6

6.2 Factors Associated with Higher Risk of Weaning Failure

Some physiological factors, such as respiratory muscle weakness and abnormal lung mechanics, may be associated with prolonged ventilation in COPD patients, with increased intrinsic PEEP (PEEPi) and pulmonary resistance, which can lead to ventilator dependency [7]. In addition, an imbalance between increased respiratory workload and reduced inspiratory muscle capacity may lead to respiratory distress and CO_2 retention, further complicating weaning from mechanical ventilation.

6.2.1 Respiratory Muscle Weakness

The biomechanical changes resulting from the pathophysiological process of COPD primarily affect the efficiency of the respiratory muscles and are one of the determining factors for prolonged stays on the ventilator. Pulmonary hyperinflation puts the diaphragm at a biomechanical disadvantage, flattening it and reducing its ability to generate pressure and force. The altered shape and position of the diaphragm result in a reduced apposition zone, impairing its function as a pressure generator [8]. This chronic process results in changes in the diaphragm, such as an increased proportion of slow, fatigue-resistant fiber types, and a greater oxidative capacity. However, these adaptations are generally not sufficient to overcome the mechanical disadvantages imposed by hyperinflation and the increased demands of the respiratory system.

Prolonged controlled mechanical ventilation is another factor associated with ventilator-induced diaphragmatic dysfunction. Levine et al. demonstrated that as little as 18 h of total diaphragmatic inactivity and controlled ventilation results in atrophy of diaphragmatic slow and fast myosin fibers [9]. Even assisted ventilation is capable of causing diaphragmatic myotrauma if there is under- or over-assistance. Excessive respiratory effort caused by under-assistance can lead to effort-induced myotrauma, causing a diaphragmatic inflammatory process and proteolysis [10]. On the other hand, excessive ventilatory support (over-assistance), which reduces the intensity of inspiratory effort, is also capable of causing diaphragmatic atrophy [11]. Patient ventilator asynchronies that produce eccentric contraction of the diaphragm, such as ineffective triggering, premature cycling, and some phenotypes of reverse triggering, are also capable of causing muscle fiber injury and potentiating diaphragm dysfunction. It is not known whether these effects are potentiated by mechanical ventilation in COPD patients, given the chronic changes in the diaphragm.

Diaphragmatic muscle weakness caused by structural changes, changes in respiratory mechanics, or diaphragmatic dysfunction induced by mechanical ventilation leads to neuromechanical uncoupling when the respiratory muscles are unable to increase their activity in proportion to the neural drive, further complicating weaning from mechanical ventilation.

6.2.2 Increased Inspiratory Load

Another factor associated with prolonged IMV in these patients is the increased resistive load resulting from high airway resistance due to mechanisms such as bronchoconstriction, loss of elastic fibers in the small airways, and mucus hypersecretion. The increased collapsibility of the small airways leads to a phenomenon known as expiratory flow limitation (EFL), which is characterized by a lack of increase in expiratory flow despite an increase in expiratory driving pressure and can be easily detected by a PEEP test (Fig. 6.1) [12]. EFL is exacerbated by dynamic hyperinflation, and both factors are closely related, so that one perpetuates the existence of the other. This leads to an increase in the end-expiratory lung volume (EELV) and PEEPi, which determines a greater mechanical disadvantage for the respiratory muscles [13]. The increase in the additional elastic load promoted by the presence of PEEPi, together with the increase in the resistive load, causes an imbalance between an increase in workload and a reduction in respiratory muscle strength, which determines a greater dependence of the patient on the ventilator and makes weaning more difficult [7].

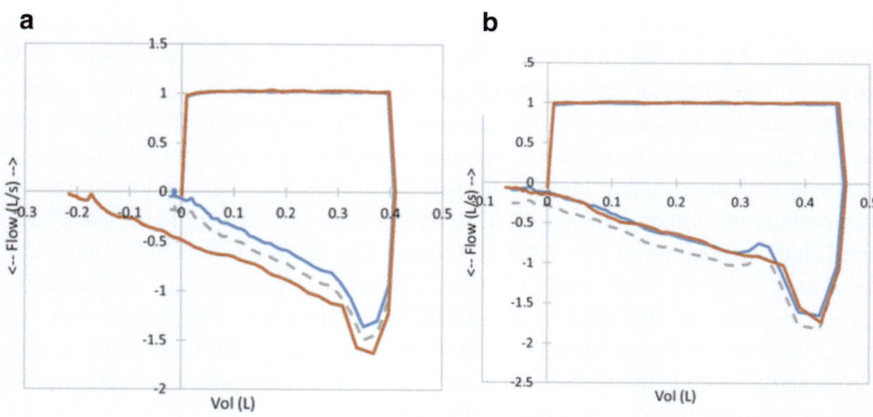

Fig. 6.1 Variation in expiratory flow and volume as PEEP is reduced from a higher to a lower value (increase in expiratory driving pressure). In the flow-volume curve (**a**), the increase in expiratory driving pressure produced an increase in peak expiratory flow and expiratory volume, indicating no EFL. In curve (**b**), the increase in expiratory driving pressure produced no increase in expiratory flow or expiratory volume, showing that the curves before and after the reduction in PEEP are completely overlapping. This indicates the presence of EFL. *PEEP* positive end-expiratory pressure, *EFL* expiratory flow limitation. (Adapted from Junhasavasdikul et al. [12] with permission)

6.2.3 Other Associated Factors

Other systemic factors such as inflammation, oxidative stress, age, and comorbidities may be added to increased work of breathing and respiratory muscle weakness as possible complicators of the weaning process in COPD patients. Comorbidities play an important role in the risk of prolonged mechanical ventilation and weaning failure. Liao et al. [14] found that comorbidities such as diabetes mellitus, hypertension, dyslipidemia, congestive heart failure, coronary artery disease, stroke, chronic kidney disease, and dementia were significantly associated with the risk of prolonged mechanical ventilation. Another study found that COPD patients aged 70 years or older had a significantly higher risk of prolonged mechanical ventilation compared to patients aged 40–49 years [15].

All of these factors, alone or in combination, highlight the complex interaction between respiratory muscle mechanics and the pathophysiology of COPD that can have a significant impact on weaning from mechanical ventilation. Understanding these factors is important for developing effective weaning strategies and optimizing respiratory support in this patient population.

6.3 Weaning Predictors

A few studies have evaluated the use of weaning predictor indices in a specific population of patients with COPD. Alvisi et al. [16] observed in a population of 81 patients undergoing an initial spontaneous breathing test that the occluded inspiratory pressure/maximum inspiratory pressure oscillation index (deltaPI/Pimax) and the compliance, rate, oxygenation, pressure (CROP) index were promising predictors with high areas under the ROC curves, suggesting their potential usefulness in this population. Other indices, such as maximal inspiratory pressure (MIP) and rapid shallow breathing index (RSBI), showed significant disagreement, with MIP set at a cut-off point of 44 cmH_2O in COPD patients compared to 15 cmH_2O in the general population. In addition, the classification error for most indices was less than 20% only for PImax, deltaPI, and CROP, highlighting that these indices differ significantly in their predictive value for COPD in a heterogeneous population of patients weaning from mechanical ventilation.

However, it is important to highlight the limitations of the study: In addition to the small sample size, Alvisi et al. chose to include only patients who failed their first weaning attempt or who were later successfully weaned, which may introduce selection bias since the characteristics that influence initial weaning outcomes (such as severity or comorbidities) may be different from those who never failed a weaning attempt.

Given the peculiarities of respiratory mechanics and the biomechanical disadvantage of the respiratory muscles in patients with COPD, it is possible that traditional predictive indices such as the RSBI may not have the same accuracy as in the general population. However, there is no robust evidence as to which indices can most reliably predict the likelihood of successful/failed extubation in COPD patients. In general, predictive indices, if used, should respect the limits established in the literature for the general population and discussed in other chapters of this book, and, not least, they should be complementary to clinical judgment. The variability in predictive power highlights the complexity of weaning COPD patients and the need for individual assessment.

6.4 Spontaneous Breathing Test in COPD Patients

The Spontaneous Breathing Test (SBT) is a clinical tool used to assess the patient's ability to breathe independently without ventilator support and to determine readiness for extubation. SBT consists of allowing the patient to breathe spontaneously with minimal or no ventilator support, usually using methods such as the T-piece, continuous positive airway pressure (CPAP), pressure support ventilation (PSV), or the use of automatic tracheal tube compensation (ATC) [17, 18]. Details of these tests are beyond the scope of this chapter and are discussed elsewhere in this book.

The search for the SBT method with the greatest accuracy in predicting successful extubation is the "Holy Grail" of mechanical ventilation. Although several studies have compared different methods in different populations, the "ideal" method for performing SBT remains an unanswered question. In a randomized controlled trial, Pellegrini et al. [19] compared PSV versus T-piece SBT in 190 COPD patients who had been on IMV for at least 48 h, divided into two groups (PSV = 91; T-piece = 99). The results showed that extubation was successful in 78% of cases in the first SBT (simple weaning), but the mean duration of mechanical ventilation was significantly longer in the T-piece group (10.82 days) compared to the PSV group (7.31 days, $p < 0.001$). However, this longer MV stay was determined by a longer pre-SBT interval due to an imbalance at baseline, with no effect of the intervention on this variable. In patients with difficult or prolonged weaning, the time to discharge was also longer in the T-piece group (8.36 days) than in the PSV group (4.06 days, $p = 0.003$). The results suggest that the type of SBT did not significantly influence the total duration of mechanical ventilation in general, but for patients in the difficult/prolonged weaning subgroup, the use of the T-piece may be associated with longer weaning times.

The GLOBAL WEAN study [20] was designed to evaluate which methods best simulate inspiratory effort after extubation in critically ill patients following abdominal surgery, brain injury, chest trauma, COPD, and various other conditions. This multicenter, randomized, cross-over study included 100 patients who underwent three different SBT methods: PSV 7 cmH_2O and PEEP 0 (PSV7PEEP0), PSV 0 and PEEP 0 (PSV0PEEP0), and a T-piece test. The results showed that unassisted tests, especially PSV0PEEP0 and the T-piece, were more effective in reproducing post-extubation respiratory effort. In the subgroup analysis, there was no significant difference between the inspiratory effort assessed by the three SBT methods and that verified after extubation in patients with COPD exacerbation, demonstrating the applicability of the three assessed methods in this specific patient population.

In a retrospective study, Liu et al. [21] evaluated the impact of spontaneous breathing tests on extubation in patients with acute exacerbations of COPD undergoing mechanical ventilation. Sixty-four patients were included, 32 of whom received SBT for 60 min prior to extubation and 32 of whom were extubated without SBT. There was no statistically significant difference in reintubation rates (12.5% in the SBT group vs 15.6% in the no SBT group, $p = 0.821$) and 28-day mortality (3.1% in the SBT group vs. 6.3% in the no SBT group, $p = 0.554$). The study concluded that SBT did not significantly affect extubation success or hospital mortality in mechanically ventilated COPD patients. However, given the inherent limitations of retrospective studies, SBT is still recommended for all patients who remain on IMV for more than 24 h [17].

Considering the currently available evidence, it is not possible to suggest the superiority of any SBT method in COPD patients, as extubation failure rates do not seem to be significantly affected by the method. Trials performed on PSV allow the patient to remain connected to the ventilator with graphic monitoring and alarms activated, which increases the level of safety of the weaning process, and this is a possible advantage of performing SBT on PSV.

The duration of SBT is also controversial, with studies ranging from 30 to 120 min. Subirà et al. [22] compared a 30-min SBT in PSV with a 2-h SBT in T-piece in mechanically ventilated patients with heterogeneous underlying disease and found that SBT in PSV (shorter and less demanding) resulted in higher rates of successful extubation. This suggests that 30 min may be sufficient in most contexts, potentially including COPD patients, although the study was not specific to this population.

6.5 Weaning Strategies for COPD Patients

6.5.1 Establishing Weaning Protocols

To avoid the adverse effects of IMV, it is recommended that patients with COPD be weaned as soon as possible. These patients suffer a progressive decline in pulmonary, physical, and cognitive function and are also more prone to ventilator-associated pneumonia (VAP) [23]. Establishing protocols to guide the weaning process is a valid strategy to reduce the length of stay on mechanical ventilation. Studies suggest that protocol-guided weaning may lead to better outcomes in terms of reduced duration of mechanical ventilation and shorter length of stay in the intensive care unit (ICU). Kollef et al. demonstrated that protocol-guided weaning performed by nurses and respiratory therapists resulted in a shorter duration of mechanical ventilation compared with physician-guided weaning [24]. Specifically in COPD patients, Kirakli et al. [25] found that a protocol-guided strategy of mechanical ventilation and respiratory therapist-guided weaning improved extubation success rates and reduced mechanical ventilation and ICU length of stay.

Protocols generally include daily assessments to determine the patient's readiness for weaning, and the criteria to be considered are described in Table 6.1. As mentioned previously, there are no specific criteria for the COPD patient population, and in general, the criteria considered for other populations can be applied. After evaluating the criteria and determining weaning readiness, spontaneous breathing tests should be performed.

6.5.2 Prophylactic Noninvasive Ventilation After Extubation

Patients with COPD who successfully undergo SBT should be extubated and then prophylactically placed on noninvasive ventilation (NIV) because of the high risk of extubation failure [18]. Evidence suggests that prophylactic NIV is beneficial in reducing the risk of respiratory failure, particularly in patients with hypercapnia (PaCO2 > 45 mmHg), and may improve outcomes. Ferrer et al. showed in a randomized controlled trial that preventive NIV after extubation significantly reduced the incidence of respiratory failure and 90-day mortality in hypercapnic patients with chronic respiratory disease compared with conventional oxygen therapy [27].

The role of high-flow nasal cannula (HFNC) in preventing reintubation in COPD patients after extubation has been studied. Studies suggest that HFNC may be comparable to NIV in this context, but the certainty of the evidence is still low. A post hoc analysis of a randomized controlled trial [28] showed that preventive NIV alternating with oxygen therapy via HFNC reduced reintubation rates in COPD patients compared with HFNC alone. Tan et al. [29]showed that HFNC was not inferior to NIV in preventing extubation failure in hypercapnic COPD patients, with better tolerability and comfort reported in the NFC group.

Table 6.1 Patients on invasive mechanical ventilation for 7 days, ventilator dependent, consider inspiratory muscle training if

Alert and cooperative
PEEP $\leq$10 cmH_2O
$FiO_2 < 0.6$
Respiratory rate < 25/min
Able to trigger the mechanical ventilator
Evidence of inspiratory muscle weakness (low MIP/FIN)

Reproduced with permission from Bisset [26]

PEEP positive end-expiratory pressure, *FiO_2* fraction of inspired oxygen, *MIP* maximal inspiratory pressure, *FIN* negative inspiratory force

Considering the potential non-inferiority of HFNC over NIV in preventing reintubations, a systematic review and meta-analysis found that although HFNC reduced reintubations compared with conventional oxygen therapy, it did not show a significant difference in reintubation rates compared with NIV [30]. However, only one of the studies in the meta-analysis included only COPD patients.

Robust evidence supports the use of prophylactic NIV in COPD patients at high risk of extubation failure, particularly those with hypercapnic respiratory failure, to reduce the risk of reintubation. HFNC may be used as an alternative, especially in patients with NIV intolerance. Therefore, individual patient characteristics and risk factors should be considered when choosing the type of noninvasive respiratory support to be used after extubation.

6.5.3 Noninvasive Ventilation to Facilitate Weaning from Invasive Ventilation

Patients with COPD are more likely to experience difficult or prolonged weaning due to the characteristics of the disease itself and the complications associated with prolonged mechanical ventilation. One of the factors contributing to weaning difficulties is the increased risk of VAP. COPD patients are often colonized with bacteria such as *Haemophilus influenzae*, *Streptococcus pneumoniae*, and *Pseudomonas aeruginosa*, which increases the likelihood of bacterial translocation and subsequent VAP. Studies in the general population show that the risk of VAP is approximately 1%–3% per day on the first day, increasing cumulatively to 10%–20% on the fifth day and up to 20%–30% on the tenth day [31–34]. However, the daily risk of VAP in patients with COPD can be 1.5–2 times higher than in patients without COPD [35, 36]. This is one of the main reasons for the need for strategies that allow earlier extubation in patients with COPD.

For patients who fail an SBT, NIV serves as a bridge to successful weaning from invasive ventilation, enabling extubation, reducing the time spent on mechanical ventilation, and improving overall outcomes. This approach, often referred to as "facilitative" NIV, is particularly beneficial in patients with COPD who are at high risk of extubation failure due to underlying respiratory impairment [37]. The use of facilitative NIV has been shown in studies to reduce mortality, the incidence of ventilator-associated pneumonia, and shorten ICU and hospital stays [38, 39]. Other associated benefits include shorter mechanical ventilation duration and lower tracheostomy rates [40]. This approach is therefore supported by evidence in COPD and recommended by clinical guidelines [37] and should be considered as a feasible strategy to reduce the length of stay on IMV.

6.5.4 Inspiratory Muscle Training and Early Mobilization

Inspiratory muscle training (IMT) has been proposed as a strategy to facilitate weaning by increasing inspiratory muscle strength and endurance and helping patients maintain spontaneous breathing. Various IMT methods and protocols have been proposed in the literature, and this heterogeneity in study methodology has led to conflicting results and made it difficult to establish evidence to support routine IMT as a standard of care in patients with difficult or prolonged weaning.

A systematic review and network meta-analysis comparing different physiotherapy interventions found that IMT in combination with conventional physiotherapy significantly reduced weaning time in mechanically ventilated patients. However, as there are no studies evaluating the impact of IMT on weaning exclusively in a population of patients with COPD, it is uncertain whether the addition of this therapy can reduce the length of stay in IMV or promote successful weaning/extubation [41].

Given the physiological plausibility that respiratory muscle weakness is more pronounced in patients with COPD, and that this is a factor associated with longer duration of mechanical ventilation, it is feasible to introduce IMT in patients with prolonged weaning, as shown in Table 6.1.

Therefore, IMT may be an adjuvant therapy in the weaning process, especially in patients with significant respiratory muscle weakness. Future research should focus on standardizing protocols and conducting high-quality randomized controlled trials, especially in COPD patients, to establish its role as a routine in clinical practice.

References

1. Galerneau LM, Bailly S, Terzi N, et al. Management of Acute Exacerbations of chronic obstructive pulmonary disease in the ICU: an observational study from the OUTCOMEREA database, 1997–2018. Crit Care Med. 2023;51(6):753–64.
2. Stefan MS, Shieh MS, Pekow PS, Hill N, Rothberg MB, Lindenauer PK. Trends in mechanical ventilation among patients hospitalized with acute exacerbations of COPD in the United States, 2001 to 2011. Chest. 2015;147(4):959–68.
3. de Miguel-Diez J, Jiménez-García R, Hernández-Barrera V, et al. Trends in the use and outcomes of mechanical ventilation among patients hospitalized with acute exacerbations of COPD in Spain, 2001 to 2015. J Clin Med. 2019;8(10)
4. Osadnik CR, Tee VS, Carson-Chahhoud KV, Picot J, Wedzicha JA, Smith BJ. Non-invasive ventilation for the management of acute hypercapnic respiratory failure due to exacerbation of chronic obstructive pulmonary disease. Cochrane Database Syst Rev. 2017;7
5. Nevins M, Epstein S. Predictors of outcome for patients with COPD requiring invasive mechanical ventilation. Chest. 2001;119(6):1840–9.
6. Liu H, Zhang T, Ye J. Analysis of risk factors for hospital mortality in patients with chronic obstructive pulmonary diseases requiring invasive mechanical ventilation. Chin Med J. 2007;120(4):287–93.
7. Purro A, Appendini L, De Gaetano A, Gudjonsdottir M, Donner CF, Rossi A. Physiologic determinants of ventilator dependence in long-term mechanically ventilated patients. Am J Respir Crit Care Med. 2000;161(4 Pt 1):1115–23.

8. Tobin MJ, Laghi F, Brochard L. Role of the respiratory muscles in acute respiratory failure of COPD: lessons from weaning failure. J Appl Physiol (Bethesda, Md: 1985). 2009;107(3):962–70.
9. Levine S, Nguyen T, Taylor N, et al. Rapid disuse atrophy of diaphragm fibers in mechanically ventilated humans. N Engl J Med. 2008;358(13):1327–35.
10. Goligher EC. Myotrauma in mechanically ventilated patients. Intensive Care Med. 2019;45(6):881–4.
11. Goligher EC, Brochard LJ, Reid WD, et al. Diaphragmatic myotrauma: a mediator of prolonged ventilation and poor patient outcomes in acute respiratory failure. Lancet Respir Med. 2019;7(1):90–8.
12. Junhasavasdikul D, Telias I, Grieco DL, et al. Expiratory flow limitation during mechanical ventilation. Chest. 2018;154(4):948–62.
13. Rossi A, Ganassini A, Polese G, Grassi V. Pulmonary hyperinflation and ventilator-dependent patients. Eur Respir J. 1997;10(7):1663–74.
14. Liao KM, Lu HY, Chen CY, Kuo LT, Tang BR. The impact of comorbidities on prolonged mechanical ventilation in patients with chronic obstructive pulmonary disease. BMC Pulm Med. 2024;24(1):257.
15. Liao KM, Lin WC, Lin TC, Li CY, Yang YH. Disease severity at the first hospitalization as a predictor for mechanical ventilation dependency in elderly patients with chronic obstructive pulmonary disease. Tohoku J Exp Med. 2014;234(4):263–9.
16. Alvisi R, Volta C, Righini E, et al. Predictors of weaning outcome in chronic obstructive pulmonary disease patients. Eur Resp J. 15(4):656–62.
17. Thille AW, Arrivé F, Le Pape S. Spontaneous breathing trials: how and for how long? Curr Opin Crit Care. 2025;31(1):86–92.
18. Ouellette DR, Patel S, Girard TD, et al. Liberation from mechanical ventilation in critically ill adults: an official American College of Chest Physicians/American Thoracic Society clinical practice guideline: inspiratory pressure augmentation during spontaneous breathing trials, protocols minimizing sedation, and noninvasive ventilation immediately after extubation. Chest. 2017;151(1):166–80.
19. Santos Pellegrini JA, Boniatti MM, Boniatti VC, et al. Pressure-support ventilation or T-piece spontaneous breathing trials for patients with chronic obstructive pulmonary disease – a randomized controlled trial. PLoS One. 2018;13(8):e0202404.
20. Capdevila M, Aarab Y, Monet C, et al. Spontaneous breathing trials should be adapted for each patient according to the critical illness. A new individualised approach: the GLOBAL WEAN study. Intensive Care Med. 2024;50(12):2083–93.
21. Liu W, Guo H, Wang J, Ding F. Effect of spontaneous breathing trial on extubation in patients with acute exacerbation of chronic obstructive pulmonary disease under mechanical ventilation. BMC Emerg Med. 2022;22(1):112.
22. Subirà C, Hernández G, Vázquez A, et al. Effect of pressure support vs T-piece ventilation strategies during spontaneous breathing trials on successful extubation among patients receiving mechanical ventilation: a randomized clinical trial. JAMA. 2019;321(22):2175–82.
23. Yin M, Liu M. Effect of chronic obstructive pulmonary disease combined with ventilator-associated pneumonia on patient outcomes: a systematic review and meta-analysis. Exp Ther Med. 2020;20(6):273.
24. Kollef MH, Shapiro SD, Silver P, et al. A randomized, controlled trial of protocol-directed versus physician-directed weaning from mechanical ventilation. Crit Care Med. 1997;25(4):567–74.
25. Kirakli C, Ediboglu O, Naz I, Cimen P, Tatar D. Effectiveness and safety of a protocolized mechanical ventilation and weaning strategy of COPD patients by respiratory therapists. J Thorac Dis. 2014;6(9):1180–6.
26. Bissett B, Leditschke IA, Green M, Marzano V, Collins S, Van Haren F. Inspiratory muscle training for intensive care patients: a multidisciplinary practical guide for clinicians. Aust Crit Care Off J Confede Aust Crit Care Nur. 2019;32(3):249–55.

27. Ferrer M, Sellarés J, Valencia M, et al. Non-invasive ventilation after extubation in hypercapnic patients with chronic respiratory disorders: randomised controlled trial. Lancet. 2009;374(9695):1082–8.
28. Thille AW, Coudroy R, Nay MA, et al. Non-invasive ventilation alternating with high-flow nasal oxygen versus high-flow nasal oxygen alone after extubation in COPD patients: a post hoc analysis of a randomized controlled trial. Ann Intensive Care. 2021;11(1):30.
29. Tan D, Walline JH, Ling B, et al. High-flow nasal cannula oxygen therapy versus non-invasive ventilation for chronic obstructive pulmonary disease patients after extubation: a multicenter, randomized controlled trial. Crit Care. 2020;24(1):489.
30. Granton D, Chaudhuri D, Wang D, et al. High-flow nasal cannula compared with conventional oxygen therapy or noninvasive ventilation immediately Postextubation: a systematic review and meta-analysis. Crit Care Med. 2020;48(11):e1129–36.
31. Cook DJ, Walter SD, Cook RJ, et al. Incidence of and risk factors for ventilator-associated pneumonia in critically ill patients. Ann Intern Med. 1998;129(6):433–40.
32. Chastre J, Fagon JY. Ventilator-associated pneumonia. Am J Respir Crit Care Med. 2002;165(7):867–903.
33. Kollef MH. Ventilator-associated pneumonia. A multivariate analysis. JAMA. 1993;270(16):1965–70.
34. Li W, Cai J, Ding L, Chen Y, Wang X, Xu H. Incidence and risk factors of ventilator-associated pneumonia in the intensive care unit: a systematic review and meta-analysis. J Thorac Dis. 2024;16(9):5518–28.
35. Restrepo MI, Anzueto A, Arroliga AC, et al. Economic burden of ventilator-associated pneumonia based on total resource utilization. Infect Control Hosp Epidemiol. 2010;31(5):509–15.
36. Torres A, Peetermans WE, Viegi G, Blasi F. Risk factors for community-acquired pneumonia in adults in Europe: a literature review. Thorax. 2013;68(11):1057–65.
37. Rochwerg B, Brochard L, Elliott MW, et al. Official ERS/ATS clinical practice guidelines: noninvasive ventilation for acute respiratory failure. Eur Respir J. 2017;50(2):1602426.
38. Burns KEA, Stevenson J, Laird M, et al. Non-invasive ventilation versus invasive weaning in critically ill adults: a systematic review and meta-analysis. Thorax. 2022;77(8):752–61.
39. Burns KE, Meade MO, Premji A, Adhikari NK. Noninvasive ventilation as a weaning strategy for mechanical ventilation in adults with respiratory failure: a Cochrane systematic review. CMAJ Can Med Assoc J journal de l'Association medicale canadienne. 2014;186(3):E112–22.
40. Burns KE, Adhikari NK, Keenan SP, Meade M. Use of non-invasive ventilation to wean critically ill adults off invasive ventilation: meta-analysis and systematic review. BMJ. 2009;338:b1574.
41. Worraphan S, Thammata A, Chittawatanarat K, Saokaew S, Kengkla K, Prasannarong M. Effects of inspiratory muscle training and early mobilization on weaning of mechanical ventilation: a systematic review and network meta-analysis. Arch Phys Med Rehabil. 2020;101(11):2002–14.

Chapter 7
Weaning in Cardiac Patients

André Luiz Lisboa Cordeiro

7.1 Heart Failure

Heart failure (HF) is a systemic clinical syndrome characterized by cardiac dysfunction resulting in inadequate blood flow to meet tissue metabolic demands [1]. Acute decompensation of HF often results in hospitalization requiring admission to an intensive care unit (ICU).

ICU admission is necessary for acute respiratory failure, cardiogenic shock, malignant arrhythmias, renal complications, and continuous hemodynamic monitoring [2]. The causes of HF decompensation are diverse and include nonadherence, worsening comorbidities, poor medication adjustment, acute events, and environmental factors [3].

Patients with HF may present with left ventricular dysfunction; therefore, it is necessary to understand the impact on pathophysiology and how positive pressure ventilation may be beneficial in this patient profile.

Cardiac dysfunction results in increased left ventricular filling pressures and pulmonary congestion [4]. Left ventricular contraction is closely linked to oxidative energy generation, so any interference with energy availability or utilization is detrimental, leading to ventricular systolic impairment and increased left ventricular end-diastolic volume (EDV) [4, 5].

The increase in left ventricular and atrial pressures, together with mitral valve regurgitation, increases pulmonary capillary pressure and accelerates pulmonary lymphatic filtration into the interstitial space. At the onset of pulmonary edema, there is an increased transfer of fluids and colloids from the capillaries into the interstitium without a significant increase in interstitial volume due to the increase

A. L. L. Cordeiro (✉)
Nobre University Center, University Center of Excellence, Feira de Santana, BA, Brazil

Bahiana School of Medicine and Public Health, Salvador, BA, Brazil

A. R. Baptistella et al. (eds.), *Weaning from Mechanical Ventilation*,
https://doi.org/10.1007/978-3-032-01145-9_7

in lymphatic flow. Even in the early stages, distension of peripheral pulmonary receptors results in an increase in respiratory rate (RR), which contributes to lymphatic pumping [6].

This edema can occur during weaning from mechanical ventilation, making the withdrawal of ventilatory support a challenge. A multidimensional approach is essential to address the complexities of HF with the goal of stabilizing and optimizing treatment, resulting in improved prognosis and quality of life for patients.

7.2 Difficulty in Weaning Patients with HF

Ventilatory weaning in patients with heart failure is often complicated by several factors, including impaired lung function, the presence of pulmonary edema, changes in respiratory mechanics, and the coexistence of comorbidities. In addition, the hemodynamic instability characteristic of heart failure can adversely affect weaning tolerance, making an individualized and careful approach essential.

Weaning is the transition from mechanical ventilation to spontaneous breathing. During inspiratory efforts, intrathoracic pressure decreases, leading to increased venous return, decreased left ventricular ejection volume, and increased intrathoracic blood volume [7]. The transition from positive to negative pressure overloads the heart (increased preload and right and left ventricular overload) and potentially induces myocardial ischemia [8]. This mechanism is associated with weaning-induced pulmonary edema, a major cause of procedural failure.

The negative pressure and increase in intrathoracic blood volume may be more pronounced in patients who exhibit increased respiratory effort during the spontaneous breathing test [9]. Recommendations suggest that a respiratory rate greater than 35 breaths per minute or a 20% increase from baseline is associated with weaning failure. This assessment is particularly important in patients with left ventricular dysfunction.

Goudelin et al. [10] demonstrated that weaning-induced pulmonary edema appears to be related to left ventricular overload associated with excessive fluid balance. Objectively, with the transition from positive pressure to spontaneous negative pressure, there is an increase in preload and afterload, resulting in increased left ventricular pressure and pulmonary artery occlusion pressure. Pulmonary edema results in increased respiratory effort and myocardial oxygen consumption. Figure 7.1 illustrates these events.

An alternative to assess and determine the potential for weaning-induced pulmonary oedema (WIPO) is echocardiography to evaluate the left ventricle. Goudelin et al. [10] demonstrated that left ventricular overload in high-risk patients was associated with the presence of WIPO and failure of the spontaneous breathing test. Vignon [11] suggests that this noninvasive approach is better suited to identify high-risk patients, describe the origin of WIPO, and tailor individual management, despite the traditional method of measuring pulmonary artery occlusion pressure.

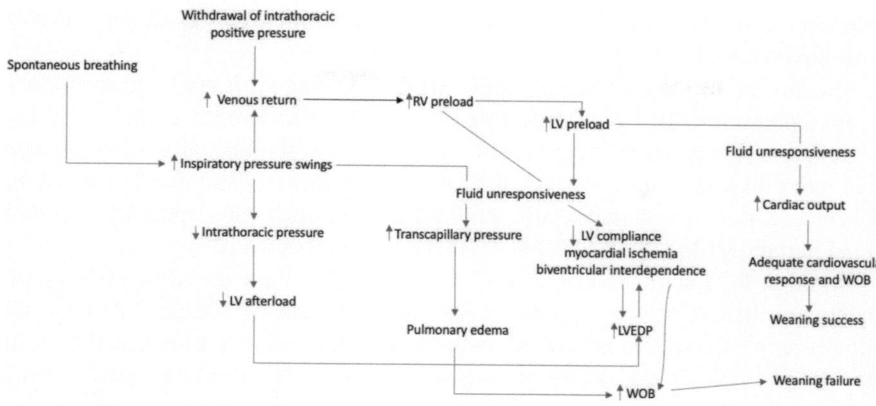

Fig. 7.1 Association between pulmonary edema and weaning

In addition to WIPO, another factor associated with weaning failure in patients with heart failure is inspiratory muscle weakness. As a result of heart failure, cardiac output is reduced, resulting in decreased blood supply to the diaphragm. Deprived of oxygen, the diaphragm undergoes metabolic changes, becoming weaker and more susceptible to fatigue. Dres et al. [12] found that diaphragm dysfunction associated with weaning-induced pulmonary edema was common in patients experiencing difficult weaning. It is worth noting that diaphragmatic dysfunction is associated with heart disease and also with the duration of invasive mechanical ventilation.

7.3 How to Wean Cardiac Patients

Noninvasive ventilation and the manner in which the spontaneous breathing test is performed are some of the strategies used to manage and increase the chances of successful weaning in patients with heart disease.

As seen above, patients with heart disease may develop pulmonary edema during weaning. There are two most common ways to perform the spontaneous breathing test: pressure support ventilation (PSV) and the T-tube [13]. Although controversial and with divided evidence, the T-tube test has better results in cardiac patients when we consider pulmonary edema and test failure for this reason. During the PSV test, PEEP is set on the mechanical ventilator. Positive pressure tends to bring the alveolus closer to the capillary, redistributing interstitial fluid, improving gas exchange, maintaining work of breathing, and producing a false positive on the SBT [14].

When testing in a T-tube, there is no positive pressure. If there is fluid in the interstitial space, the alveolar-capillary distance will increase, resulting in decreased exchange, respiratory discomfort, and SBT failure. At this point, the patient can be reconnected to the ventilator, reducing the negative impact of extubation after a false-positive SBT.

Gacouin et al. [15] compared T-tube to PSV testing with zero end-expiratory positive pressure (ZEEP) and found that there was no difference in the seven-day reintubation rate between the groups. In the study by Cabello et al. [16] in patients with heart disease, T-tube testing failed in 11/14 patients (79%) due to LV failure (PAOP >18 mmHg), whereas SBT with positive or zero end-expiratory pressure failed in only 3/14 (21%) and 6/14 (43%) patients, respectively.

Na et al. [17] compared SBT in PSV with T-tube. Patients in the PSV group underwent the test with a support pressure of 8 cmH2O and ZEEP. There was no difference in weaning success between the groups, but weaning time was shorter in the PSV group. It should be noted that some of the patients studied had heart disease.

In another study, Subirà et al. [18] compared the extubation success of patients undergoing T-tube SBT with a support pressure of 8 cmH_2O and zero positive end-expiratory pressure. The success rate was higher in the PSV group, but they completed the test in 30 min while the T-tube group took 2 h. This suggests that time is another factor influencing the success of SBT. The latest Brazilian guidelines on mechanical ventilation recommend the use of noninvasive ventilation in three ways during weaning from MV [19]: facilitative NIV, curative NIV, and preventive NIV. The first two are not suitable for patients with heart disease, but the last (preventive) is fully associated with this patient profile. Preventive NIV is used in patients who have passed the spontaneous breathing test but have some risk factors for post-extubation failure. The list of risk factors is shown in Table 7.1.

According to Table 7.1, it can be seen that patients with heart failure and heart failure as the cause of intubation are indicated for the use of preventive NIV, in order to increase the chances of successful weaning.

Table 7.1 Caption

Hypercapnia after extubation (>45 mmHg)
Cardiac insufficiency
Ineffective cough
Copious secretions
More than one consecutive weaning failure
More than one comorbidity
Upper airway obstruction
Age over 65 years
Heart failure as the cause of intubation
APACHE >12 on the day of extubation
Patients with more than 72 h of IMV

Fonte: Barbas et al. [19]

Another point to consider is fluid balance. Patients with a positive fluid balance tend to have higher capillary pressures and fluid extravasation, causing all the effects described above. For this reason, it is recommended that the balance be zero or negative in 24 h prior to the spontaneous breathing test.

7.4 Conclusion

It is important to monitor the clinical response to treatment and adjust the weaning strategy according to the patient's tolerance. In addition, consideration of various methods of assessing spontaneous breathing, such as the spontaneous breathing test (SBT) and other forms of respiratory monitoring, is critical to ensure the safety of the process. These tests provide valuable information about the patient's respiratory capacity and readiness for extubation, allowing for a smoother transition and avoiding complications. Therefore, a comprehensive assessment and collaboration among the healthcare team are essential to optimize weaning and improve the patient's quality of life.

References

1. McMurray JJV, Pfeffer MA. Heart failure. Lancet. 2005;365(9474):1877–89.
2. Ponikowski P, Voors AA, Anker SD, et al. 2016 ESC guidelines for the diagnosis and treatment of acute and chronic heart failure: the task force for the diagnosis and treatment of acute and chronic heart failure of the European Society of Cardiology (ESC) developed with the special contribution of the heart failure association (HFA) of the ESC. Eur Heart J. 2016;37(27):2129–200. https://doi.org/10.1093/eurheartj/ehw128.
3. Ambrosy AP, Fonarow GC, Butler J, et al. The global health and economic burden of hospitalizations for heart failure: lessons learned from hospitalized heart failure registries. J Am Coll Cardiol. 2014;63(12):1123–33. https://doi.org/10.1016/j.jacc.2013.11.053.
4. Schwinger RHG. Pathophysiology of heart failure. Cardiovasc Diagn Ther. 2021 Feb;11(1):263–76. https://doi.org/10.21037/cdt-20-302.
5. Martinez-Garcia G, Rodriguez-Ramos M, Santos-Medina M, Carrero-Vazquez AM, Chipi-Rodriguez Y. New model predicts in-hospital complications in myocardial infarction. Discover. 2022 Mar;10(1):e142. https://doi.org/10.15190/d.2022.1.
6. Boorsma EM, Ter Maaten JM, Damman K, Dinh W, Gustafsson F, Goldsmith S, Burkhoff D, Zannad F, Udelson JE, Voors AA. Congestion in heart failure: a contemporary look at physiology, diagnosis and treatment. Nat Rev Cardiol. 2020;17(10):641–55. https://doi.org/10.1038/s41569-020-0379-7. Epub 2020 May 15
7. Dres M, Teboul JL, Anguel N, et al. Passive leg raising performed before a spontaneous breathing trial predicts weaning-induced cardiac dysfunction. Intensive Care Med. 2015;41(3):487–94. https://doi.org/10.1007/s00134-014-3637-8.
8. Jaber S, Petrof BJ, Jung B, et al. Rapidly progressive diaphragmatic weakness and injury during mechanical ventilation in humans. Am J Respir Crit Care Med. 2011;183(3):364–71. https://doi.org/10.1164/rccm.201004-0670OC.

9. Sinderby C, Navalesi P, Beck J, Skrobik Y, Comtois N, Friberg S, Gottfried SB, Lindström L. Neural control of mechanical ventilation in respiratory failure. Nat Med. 1999 Aug;5(8):1433–6. https://doi.org/10.1038/71012.
10. Goudelin M, Champy P, Amiel JB, Evrard B, Fedou AL, Daix T, François B, Vignon P. Left ventricular overloading identified by critical care echocardiography is key in weaning-induced pulmonary edema. Intensive Care Med. 2020;46(7):1371–81. https://doi.org/10.1007/s00134-020-06061-y. Epub 2020 May 6. PMID: 32377766; PMCID: PMC7223421
11. Vignon P. Cardiopulmonary interactions during ventilator weaning. Front Physiol. 2023;14:1275100. https://doi.org/10.3389/fphys.2023.1275100. PMID: 37745230; PMCID: PMC10512459
12. Dres M, Rozenberg E, Morawiec E, Mayaux J, Delemazure J, Similowski T, et al. Diaphragm dysfunction, lung aeration loss and weaning-induced pulmonary oedema in difficult-to-wean patients. Ann Intensive Care. 2021;11(1):99. https://doi.org/10.1186/s13613-021-00886-6. PMID: 34181105; PMCID: PMC8237539
13. Smith AB, Jones CD. Spontaneous breathing trial in cardiac patients: a comparative study. J Cardiol. 2020;45(3):123–35. https://doi.org/10.10123/jcard.2020.12345.
14. Brown EF, Johnson GH. Pulmonary edema during weaning: strategies and controversies. Crit Care Med. 2019;27(6):789–801. https://doi.org/10.10456/ccm.2019.45678.
15. Gacouin A, Lesouhaitier M, Reizine F, Painvin B, Maamar A, Camus C, et al. 1-hour t-piece spontaneous breathing trial vs 1-hour zero pressure support spontaneous breathing trial and reintubation at day 7: a non-inferiority approach. J Crit Care. 2022;67:95–9. https://doi.org/10.1016/j.jcrc.2021.10.016. Epub 2021 Nov 2
16. Cabello B, Thille AW, Roche-Campo F, Brochard L, Gómez FJ, Mancebo J. Physiological comparison of three spontaneous breathing trials in difficult-to-wean patients. Intensive Care Med. 2010;36(7):1171–9. https://doi.org/10.1007/s00134-010-1870-0. Epub 2010 Mar 30
17. Na SJ, Ko RE, Nam J, Ko MG, Jeon K. Comparison between pressure support ventilation and T-piece in spontaneous breathing trials. Respir Res. 2022;23(1):22. https://doi.org/10.1186/s12931-022-01942-w. PMID: 35130914; PMCID: PMC8822807
18. Subirà C, Hernández G, Vázquez A, Rodríguez-García R, González-Castro A, García C, et al. Effect of pressure support vs T-piece ventilation strategies during spontaneous breathing trials on successful Extubation among patients receiving mechanical ventilation: a randomized clinical trial. JAMA. 2019;321(22):2175–82. https://doi.org/10.1001/jama.2019.7234. Erratum in: JAMA. 2019, Aug 20;322(7):696. PMID: 31184740; PMCID: PMC6563557
19. Mechanical Centilation Committee of the Brazilian Intensive Care Medicine Association; Commission of Intensive Therapy of the Brazilian Thoracic Society. Brazilian recommendations of mechanical ventilation 2013. Part I. J Bras Pneumol. 2014;40(4):327–63. https://doi.org/10.1590/s1806-37132014000400002. PMID: 25210957; PMCID: PMC4201165

Chapter 8
Weaning in Neurological Patients

Sergio Nogueira Nemer

8.1 Introduction

Neurological patients often require admission to the intensive care unit (ICU) and, when possible, in a neurological intensive care unit (NICU), in addition to invasive mechanical ventilation [1], often due to a decreased level of consciousness. Glasgow Coma Scale less (GCS) or equal eight is used as a criterion for intubation of these patients [2]. Neurological patients may have a direct influence on the respiratory pump system, requiring prolonged mechanical ventilation [3, 4]. Rates of weaning failure, prolonged weaning, re-intubation, ventilation-associated pneumonia (VAP), and mortality are higher in neurological patients than in non-neurological [3]; therefore, specific care and approaches are necessary in this population [4].

8.2 Complications Related to Neurological Patients Weaning

Due to the decreased level of consciousness, the risk of aspirative pneumonia is eminent in some neurological patients, increasing the rate of acute respiratory failure and invasive mechanical ventilation. In addition, noninvasive ventilation (NIV), which can avoid intubation in non-neurological [5] and some neurological patients [6], should not be used in the absence of airway protection. This way, one of the effective approaches to avoid intubation in non-neurological patients has extreme limitations in neurological patients.

The weaning indexes, often used to predict the outcome of this process [7], can also be used in neurological patients [8, 9] but are not always accurate [10], becoming the weaning prognosis, sometimes uncertain in this population.

S. N. Nemer (✉)
Niterói Hospital Complex, Rio de Janeiro, Brazil

A. R. Baptistella et al. (eds.), *Weaning from Mechanical Ventilation*,
https://doi.org/10.1007/978-3-032-01145-9_8

Brain hypoxemia, seen in severe brain injury patients, can lead to hypoxic encephalopathy, worsening the outcomes [11]. Brain hypoxemia can be accurately monitored by brain tissue oxygen pressure (PbrO2), and maneuvers that improve systemic oxygenation (such as increased fraction of inspired oxygen and positive end expiratory pressure) can also improve brain oxygenation in selected patients [12].

In severe neurological patients, with brainstem damage and respiratory drive impairment, respiratory arrythmias, desynchronies, tachypnea, and central neurogenic hyperventilation can be observed, making the weaning process more difficult and sometimes prolonged [13].

8.3 Airway Protection Capacity

Even in patients who have respiratory failure, NIV should not be used in those with GCS $\leq$ 8, due to the reduced protective capacity of the airways [2]. Not even a presence of physician or a physiotherapist close to the patient makes this approach safe, mainly in case of vomiting, due to the high risk of aspiration.

However, high-flow nasal canula (HFNC) can be used (with high attention) in case of hypoxemic respiratory failure in neurological patients with adequate airway protection capacity.

Patients with GCS $\leq$ 8, high intracranial pressure, brain herniation, combative or with severe agitation should be intubated due to the reduced airway protection capacity and possible neuroworsening.

The risk of extubation failure should be considered in the presence of reduced airway protective capacity. Therefore, judicious assessment of the airway's protective capacity must be carried out before extubation.

8.4 What Is Important to Wean a Neurological Patient?

Weaning includes the process of liberating the patient from mechanical ventilation and endotracheal tube, although weaning and extubation require different assessments and have distinct causes of failure.

Successful weaning can be defined as the absence of ventilatory support after 48 h of extubation or disconnection from mechanical ventilation.

Weaning failure can be defined as the failure of a spontaneous breathing trial (SBT), or the need for reintubation, *or still, the need of return to mechanical ventilation* within 48 h following disconnection in tracheostomized patients.

Since 2007, weaning has generally been divided into three categories: simple, difficult, and prolonged weaning [14].

Extubation failure is related to airway obstruction, excessive secretions, laryngeal edema, or decrease in airway protection capacity [14]. Although extubation is recommended after a successful SBT, 10%–20% of patients who successfully complete this test experience extubation failure [15].

In addition to the usual care for any patient undergoing weaning, neurological patients have specific characteristics, which make them different in this process. One of the basic and essential criteria, which is the resolution of the cause for beginning mechanical ventilation (such as pneumonia in a patient with chronic obstructive pulmonary disease), cannot always be resolved in a neurological patient, as some diseases are difficult to control (as myasthenia gravis), or not even curable (as amyotrophic lateral sclerosis).

Several neurological patients can tolerate the SBT but cannot be extubated due to the inability to protect the airway. For this reason, some scores have been proposed, such as VISAGE score [16], semiquantitative cough strength (SCSS) [17], STAGE score [18] (Table 8.1), and GCS > 8 [4], among others, in order to minimize the risk of extubation failure in neurological patients.

A VISAGE score of 3 or greater was associated with 90% extubation success in the study of Asehnoune et al. Extubation success was significantly associated with shorter duration of mechanical ventilation (11 vs 22 days; $p < 0.0001$), shorter intensive care unit length of stay (15 vs 27 days; $p < 0.0001$), and lower in-intensive care unit mortality (4 vs 11.1%, $p < 0.0001$). The authors conclude that VISAGE score, exploring both airway functions and neurologic status, may increase the probability of successful extubation in patients with severe brain injury. However, the area under the receiver operating characteristic curve (AUROC) of VISAGE score was 0.73 [16], which means only moderate accuracy in predicting extubation outcome. One question to be questioned would be, is age over 40 really an appropriate cutoff point to differentiate patients at higher risk of extubation failure, or should this age be higher?

The SCSS evaluates the patient's ability to generate a cough for predicting reintubation after planned extubation (Table 8.2). The SCSS was used in the study of Ibrahim et al. in 80 patients with traumatic brain injury (TBI), with a median admission GCS of 8. If the patient does not obey the command to cough (SCSS = 0), the authors examined the cough response by introducing a catheter into the tracheal tube and stimulating the carina. Odds ratio for SCSS in predicting extubation success was 2.99 ($p < 0.001$), higher than GCS (1.85; $p = 0.03$), and still higher than rapid shallow breathing and PaO_2/FiO_2 ratio (1.01 and 1.0; $p = 0.405$ and $p = 0.47$, respectively). Although SCSS showing promise in predicting successful extubation in TBI patients, the authors recommend further research to help determine accurate predictors of extubation success or failure in TBI patients [17].

Table 8.1 VISAGE score calculation

Extubation success score	Assigned points according to items
Age < 40 years old (yes/no)	1/0
Visual pursuit (yes/no)	1/0
Swallowing attempts (yes/no)	1/0
Glasgow Coma Scale (yes/no)	1/0

Table 8.2 Semiquantitative cough strength (SCSS)

Cough score	Response
Zero	No cough on command
1	Audible movement of air through the endotracheal tube, but no audible cough
2	Weakly (barely) audible cough
3	Clearly audible cough
4	Stronger cough
5	Multiple sequential strong cough

Table 8.3 STAGE score

Result	Score
Swallowing (strong/poor)	3/0
Tongue protrusion (strong/poor)	2/0
Spontaneous cough (strong/poor)	2/0
Suctioning cough (strong/poor)	3/0
Motor response in GCS (≥5/<5)	2/0
Total STAGE score	12/0

Another score recently proposed by Xu Shan-Shan et al., developed to predict the extubation outcome in neurosurgical patients, was the STAGE score (swallowing, tongue protrusion, airway protection reflected by spontaneous and suctioning cough, and GCS) (Table 8.3). STAGE score was evaluated in 226 neurosurgical patients with a GCS of 10 on ICU admission. At STAGE score in 6, presented 59% of sensitivity, 74% of specificity, 90% positive predictive value, and only 30% of negative predictive value. At STAGE score of 9 or higher, specificity and positive predictive value were 100% for predicting extubation success [18]. The STAGE score evaluates four of its five topics as strong or weak, which may result in subjective results. The STAGE core is promising, but as it is still recent and little explored, more studies may be needed before it can be used in daily routine.

Other evaluations used to determine extubation readiness in the general population, such as an expiratory peak cough flow 60 L/min [19] may be used with neurological patients but, require further study in this population.

A common but unfortunate thought that says: “let extubate and see what happens, anything, we’ll reintubate later,” should not be taken into consideration, as reintubation is associated with several complications, such as increased mechanical ventilation time and mortality [4]. So, extubation should be well planned in order to minimize the risk of failure.

In the absence of criteria that allow extubation, or in patients who presented extubation failure, tracheostomy should be performed, but not earlier than 4 days after intubation [4].

8.5 Preexisting Neuromuscular Disease

Neuromuscular diseases (NMD) are different syndromes that affect nerve, muscle, and/or neuromuscular junction [20]. NMD result in deteriorating respiratory muscle function (decrease in vital capacity, inspiratory muscle strength, and tidal volume with possible tachypnea) and mobility over time, with impairment and disability [21]. Guillain-Barre syndrome (GBS) and myasthenia gravis are the most frequent causes of respiratory failure in NMD patients.

8.5.1 Guillain-Barre Syndrome (GBS)

GBS is an acute immune-mediated polyradiculopathy that can affect all myelinated nerves and is the most common cause of acute flaccid paralysis [22]. It is a rare immune-mediated peripheral nerve disease often preceded by infections [23], with an incidence of about 0.62–2.66 person-years in Europe and North America [24]. Patients with GBS may develop acute respiratory failure as a result of progressive weakness of respiratory muscles and bulbar dysfunction [24], mainly in axonal GBS. Myelinic GBS (without axonal damage) is less likely to develop respiratory failure.

About 30% become ventilator dependent, with a subsequent increased risk of difficult/prolonged weaning and death, that ranges between 5% and 12% [24]. Criteria proposed for intubation in GBS patients include significant distress, time from the onset of symptoms to hospitalization less than 7 days, fatigue, tachycardia, functional vital capacity (FVC) of 10–12 ml/kg (<30%–35% of predicted), maximal inspiratory pressure (MIP) higher than −30 cmH_2O and $PaCO_2$ greater than 50 mmHg [25]. NIV can be attempted to facilitate weaning [26] and avoid intubation, emphasizing inspiratory pressure enough to remove CO_2, as respiratory failure in these patients is often hypercapnic. NIV should not be considered in the presence of bulbar dysfunction. Cough assist can be used both to clear secretions [27, 28] and avoid intubation, as to facilitate weaning in GBS patients, in NMD patients, or in any patient with an ineffective cough. Parameters must be individualized, although median inspiratory and expiratory pressure are generally set around +25 and − 35 cmH_20, respectively, but can reach +50 and − 50 cmH_2O [28].

In GBS patients, recovery often begins after 2–4 weeks [29]. After this period, or resolution of the acute phase of the disease, weaning should be attempted. Tracheostomy should be done to facilitate weaning, mainly if mechanical ventilation time is higher than 10–14 days [14].

Inspiratory muscle training (IMT) can be used to facilitate weaning in several situations, and also in GBS patients [23], especially in the case of difficult/prolonged weaning. IMT can be done with a resistive load between 30% and 70%, from one to six sessions of up to 1 min (or a number of repetitions that are close to this period), one to two times a day for 1–2 weeks [30]. Several training protocols are proposed, and there seems to be no consensus on which, among them, is the best [31], mainly in NMD.

8.5.2 *Myasthenia Gravis*

Myasthenia gravis (MG) is a disorder of neuromuscular transmission, resulting from binding of autoantibodies to components of the neuromuscular junction, most commonly the acetylcholine receptor (AChR) [32], and also autoantibody against muscle-specific receptor tyrosine kinase (anti-MusK) [20]. MG is characterized by fatigable weakness of voluntary muscles, including facial and oropharyngeal muscles [20]. The incidence of MG ranges from 0.3 to 2.8 per 100.000 people, and it is estimated to affect more than 700,000 people worldwide [32].

Generalized MG is a frequent cause of respiratory failure in NMD [25]. Myasthenic and cholinergic crises are exacerbations of the generalized weakness, with associated respiratory failure and need for NIV and invasive mechanical ventilation [25]. About 30% of patients with generalized MG will require invasive mechanical ventilation [26]. NIV can reduce the need for intubation in 60%–70% in patients with generalized MG (without bulbar dysfunction), but hypercapnia, with $PaCO_2 > 45–50$ mmHg, is a strong predictor of NIV failure. Hospital mortality rate is around 2.2%, being higher in MG crisis (4, 47%) [33].

Criteria for intubation and extubation in MG patients are almost the same used in GBS. As in GBS, NIV can also be attempted to facilitate weaning [26] and avoid intubation in MG, emphasizing inspiratory pressure enough to remove CO_2. NIV should not be considered in the presence of bulbar dysfunction. Weaning should be attempted after the acute phase of the disease and resolution of myasthenic/cholinergic crisis. Since effort predisposes to fatigue with greater intensity in MG, and there is a lack of high-quality studies on IMT in these patients, this approach should be avoided in this population. In the same way, long periods of SBT and greater efforts during weaning attempts should be avoided during this process in patients with MG [25]. Tracheostomy should be done to facilitate weaning, mainly if mechanical ventilation time is higher than 10–14 days [14].

8.5.3 *Amyotrophic Lateral Sclerosis*

Amyotrophic lateral sclerosis (ALS) is a progressive neurodegenerative disease, or a motor neuron disease, characterized by death of upper motor neurons and lower motor neurons [34], which leads to muscle weakness and eventual paralysis [35]. Patients with ALS often die from respiratory failure within 2–5 years of symptom onset [34]. Nowadays, ALS is classified as motor neuron disease, and no more as NMD, once new imaging and neuropathological data have indicated the involvement of the non-motor neuraxis in disease pathology [35]. There is no damage to the neuromuscular junction in ALS, and peripheral nerves are also preserved. The mean time from the onset of symptoms to confirmation of the diagnosis is 10–18 months [34]. The etiology of 90%–95% of ALS remains unknown, while 5%–10% of ALS patients have inherited familial forms of the disease [36]. The current diagnosis of ALS depends mainly on clinical symptoms (of impaired upper and lower motor neurons) and signs observed through clinical visits and various examinations [36]. As the inspiratory and expiratory muscles are affected, the use of NIV and cough assist is highly used in ALS, except in patients with bulbar dysfunction (bulbar ALS). NIV should emphasize inspiratory pressure in order to keep adequate tidal volume and avoid CO_2 retention. Parameters during the use of cough assist must be individualized, although median inspiratory and expiratory pressure are generally set around +25 and − 35 cmH_2O respectively, but can reach +50 and − 50 cm H_2O [28].

NIV should begin as soon as signs of orthopnea appear [37] and MIP decreases in less than −40 cm H_2O [38], mainly at night, where respiratory distress are more frequent. Impairment in inspiratory force appears to be the most common reason for NIV initiation and often preceded significant declines in forced vital capacity [38].

As ALS is a progressive and degenerative disease, with no cure, weaning becomes extremely rare in the advanced stage, with a lack of high-quality studies that demonstrate the success of this process. As patients with ALS generally become dependent on mechanical ventilation, tracheostomy often becomes unavoidable, and home mechanical ventilation becomes an option in chronic situations, of course, with all the care of a multidisciplinary team.

8.6 Conclusion

As the pathophysiology is completely distinct, neurological patients should be divided into patients with brain injury and neuromuscular patients. Patients with brain injury are generally intubated due to reduced level of consciousness, while NMD or MND patients are often intubated due to respiratory failure, almost always awake.

Due to the comatose or vegetative state, often found in patients with severe brain injury, weaning may become difficult or prolonged in these patients. On the other hand, in NMD or MND patients, weaning generally becomes difficult or prolonged due to respiratory muscle failure or bulbar dysfunction.

Adequate airway protection is essential to carry out a safe extubation in neurological patients. Weaning indexes can be evaluated, but they are less accurate in patients with brain injury, since the reason for mechanical ventilation was the reduction in the level of consciousness, and not respiratory failure.

Because each neurological disease has its own pathophysiology, there is no generic approach for all patients. There is no one-size-fits-all solution; each disease requires a specific approach.

References

1. Sanfilippo F, Urygaz A, Ball L, Battaglini D, Giorgia I, Smielewski P, et al. The effect of recruitment maneuvers on cerebrovascular dynamics and right ventricular function in patients with acute brain injury: a single-center prospective study. Neurocrit Care. 2024;41 https://doi.org/10.1007/s12028-024-01939-x.
2. Robba C, Poole D, McNett M, Asehnoune K, Boesel J, Bruder N, et al. Mechanical ventilation in patients with acute brain injury: recommendations of the European Society of Intensive Care Medicine consensus. Intensive Care Med. 2020;46:2397–410.
3. Fan L, Su Y, Elmadhoun OA, Zhang Y, Zhang Y, Daiquan G, Ye H, Chen W. Protocol-directed weaning from mechanical ventilation in neurological patients: a randomized controlled trial and subgroup analyses based on consciousness. Neurol Res. 2015;37:1006–14.
4. Bureau C, Demoule A. Weaning from mechanical ventilation in neurocritical care. Rev Neurol. 2022;178:111–20.
5. Brett H, Nicole H, Tran A, Shannon F, Bram R, Karen B, Andrew S. Predictors of non-invasive ventilation failure in the post extubation period: a systematic review and meta-analysis. Crit Care Med. 2023;51(7):872–80.
6. Weiss N. Should we assess diaphragmatic function during mechanical ventilation weaning in Guillain-Barré syndrome and myasthenia gravis patients? Neurocrit Care. 2021;34:371. https://doi.org/10.1007/s12028-020-01159-z.
7. Nemer S, Barbas CS, Caldeira JB, Cárias T, Santos R, Almeida L, Azeredo L, Noé R, Guimarães B, Souza P. A new integrative weaning index of discontinuation from mechanical ventilation. Crit Care. 2009;13:R152.
8. Lazardis C, DeSAntis S, McLawhorn M, Krishna V. Liberation on neurosurgical patients from mechanical ventilation and tracheostomy in neurocritical care. J Crit Care. 2012;27:417.e1–8.
9. El-Baradey GF, El-Shmaa NS, Ganna SA. Can integrative weaning index be a routine predictor for weaning success? Indian J Crit Care Med. 2015;19:703–7.
10. Ko R, Ramos L, Chaleta J. Conventional weaning parameters do not predict extubation failure in neurocritical care patients. Neurocrit Care. 2009;10:269–73.
11. Bernard F, Barsan W, Diaz-Arrastia R, Merck LH, Yeatts S, Shutter LA. Brain oxygen optimization in severe traumatic brain injury (BOOST-3): a multicentre, randomized, blinded-endpoint, comparative effectiveness study of brain tissue oxygen and intracranial pressure monitoring versus intracranial pressure alone. BMJ Open. 2022;12:e060188.
12. Nemer SN, Caldeira JB, Santos RG, Guimarães BL, Garcia JM, Prado D, Silva RT. Effects of positive end-expiratory pressure on brain tissue oxygen pressure of severe traumatic brain injury patients with acute respiratory distress syndrome. J Crit Care. 2015;30:1263–6.
13. Jonkman AH, Vries HJ, Heunks ML. Physiology of respiratory drive in ICU patients: implications for diagnosis and treatment. Crit Care. 2020;24:104.
14. Boles JM, Connors BA, Herridge M, Melot MC, Pearl R, Silverman H, et al. Weaning from mechanical ventilation. Statement of the sixth international consensus conference on intensive care medicine. Eur Respir J. 2007;29:1033–56.
15. Duan J, Zhang X, Song J. Predictive power of extubation failure diagnosed by cough strength: a systematic review and meta-analysis. Crit Care. 2021;25:357.
16. Asehnoune K, Seguin P, Lasocki S, Roquiliy A, Delater A, Gros A, et al. Extubation sucess prediction in a multicenter cohort of patients with severe brain injury. Anesthesiology. 2017;127:338–46.
17. Ibrahim AS, Aly MG, Abdel-Rahman KA, Mohamed MA, Mehany MM, Aziz EM. Semi-quantitative cough strength score as a predictor for extubation outcome in traumatic brain injury: a prospective observational study. Neurocrit Care. 2018;29 https://doi.org/10.1007/s12028-018-0539-3.
18. Xu SS, Tian Y, Ma YJ, Zhou YM, Tian Y, Gao R, et al. Development of a prediction score for evaluation of extubation in neurosurgical patients with mechanical ventilation. Anesthesiology. 2023;139:614–27.

19. Thille AW, Cortés-Puch I, Esteban A. Weaning from mechanical ventilation in ICU. Curr Opin Crit Care. 2013;19:57–64.
20. Crespo V, James MLL. Neuromuscular disease in the neurointensive care unit. Anesthesiology Clin. 2016;34:601–19.
21. Watson K, Egerton T, Sheers N, Reticas S, McGaw R, Clohessy T, et al. Respiratory muscle training in neuromuscular disease: a systematic review and meta-analysis. Eur Respir Rev. 2022;31:220065.
22. Bust KM, Fried H, Muehischlegel S, Wartenberg KE, Rajajee V. Guidelines for neuroprognostication in adults with Guillain-Barré syndrome. Neurocrit Care. 2023;38:564–83. https://doi.org/10.1007/s12028-023-01707-3.
23. Almeida MP, Winck JC, Marques A. InspireGBS – inspiratory muscle training with Guillain-Barré syndrome: a feasibility study. PM&R. 2024;17 https://doi.org/10.1002/pmrj.13251.
24. Melone MA, Heming N, Meng P, Mompoint D, Aboab J, Clair B, et al. Early mechanical ventilation in patients with Guillain-Barre syndrome at high risk of respiratory failure: a randomized trial. Ann Intensive Care. 2020;10:128.
25. Rezania K, Goldenberg FD, White S. Neuromuscular disorders and acute respiratory failure: diagnosis and management. Neurol Clin. 2012;30:161–85.
26. Weiss N. Should we assess diaphragmatic function during mechanical ventilation weaning in Guillain-Barré syndrome and myasthenia gravis? Neurocrit care, vol. 34; 2021. https://doi.org/10.1007/s12028-020-01159-z.
27. Sheers NL, Andersen T, Chatwin M. Airway clearance in neuromuscular disease. Sleep Med. 2024;19:485–96.
28. Chatwin M, Simonds AK. Long-term mechanical insufflation-exsufflation cough assistance in neuromuscular disease: patterns of used and lessons for application. Respir Care. 2020;65:135–43.
29. Mirian A, Nicolle MW, Budhram A. Syndrome de Guillain-Barré. CMAJ. 2021;193:E378.
30. Bisset BM, Wang J, Neeman T, Leditschke IA, Boots R, Paratz J. Which ICU patients benefit most from inspiratory muscle training? Retrospective analysis of a randomized trial. Physiother Theory Pract. 2019;36:1316–21.
31. Worraphan S, Thammata A, Chittawatanarat K, Pharmd SS. Effects of inspiratory muscle training and early mobilization on weaning of mechanical ventilation. Arch Phys Med Rehabil. 2020;101:2002–14.
32. Sanders DB, Wolfe GI, Benatar M, Evoli A, Gilhus NE, Illa I, et al. International consensus guidance of myasthenia gravis. Neurology. 2016;87:419–25.
33. Alshekhlee A, Miles JD, Katirji B, Preston DC, Kaminski HJ. Incidence and mortality rates of myasthenia gravis and myasthenic crisis in US hospitals. Neurology. 2009;72:1548–54.
34. Tao QQ, Wu ZY. Amyotrophic lateral sclerosis: precise diagnosis and individualized treatment. Chin Med J. 2017;130:2269–72.
35. Hardiman O, Al-Chalabi A, Chio A, Corr EM, Logroscino G, Robbererecht W, et al. Nat Rev Dis Primers. 2017;3:1701. https://doi.org/10.1038/nrdp.2017.71.
36. Yuan M, Xu RS. Considerations on the concept, definition, and diagnosis of amyotrophic lateral sclerosis. Neural Regen Res. 2021;16:1723–9.
37. D'Cruz RF, Murphy PB, Kaltsakas G. Sleep disordered breathing in motor neuron disease. J Thorac Dis. 2018;10:S86–93.
38. Jimenez JV, Tang MJ, Wilson MW, Morrison AH, Ackrivo JA, Choi PC. Initiation of noninvasive ventilation in patients with amyotrophic lateral sclerosis. Mescle Nerve. 2024;70:1–5.

Chapter 9
The Use of Noninvasive Ventilation and High-Flow Nasal Cannula in the Weaning

Aline Almeida Gulart, Karoliny dos Santos Isoppo, and Isabela Julia Cristiana Santos Silva

9.1 Introduction

Prolonged mechanical ventilation (MV) can lead to serious complications and side effects. Therefore, early extubation is recommended whenever possible. However, approximately 15% of patients may develop respiratory failure and require reintubation, of which 25%–30% are at high risk [1].

The development of respiratory failure after extubation is a factor associated with high mortality in the intensive care unit (ICU). The main causes of respiratory failure after extubation include respiratory muscle fatigue or increased work of breathing due to reduced lung compliance or increased airway resistance. In addition, airway obstruction, excessive secretions, ineffective coughing, and neurological impairment are common in patients who cannot tolerate extubation [1, 2].

There are three ways to improve oxygenation after extubation: conventional oxygen therapy (COT), high-flow nasal cannula (HFNC), and noninvasive ventilation (NIV). COT is the most commonly used, but in recent years HFNC and NIV have been increasingly used. These methods have the potential to prevent or treat extubation failure by promoting alveolar recruitment, preventing collapse and reducing the workload on the respiratory muscles [2, 3].

A. A. Gulart (✉)
Physical Therapy Graduate Program, University of the State of Santa Catarina, Florianópolis, Brazil
e-mail: aline.gulart@udesc.br

K. dos S. Isoppo
Department of Health Sciences, Federal University of Santa Catarina, Araranguá, Brazil
e-mail: karoliny.isoppo@ufsc.br

I. J. C. S. Silva
School of Rehabilitation Science, McMaster University, Hamilton, Canada
e-mail: santoi2@mcmaster.ca

A. R. Baptistella et al. (eds.), *Weaning from Mechanical Ventilation*,
https://doi.org/10.1007/978-3-032-01145-9_9

In this chapter, we will look at when the use of NIV or HFNC can be considered to optimize weaning from MV.

9.2 The Role of NIV Post-Extubation

NIV is a form of noninvasive respiratory support that can provide pressure at one level (known as continuous positive airway pressure—CPAP) or at two levels. CPAP provides pressure that is equivalent to positive end-expiratory pressure (PEEP) because it maintains only one level of pressure throughout the respiratory cycle. In contrast, NIV with two levels provides one during the expiratory phase (PEEP) and another during the inspiratory phase.

NIV can be used in different post-extubation contexts: to facilitate weaning, to treat acute respiratory failure, and as a preventive therapy. The key practical issues in the use of NIV in the context of weaning from MV are described in Table 9.1.

9.2.1 NIV to Facilitate Weaning

NIV may be used to facilitate weaning when a patient fails the spontaneous breathing trial (SBT) but is still extubated [4]. It may also be used when an SBT is not performed [5]. In this setting, NIV is adjusted after extubation to reduce the respiratory muscle overload after extubation without a successful SBT [4].

9.2.2 NIV as a Treatment for Acute Respiratory Failure.

NIV may be used as a curative strategy when the patient successfully passes the SBT but presents with acute respiratory failure after extubation [4]. In this context, NIV may help to treat the cause or alleviate the symptoms of acute respiratory failure [3]. This could reduce the need for reintubation and the adverse effects of invasive MV [4].

9.2.3 NIV as a Preventive Therapy

NIV can be instituted immediately after extubation in patients at high risk for extubation failure who have been mechanically ventilated for more than 24 h and have passed an SBT [6].

Table 9.1 Key points when using NIV in the context of weaning from mechanical ventilation

	Indications	Parameters	Reintubation/failure of NIV criteria	Practical aspects
NIV to facilitate weaning	COPD/hypercapnic patients Hypoxemic patients (especially the postoperative population)	Initial parameters: Same inspiratory pressure and positive end-expiratory pressure as in the invasive mechanical ventilation If necessary, adjust inspiratory pressure to obtain tidal volume between 6 and 8 mL/kg (ideal body weight) and RR < 30 bpm Weaning parameters: Gradual reduction of parameters after 6–24 h of continuous NIV When minimum parameters are achieved, perform an SBT	Cardiac/respiratory arrest New acute respiratory failure: RR > 30 bpm RR < 12 bpm $FiO_2 > 50\%$ or oxygen therapy flow >6 L/min Increase of $pCO_2 > 10\%$ from pre-extubation value and arterial pH < 7.35 $pO_2/FiO_2 < 200$ mmHg Signs of respiratory distress Incompatible level of consciousness Inability to protect the airway Irresponsive hemodynamic instability Difficult to manage psychomotor agitation Intolerance to all NIV interfaces Septic shock and multiple organ failure	Reduction of parameters and possibility of SBT are evaluated at least once a day SBT can be performed with or without oxygen support
NIV as a treatment	Postoperative patients	Inspiratory pressure set to achieve 6–8 ml/kg (predicted body weight) and RR < 25 bpm PEEP of 4–10 cmH_2O Consider patient comfort	Signs of respiratory failure after 2 h trial Respiratory or cardiac arrest Incompatible consciousness level Inability to protect the airways Irresponsive hemodynamic instability Severe encephalopathy Difficult to manage psychomotor agitation Shock Gas exchange deterioration	In postoperative patients, any potential surgical complications should be considered and the interface used should be the one that best suits the patient's needs The duration of therapy should be 1–2 h. If the patient continues to show signs of respiratory failure after this time, reintubation should be considered

(continued)

Table 9.1 (continued)

	Indications	Parameters	Reintubation/failure of NIV criteria	Practical aspects
NIV as a preventive strategy	Age >65 years HF as the cause of intubation APACHE II score >12 at the time of extubation Acute exacerbation of COPD Chronic respiratory disease with ventilation >48 h and hypercapnia during SBT More than one of the following: Failure of consecutive SBT Chronic HF $pCO_2 > 45$ mmHg after extubation Multiple comorbidities Weak cough or stridor after extubation	Inspiratory pressure set to achieve 6–8 ml/kg (predicted body weight) and RR <25 bpm PEEP of 5–10 cmH_2O Adjust parameters for adequate gas exchange (SpO_2 92% and pH > 7.35) Consider patient comfort	Arterial pH < 7.35 with $pCO_2 > 45$ mmHg $SpO_2 < 90\%$ or $pO_2 < 60$ mmHg at an $FiO_2 > 50\%$ RR > 35 bpm Decreased consciousness, agitation or diaphoresis Clinical signs suggestive of respiratory muscle fatigue and/or increased work of breathing, such as the use of respiratory accessory muscles, paradoxical motion of the abdomen, retraction of the intercostal spaces, expiratory pauses with loss of consciousness or gasping for air Persistent inability to clear respiratory secretions HR < 50/min with loss of alertness Hemodynamic failure with the need for vasopressors Cardiac or respiratory arrest	Prophylactic NIV should preferably be used immediately after extubation, for at least 6 h per day, with the aim of maintaining therapy for 24 to 48 h after extubation

NIV Noninvasive ventilation, *COPD* Chronic obstructive pulmonary disease, *mL* milliliters, *Kg* kilogram, *RR* respiratory rate, *bpm* breaths per minute, cmH_2O centimeter of water, FiO_2 fraction of inspired oxygen, *L* liter, *min* minute, pCO_2 partial pressure of carbon dioxide, pO_2 partial pressure of oxygen, *SBT* spontaneous breathing trial, *HF* heart failure, *APACHE* Acute Physiology and Chronic Health Evaluation, SpO_2 pulse oxygen saturation, *HR* heart rate

9.3 Indication of NIV Post-Extubation

Figure 9.1 summarizes the main indications for NIV in the context of weaning from MV.

9.3.1 NIV to Facilitate Weaning

NIV to facilitate weaning is already well established in the literature. A recent systematic review and meta-analysis including patients with all diagnoses found that NIV to facilitate weaning was significantly associated with lower mortality (RR 0.57, 95% CI 0.44–0.74), incidence of ventilator-associated pneumonia (RR 0.30, 95% CI 0.22–0.41), and weaning failure (RR 0.59, 95% CI 0.43–0.81) compared with conventional weaning with invasive ventilation, and the quality of the evidence was high for all outcomes. In addition, length of stay in the ICU (MD −4.62 days, 95% CI −5.91 to −3.34) and hospital (MD −6.29 days, 95% CI −8.90 to −3.68), days of invasive ventilation (MD −7.75 days, 95% CI −9.86 to −5.64) and total ventilation (MD −5.26 days, 95% CI −7.86 to −2.67) were significantly reduced in

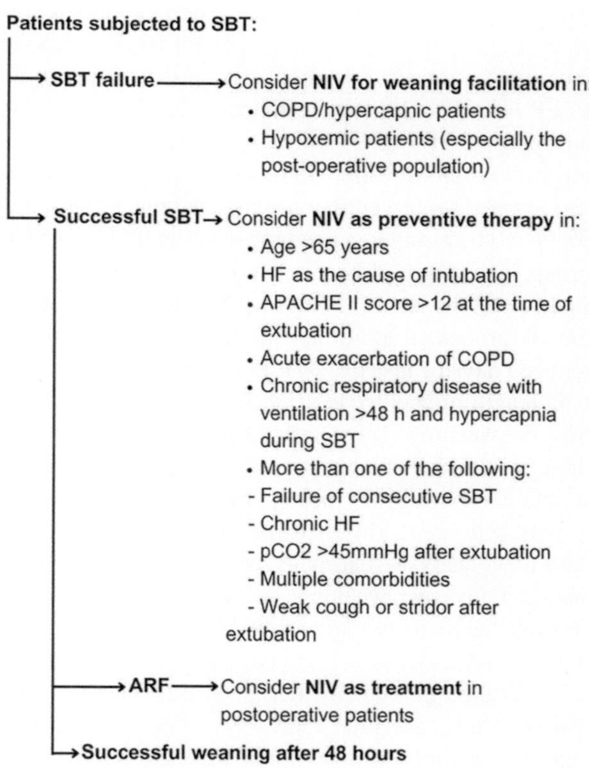

Fig. 9.1 Schematic representation of the use of noninvasive ventilation (NIV) application during the different weaning phases, based on Ferreyra et al. [4] and the recent recommendations [6–11]. *SBT* spontaneous breathing trial, *ARF* acute respiratory failure, *COPD* chronic obstructive pulmonary disease, *HF* heart failure, *APACHE* Acute Physiology and Chronic Health Evaluation

the NIV group. However, when the authors analyzed the COPD subgroup compared with mixed populations (any non-COPD), they found that these effects were even higher [8].

Since the 2017 ATS/ERS guideline [10], hypercapnic patients have been known to be the population with the most evidence that NIV is effective in facilitating weaning. The 2022 systematic review confirms this [8]. Mortality (COPD: RR 0.36, 95% CI 0.25 to 0.51 vs. mixed population: RR 0.81, 95% CI 0.62–1.05), ventilator-associated pneumonia (COPD: RR 0.22, 95% CI 0.15–0.33 vs. mixed population: RR 0.42, 95% CI 0.28–0.64), ICU length of stay (COPD: MD −6.1, 95% CI −8.1 to −4.0 vs. mixed population: MD −3.1, 95% CI −5.0 to −1.1) and reintubation (COPD: RR 0.48, 95% CI 0.34–0.67 vs. mixed population: RR 0.89, 95% CI 0.59–1.35) were lower in COPD patients when NIV was used to facilitate weaning compared to studies that included mixed populations ($p < 0.05$ for all variable subgroup differences).

The 2017 ERS/ATS guideline does not recommend this type of NIV in hypoxemic patients because of a lack of studies in this population at that time [10]. However, since the publication of this guideline, two large studies have been published using NIV to facilitate weaning in hypoxemic patients.

One of these studies was published by Vaschetto et al. [5], who compared weaning with NIV to weaning with invasive MV in non-hypercapnic patients who had not been tested with the SBT. In the NIV group, the protocol was to extubate the patient as soon as he/she met the criteria and then apply the NIV with decreasing parameters every 2 h. Once the patient reached predefined criteria (arterial partial pressure of oxygen / fraction of inspired oxygen ratio—pO_2/FiO_2 > 250 mmHg; PEEP = 8 cmH_2O; pressure support - PS = 10 cmH_2O), he or she was tested by an unsupported SBT (COT only). If the patient passed the test and did not experience respiratory failure within 48 h, weaning was considered successful. The NIV group had lower rates of ventilator-associated pneumonia and tracheobronchitis (25% vs. 9%; $p = 0.019$) and less need for sedation (85% vs. 57%; $p = 0.001$) than the control group. The length of hospital stay was also reduced [median (interquartile range): 27 (18–39) vs. 20 (13–32) days]. Mortality and ICU length of stay were similar in the two groups. In addition, when analyzing surgical patients, the NIV group showed reduced days of invasive MV [3.0 (2.0–6.0) days vs. 5.4 (3.8–8.9); $p = 0{,}004$] and ICU length of stay [6.0 (5.0–8.3) vs. 8.5 (6.3–13.5) days; $p = 0.036$] compared to invasive weaning. These differences were not seen in the nonsurgical patients. All these results show that hypoxemic patients may benefit from NIV as a facilitator of weaning, especially the postoperative population.

Vaschetto et al. [11] also conducted a systematic review with individual patient data meta-analysis that analyzed the efficacy of weaning with NIV compared to standard invasive weaning in hypoxemic non-hypercapnic patients. The study showed that patients who received NIV had a shorter duration of invasive MV (MD -3.43, 95% CI -5.17 to −1.69 days; $p < 0.001$), total MV (MD -2.04, 95% CI -3.82 to −0.27 days; $p = 0.024$), ICU stay (time ratio 0.81, 95%CI 0.68–0.96, $p = 0.015$), and hospital stay (time ratio 0.81, 95% CI 0.69–0.95; $p = 0.010$). The risk of ventilator-associated pneumonia was also reduced (OR 0.24, 95% CI 0.08–0.71;

$p = 0.014$), while there was no difference in the time from randomization to ICU death (time ratio: 0.75, 95% CI 0.45–1.23; $p = 0.251$). These results suggest that, in light of recent publications, hypoxemic patients may benefit from NIV to facilitate weaning.

When analyzing time to weaning (invasive or noninvasive), Perkins et al. [12], whose study included all diagnoses (hypercapnic patients were less than 10% of the sample), found no differences when comparing the group weaned with NIV and the group weaned with invasive ventilation (4.3 vs 4.5 days, respectively; adjusted hazard ratio: 1.1, 95% CI 0.89–1.40). They also found no differences in the rates of survival, reintubation, tracheostomy, and adverse events. This suggests that while NIV weaning may have an effect on reducing invasive ventilation days, it does not reduce overall ventilation use. However, this may still be of interest because invasive MV duration is associated with higher mortality, sedation use, and the rate of ventilator-associated pneumonia [11].

NIV to facilitate weaning was also tested in COVID-19 patients by Cammarota et al. [13]. In this study, the intervention group was extubated without performing SBT (but they had to meet some criteria like peak pressure < 30cmH_2O, respiratory rate < 30 bpm, effective cough, etc.). This group had a shorter duration of invasive MV [median (interquartile range): 9.0 (6.0–11.0) vs 11.0 (6.0–15.0); $p = 0.034$] and lower reintubation (18.2% vs 40%; $p = 0.009$) and extubation failure rates (18.2% vs 45.5%; $p = 0.002$). There were no differences in ICU length of stay or ICU mortality.

9.3.2 *NIV as a Treatment*

Patients who appear to benefit most from this treatment are postoperative patients who develop acute respiratory failure after extubation from surgery, particularly after thoracic, cardiac, and abdominal surgery [10].

Pulmonary complications such as atelectasis and pneumonia are common after surgery. These can lead to hypoxemia and respiratory failure [14]. Postoperative pain and anesthesia can also affect the respiratory system [15]. In this scenario, NIV can be used to treat acute respiratory failure and prevent reintubation because it helps to treat atelectasis, improves arterial oxygenation, reduces work of breathing, and does not cause adverse hemodynamic effects [3, 10].

The ATS/ERS guideline recommends NIV in these patients with moderate certainty of evidence. NIV has been shown to be effective in reducing intubation rates (RR 0.27, 95% CI 0.12–0.61; low certainty), nosocomial pneumonia (RR 0.20, 95% CI 0.04–0.88; very low certainty), and mortality (RR 0.28, 95% CI 0.09–0.84; moderate certainty) [10].

Recent studies have confirmed these good results in surgical patients. A systematic review of randomized and non-randomized controlled trials compared NIV with COT (e.g., face mask, venturi mask, nasal prongs, and non-rebreather mask) in 11,292 postoperative patients. They found that NIV for respiratory failure reduced the risk of reintubation (OR 0.23, 95% CI 0.09–0.58). When studies using CPAP were included in the analysis, the reduced risk was still observed (OR 0.25, 95% CI 0.11 to 0.60) [9].

When using NIV in surgical patients, it is important to consider some relative contraindications that may be present in this type of patient [3, 10, 16]:

- Anastomotic leak
- Intra-abdominal sepsis
- Severe upper gastrointestinal bleeding or hemoptysis
- Neurological or facial surgery
- Recent esophageal anastomosis*

*In these patients, it is important to avoid pressurization above 20 cmH_2O.

Any potential surgical complications should be considered and the interface used should be the one that best suits the patient's needs [3].

Another group of patients who appear to benefit from this therapy is hypercapnic patients. Thille et al. [17] compared mortality and reintubation rates between a group using NIV and HFNC versus HFNC alone to prevent reintubation in patients who developed respiratory failure within 7 days of extubation. They found no difference in mortality (at 28 days) or reintubation rates. However, when they stratified the sample into hypercapnic and non-hypercapnic patients, they found that the hypercapnic patients had lower reintubation rates than those without hypercapnia, regardless of which group they were in (37% vs 57%, respectively; $p = 0.03$). Also, when analyzing only the hypercapnic patients, they showed that the mortality rate was lower in the NIV + HFNC subgroup than in the HFNC-only group [difference: −28% (95% CI −54 to −6); $p = 0.006$]. This suggests that these patients may also benefit from this treatment. However, further studies are needed to confirm this.

It is important to note that although NIV is a good option, it should be used with caution because it may delay intubation and increase mortality. Thille et al. [17] attribute their lower mortality rates (than other previous studies, which we will mention below) to predefined criteria for reintubation that were strictly followed, and, therefore, the interval between the onset of respiratory failure and reintubation was shorter in the NIV group [median (interquartile range): 5.1 (1.8–18.0) h]. Although NIV has shown good results in postoperative and hypercapnic patients, these results cannot be extrapolated to other populations.

The ATS/ERS 2017 guidelines on NIV for acute respiratory failure suggest, as a conditional recommendation with low certainty of evidence, that NIV should not be used in post-extubation respiratory failure (except in the postoperative setting) [10]. One of the studies included in the guideline review evaluated patients who developed respiratory failure within 48 h of extubation and showed that NIV in this setting did not reduce ICU length of stay or reintubation rates [18]. In fact, it may be harmful, as mortality was higher in the NIV group (RR 1.78; 95% CI 1.03–3.20). The authors hypothesized that this may be because reintubation was delayed with NIV compared with COT, resulting in self-inflicted lung injury due to excessive transpulmonary pressure [19]. In the NIV group, the median time from onset of respiratory failure to reintubation was 12 h (interquartile range: 2 h 10 min–28 h), while in the COT group, the median time was 2 h and 30 min (interquartile range: 45 min–16 h 30 min, $p = 0.02$). The study included multiple diagnoses: ARDS, pneumonia, sepsis, trauma, heart failure, etc. [18]. Therefore, it is important to consider the patient's diagnosis before using NIV as a curative method for respiratory failure. The 2017 ATS/ERS guideline suggests further research due to the limitations of the studies published at that time [10].

In addition, if the patient does not show improvement in the symptoms of respiratory failure within the first 1–2 h after initiation of NIV, the patient should be reintubated [19, 20]. Again, this therapeutic use should always be questioned because, as we have seen above, it works in a very small group of individuals and in most cases it may be most beneficial to opt for reintubation [19].

9.3.3 NIV as a Preventive Therapy

Studies have shown that the use of NIV as a preventive therapy has the potential to reduce reintubation rates and mortality in well-selected patients [21–25]. In the general population of mechanically ventilated patients, there is no evidence to support the use of this strategy. Risk factors are variable across studies and include a variety of comorbidities such as COPD, chronic heart failure, hypercapnia, older age, and greater disease severity. Table 9.1 lists the main risk factors that may be considered when deciding whether or not to use NIV after extubation. A patient under 65 years of age who has passed their first SBT, has a normal pCO_2, and has no significant respiratory or cardiac comorbidities is not at potential risk of extubation failure, and there is no evidence to support the routine use of prophylactic NIV [6].

The 2017 ATS/ERS guidelines suggest that NIV should be used to prevent respiratory failure after extubation in high-risk patients and should not be used in non-high-risk patients. These recommendations were conditional, with low certainty of evidence [10]. The pooled analysis showed that NIV reduced mortality (RR 0.41, 95% CI 0.21–0.82) and the need for intubation (RR 0.75, 95% CI 0.49–1.15). In the same year, an American College of Chest Physicians/ATS clinical practice guideline on weaning from MV gave a strong recommendation and moderate quality of evidence for the use of NIV as a preventive strategy after extubation in high-risk patients [6]. NIV was favorable compared to standard care in high-risk patients for extubation success (RR 1.14, 95% CI 1.05 to 1.23), ICU length of stay (mean difference −2.48 d, 95% CI −4.03 to −0.93 d), short-term mortality (RR 0.37, 95% CI 0.19–0.70), and long-term mortality (RR 0.58, 95% CI 0.27–1.22).

Recently, a systematic review and meta-analysis showed that prophylactic NIV use was associated with lower rates of ventilator-associated pneumonia (OR 0.49, 95% CI 0.34–0.73; $p < 0.001$, moderate certainty), lower hospital mortality (OR

0.64, 95% CI 0.47–0.87; $p = 0.004$, moderate certainty), and shorter ICU stay (MD -0.72 days, 95% CI −1.44 to 0.00 days; $p = 0.049$, very low certainty), without affecting reintubation time. This last finding is important because delaying reintubation may increase the risk of death. In a subgroup analysis, prophylactic NIV reduced the risk of extubation failure compared to COT only in high-risk patients (OR 0.50, 95% CI 0.33–0.75; $p < 0.001$). In low-risk patients and postoperative ICU patients, prophylactic NIV did not reduce the incidence of extubation failure compared with COT [7].

The routine use of prophylactic NIV in postoperative patients remains uncertain. Lockstone et al. [26] included 17 studies with 6108 patients in a meta-analysis and found no significant benefit of NIV/CPAP in reducing postoperative pulmonary complications after upper abdominal surgery (RR 0.89, 95% CI 0.78–1.01; very low certainty), including in adults identified as being at higher risk of postoperative pulmonary complications (RR 0.91, 95% CI 0.77–1.07; very low certainty) [26]. In patients undergoing cardiac surgery, the use of NIV or CPAP reduced the length of ICU stay (MD −1 h, 95% CI −1.38 to −0.63 h; $p < 0.00001$) and hospital stay (MD −1 d, 95% CI −1.12 to −0.87 d; $p < 0.00001$). However, the clinical significance of these results is questionable. Furthermore, NIV or CPAP did not reduce the risk of atelectasis, pneumonia, cardiac complications, or reintubation rate [27]. It is important to emphasize that there was great variability in the use of NIV in the studies included in this review.

Another strategy that has recently been investigated to prevent extubation failure is HFNC. In addition, the use of NIV interspersed with HFNC has been widely used to increase patient tolerance to therapy, as HFNC tends to be better tolerated by patients. Thille et al. [28] conducted a clinical trial comparing a group receiving HNFC alone (control group) and a group receiving NIV interspersed with HNFC (intervention group). The control group received continuous HNFC alone for at least 48 h. The intervention group received NIV immediately after extubation with an initial session of at least 4 h and a minimum of 12 h per day during the 48 h following extubation. HNFC was administered between NIV sessions as in the control group. The reintubation rate at day 7 was lower in the NIV group (absolute difference −6.4%, 95% CI −12.0 to −0.9; $p = 0.02$). In addition, the proportion of patients with post-extubation respiratory failure at day 7 was significantly lower with NIV (absolute difference −8.7%, 95% CI −15.2% to −1.8%; $p = 0.01$). There were no differences in hospital or ICU mortality between the groups.

Recently, Thille et al. [29] performed a post-hoc analysis of these data, isolating a subgroup of obese and overweight patients. In this group, reintubation rates at day 7 (absolute difference −13% CI 95% −19 to −6; $p = 0.0002$) and ICU mortality (absolute difference −6% CI95% −11 to −2; $p = 0.006$) were significantly lower in the group receiving NIV alternating with HFNC than in the group receiving HFNC alone. There is insufficient evidence to support the routine use of prophylactic NIV in obese or overweight patients, but the results of this study demonstrate that this may be a population that should be considered for use to prevent extubation failure.

9.4 The Use and Indication of HFNC Post-extubation

Oxygen therapy is typically delivered via low-flow systems (e.g., nasal cannula or masks) or high-flow systems (e.g., venturi masks or non-rebreathers). HFNC is a method of noninvasive respiratory support that delivers heated, humidified oxygen at a FiO_2 of 0.21–1.0 and a flow rate of up to 60 L/min [30]. HFNC devices typically include a heated humidifier, a flow generator, a single-limb heated circuit, and a nasal cannula [31]. Humidification increases the mucosal water content, which moistens the airways and prevents the epithelial damage associated with airway desiccation [32]. In addition, the HFNC assists in the removal of secretions, potentially reducing the work of breathing [30].

The differences between NIV and HFNC lie in the interfaces as well as the constant pressure versus the ability to deliver different inspiratory and expiratory pressures [31]. Compared to NIV, HFNC interfaces reduce dead space [33] and have a good acceptance and tolerability due to their soft and pliable nasal prongs [30]. HFNC does not increase tidal volume but improves alveolar ventilation by washing out anatomical dead space [33].

HFNC has been increasingly studied as a strategy to prevent extubation failure, and its physiological effects are beginning to be better understood [34]. A randomized crossover study showed that HFNC resulted in significantly lower work of breathing, slightly higher oxygenation (pO_2/FiO_2 ratio), and increased end-expiratory lung volume compared to COT. On the other hand, there seems to be no differences in the tidal volume, pCO_2, hemodynamics, and cardiovascular stress biomarkers when HFNC is compared with standard oxygen [34].

9.4.1 HFNC Versus *COT*

The ERS guidelines [35] suggest HFNC over COT in nonsurgical patients after extubation at low or moderate risk of extubation failure, with low certainty of evidence. HFNC compared with COT probably reduces the rate of reintubation (RR 0.62, 95% CI 0.38–1.01; risk difference −5.1%, 95% CI −8.2% to 0.1%; moderate certainty) and the need for escalation to NIV (RR 0.38, 95% CI 0.17–0.85; risk difference −9.4%, 95% CI −12.5% to −2.3%; moderate certainty) for ICU patients. HFNC is associated with a small improvement in comfort (SMD 0.77 SD, 95% CI 0.03 SD to 1.5 SD; high certainty) and reduction of respiratory rate (MD −1.98 bpm, 95% CI −3.9 to −0.06 bpm; high certainty). However, there are no differences in mortality, length of ICU and hospital stay, and gas exchange (pO_2 and pCO_2 levels).

In postoperative patients at low risk of respiratory complications, ERS guidelines [35] suggest either COT or HFNC, with low certainty of evidence. The use of HFNC results in a smaller reduction in the risk of reintubation (RR 0.66, 95% CI 0.23–1.91;

risk difference −1.2, 95% CI −2.8 to 3.3; low certainty) and an uncertain reduction in the risk of escalation to NIV (RR 0.77, 95% CI 0.42–1.40; risk difference −2.6, −6.8 to 4.7; very low certainty). HFNC probably has little or no effect on mortality (RR 0.64, 95% CI 0.19–2.14; risk difference −0.5%, 95% CI −1.1% to 1.5%; moderate certainty). It also has a small effect on the length of ICU and hospital stay (high certainty of evidence). On the other hand, HFNC may result in a higher pO_2/FiO_2 ratio (MD 34.89 mmHg, 95% CI −15.19 mmHg to 84.96 mmHg; moderate certainty) and pO_2 values (MD 6.2 mmHg, 95%CI 3.58 mmHg to 8.28 mmHg; high certainty).

9.4.2 HFNC Versus *NIV*

In patients at very high risk of extubation failure, evidence from ERS guidelines [35] suggest the use of NIV over HFNC unless there are relative or absolute contraindications to NIV (moderate certainty of evidence). Compared with NIV, HFNC increases the rate of reintubation (RR 1.31, 95% CI 1.04–1.64; risk difference 4.4%, 95% CI 0.6%–9.2%; high certainty), with little effect on mortality (RR 1.07, 95% CI 0.84–1.36; risk difference 1.0%, 95% CI −2.3% to 5.1%; moderate certainty). Despite this, HFNC is associated with slightly shorter ICU stay (MD -1.0 day, 95% CI -1.52 to −0.47 days) and hospital stay (MD −1.44 days, 95% CI −2.63 to −0.25 days), with high certainty of evidence. No differences were observed for respiratory rate and gas exchange.

In patients with acute exacerbations of COPD, a meta-analysis of eight studies showed no statistically significant difference in reintubation rate and ICU length of stay between the HFNC group and the NIV group [36]. Compared with NIV, HFNC could significantly reduce the complications in post-extubation patients, mainly nasal-facial skin breakdown, aspiration, and flatulence. However, in the non-hypercapnic patients, the reintubation rate was significantly higher in the HFNC group (RR 2.61, 95% CI 1.41–4.83), indicating that the treatment effect was not as good as in the NIV group [36].

For postoperative patients at high risk of respiratory complications, ERS guidelines [35] suggest the use of either HFNC or NIV. HFNC results in a small increase in mortality (RR 1.22, 95% CI 0.72–2.09; risk difference 1.2%, 95% CI −1.5% to 6.0%; low certainty), with probably little to no difference in reintubation (RR 1.02, 95% CI 0.73 to 1.44; risk difference 0.3%, 95%CI −3.7% to 6.0%; moderate certainty). In addition, compared with NIV, HFNC had little or no difference in ICU and hospital length of stay, respiratory rate, and pCO_2 values. Despite this, NIV patients had more skin breakdown at 24 h than HFNC patients.

9.4.3 Predict the Success of HFNC After Planned Extubation

In recent years, the respiratory rate-oxygenation (ROX) index, defined as SpO_2/FiO_2/respiratory rate, has been proposed to predict the outcome of HFNC in pneumonia patients with acute hypoxemic respiratory failure [37]. The effectiveness of the ROX index was also evaluated to predict success or failure after planned extubation [38]. In this setting, the ROX index proved to be a more accurate predictor of success than the other respiratory variables (AUC > 0.7). Particularly, the ROX index at 12 h of HFNC showed greater accuracy in predicting success or failure (AUC = 0.729), with 10.4 as the optimal cut-off value [38].

Furthermore, low ROX index, male sex, low body mass index, and long total MV duration were significant predictors of reintubation within 72 h [38]. Thus, it is suggested that an integrated model including these variables could be used to predict HFNC success within 72 h after extubation.

9.5 Conclusions

In well-selected critically ill patients, NIV can be used to facilitate weaning from MV and to prevent and treat post-extubation respiratory failure, with the potential to improve clinically relevant outcomes. However, there is no evidence to support its indiscriminate use in all mechanically ventilated patients. Therefore, it is essential that the criteria for indication of this therapy in the ICU are well established. Regarding the use of HFNC, there is no evidence to support its use over NIV. There is some evidence that this therapy may be superior to COT in high-risk patients. In these patients, HFNC may be considered if there is a contraindication to the use of NIV or if the patient is intolerant.

References

1. Thille AW, Boissier F, Ben-Ghezala H, et al. Easily identified at-risk patients for extubation failure may benefit from noninvasive ventilation: a prospective before-after study. Crit Care. 2016;20:48.
2. Singh L. Role of prophylactic noninvasive ventilation in patients at high risk of extubation failure. Indian J Crit Care Med. 2020;24:1158–60.
3. Jaber S, Chanques G, Jung B. Postoperative noninvasive ventilation. Anesthesiology. 2010;112:453–61.

4. Ferreyra G, Fanelli V, Del Sorbo L, et al. Are guidelines for non-invasive ventilation during weaning still valid? Minerva Anestesiol. 2011;77:921–6.
5. Vaschetto R, Longhini F, Persona P, et al. Early extubation followed by immediate noninvasive ventilation vs. standard extubation in hypoxemic patients: a randomized clinical trial. Intensive Care Med. 2019;45:62–71.
6. Ouellette DR, Patel S, Girard TD, et al. Liberation from mechanical ventilation in critically ill adults: an official American College of Chest Physicians/American Thoracic Society clinical practice guideline: inspiratory pressure augmentation during spontaneous breathing trials, protocols minimizing sedation, and noninvasive ventilation immediately after extubation. Chest. 2017;151:166–80.
7. Boscolo A, Pettenuzzo T, Sella N, et al. Noninvasive respiratory support after extubation: a systematic review and network meta-analysis. Eur Respir Rev. 2023;32:220196.
8. Burns KEA, Stevenson J, Laird M, et al. Non-invasive ventilation versus invasive weaning in critically ill adults: a systematic review and meta-analysis. Thorax. 2022;77:752–61.
9. Pettenuzzo T, Boscolo A, Pistollato E, et al. Effects of non-invasive respiratory support in postoperative patients: a systematic review and network meta-analysis. Crit Care. 2024;28:152.
10. Rochwerg B, Brochard L, Elliott MW, et al. Official ERS/ATS clinical practice guidelines: noninvasive ventilation for acute respiratory failure. Eur Respir J. 2017;50:1602426.
11. Vaschetto R, Pecere A, Perkins GD, et al. Effects of early extubation followed by noninvasive ventilation versus standard extubation on the duration of invasive mechanical ventilation in hypoxemic non-hypercapnic patients: a systematic review and individual patient data meta-analysis of randomized controlled trials. Crit Care. 2021;25:189.
12. Perkins GD, Mistry D, Gates S, et al. Effect of protocolized weaning with early extubation to noninvasive ventilation vs invasive weaning on time to liberation from mechanical ventilation among patients with respiratory failure: the breathe randomized clinical trial. JAMA. 2018;320:1881–8.
13. Cammarota G, Vaschetto R, Azzolina D, et al. Early extubation with immediate non-invasive ventilation versus standard weaning in intubated patients for coronavirus disease 2019: a retrospective multicenter study. Sci Rep. 2021;11:13418.
14. Nava S, Hill N. Non-invasive ventilation in acute respiratory failure. Lancet. 2009;374:250–9.
15. Warner DO. Preventing postoperative pulmonary complications: the role of the anesthesiologist. Anesthesiology. 2000;92:1467–72.
16. Barbas CS, Isola AM, Farias AM, et al. Brazilian recommendations of mechanical ventilation 2013. Part I Rev Bras Ter Intensiva. 2014;26:89–121.
17. Thille AW, Monseau G, Coudroy R, et al. Non-invasive ventilation versus high-flow nasal oxygen for postextubation respiratory failure in ICU: a post-hoc analysis of a randomized clinical trial. Crit Care. 2021;25:221.
18. Esteban A, Frutos-Vivar F, Ferguson ND, et al. Noninvasive positive-pressure ventilation for respiratory failure after extubation. N Engl J Med. 2004;350:2452–60.
19. Kacmarek RM. Noninvasive respiratory support for postextubation respiratory failure. Respir Care. 2019;64:658–78.
20. Curtis JR, Cook DJ, Sinuff T, et al. Noninvasive positive pressure ventilation in critical and palliative care settings: understanding the goals of therapy. Crit Care Med. 2007;35:932–9.
21. Ferrer M, Sellares J, Valencia M, et al. Non-invasive ventilation after extubation in hypercapnic patients with chronic respiratory disorders: randomised controlled trial. Lancet. 2009;374:1082–8.
22. Ferrer M, Valencia M, Nicolas JM, et al. Early noninvasive ventilation averts extubation failure in patients at risk: a randomized trial. Am J Respir Crit Care Med. 2006;173:164–70.
23. Glossop AJ, Shephard N, Bryden DC, et al. Non-invasive ventilation for weaning, avoiding reintubation after extubation and in the postoperative period: a meta-analysis. Br J Anaesth. 2012;109:305–14.
24. Liang GP, Zeng YH, Chen BX, et al. Prophylactic noninvasive positive pressure ventilation in the weaning of difficult-weaning tracheotomy patients. Ann Transl Med. 2020;8:300.

25. Ou J, Chen H, Li L, et al. The role of non-invasive ventilation used immediately after planned extubation for adults with chronic respiratory disorders. Saudi Med J. 2018;39:131–6.
26. Lockstone J, Denehy L, Truong D, et al. Prophylactic postoperative noninvasive ventilation in adults undergoing upper abdominal surgery: a systematic review and meta-analysis. Crit Care Med. 2022;50:1522–32.
27. Wu Q, Xiang G, Song J, et al. Effects of non-invasive ventilation in subjects undergoing cardiac surgery on length of hospital stay and cardiac-pulmonary complications: a systematic review and meta-analysis. J Thorac Dis. 2020;12:1507–19.
28. Thille AW, Muller G, Gacouin A, et al. Effect of postextubation high-flow nasal oxygen with noninvasive ventilation vs high-flow nasal oxygen alone on reintubation among patients at high risk of Extubation failure: a randomized clinical trial. JAMA. 2019;322:1465–75.
29. Thille AW, Coudroy R, Nay MA, et al. Beneficial effects of noninvasive ventilation after extubation in obese or overweight patients: a post hoc analysis of a randomized clinical trial. Am J Respir Crit Care Med. 2022;205:440–9.
30. Park S. High-flow nasal cannula for respiratory failure in adult patients. Acute Crit Care. 2021;36:275–85.
31. Nishimura M. High-flow nasal cannula oxygen therapy devices. Respir Care. 2019;64:735–42.
32. Williams R, Rankin N, Smith T, et al. Relationship between the humidity and temperature of inspired gas and the function of the airway mucosa. Crit Care Med. 1996;24:1920–9.
33. Moller W, Feng S, Domanski U, et al. Nasal high flow reduces dead space. J Appl Physiol (1985). 2017;122:191–7.
34. Basoalto R, Damiani LF, Jalil Y, et al. Physiological effects of high-flow nasal cannula oxygen therapy after extubation: a randomized crossover study. Ann Intensive Care. 2023;13:104.
35. Oczkowski S, Ergan B, Bos L, et al. ERS clinical practice guidelines: high-flow nasal cannula in acute respiratory failure. Eur Respir J. 2022;59:2101574.
36. Feng Z, Zhang L, Yu H, et al. High-flow nasal cannula oxygen therapy versus non-invasive ventilation for AECOPD patients after extubation: a systematic review and meta-analysis of randomized controlled trials. Int J Chron Obstruct Pulmon Dis. 2022;17:1987–99.
37. Roca O, Messika J, Caralt B, et al. Predicting success of high-flow nasal cannula in pneumonia patients with hypoxemic respiratory failure: the utility of the ROX index. J Crit Care. 2016;35:200–5.
38. Lee YS, Chang SW, Sim JK, et al. An integrated model including the ROX index to predict the success of high-flow nasal cannula use after planned extubation: a retrospective observational cohort study. J Clin Med. 2021;10

Chapter 10
Ultrasound and Weaning

Marcelo Azeredo Terra and Michele Vaz Pinheiro Canena

10.1 The Pulmonary Ultrasound During Weaning

Ventilatory weaning is characterized by the gradual reduction of ventilatory support as the cause of respiratory failure improves. This process is complex and continuous and requires several criteria to assess the potential progress of weaning. Weaning success is determined by the absence of ventilatory support for 48 h after extubation [1]. Several factors may be associated with failure to wean, one of the most important being a delay in initiating weaning. This delay in weaning may be due to a lack of understanding of current practices for managing weaning from invasive ventilation [2].

Early weaning can lead to better patient outcomes, reduce the risk of complications such as infection and muscle weakness, shorten the length of hospital stay, and reduce the likelihood of developing ventilator-induced lung injury [1]. Approximately 30% of mechanically ventilated patients fail weaning, and the weaning process accounts for 42% of the total duration of mechanical ventilation [3].

Therefore, early identification of the mechanisms that lead to ventilator weaning failure allows measures to be taken to minimize failure and promote safe removal of the ventilator prosthesis. Bedside ultrasound is a valuable tool for various aspects related to the weaning process, such as identifying changes in lung aeration, respiratory muscle function, airway patency, hemodynamic stability, and the effectiveness and monitoring of respiratory physiotherapy during this process in critically ill patients [4].

M. A. Terra (✉)
MTerra Education and Consultancy LTDA, Niterói, Rio de Janeiro, Brazil

M. V. P. Canena
Federal University of Rio Grande, Rio Grande, Rio Grande do Sul, Brazil

A. R. Baptistella et al. (eds.), *Weaning from Mechanical Ventilation*,
https://doi.org/10.1007/978-3-032-01145-9_10

Lung ultrasound can detect areas of lung collapse and infection, and help diagnose acute respiratory distress syndrome (ARDS). It also detects pulmonary edema, alveolar interstitial syndrome, and the presence of fluid and air between the pleura as in pneumothorax, as well as blood clots that can block pulmonary arteries and abnormalities caused by viruses such as COVID-19 [5].

Air is an obstacle to the transmission of the ultrasound wave, which for many years made it impractical to use this method to assess lung aeration. Recently, it has been observed that ultrasound imaging can more easily detect artifacts through which the ultrasound wave propagates; these artifacts correspond to soft tissues and organs rich in water, allowing the assessment of pathological lung and pleural conditions [6].

The methods, also known as ultrasound modes, commonly used to assess pleuro-pulmonary conditions are as follows: B-mode, commonly referred to as two-dimensional (2D), and M-mode (motion). B-mode serves as the main modality for performing ultrasound assessments at the beginning of the examination, known as glow mode, and through it, we identify the structures and possible alterations found in pathological processes. Similarly, M-mode is used to confirm the dynamic nature of anatomical structures over time, such as diaphragmatic mobility, inferior vena cava thickness variations, pleural sliding, and others. This is achieved by using a fixed line displayed on the ultrasound machine, with the examiner positioning the line at the site of interest, as shown in Fig. 10.1 [6].

Pleuro-pulmonary assessment is used in the weaning process to monitor pulmonary changes and possible pleural changes. The pleural line, a hyperechoic structure

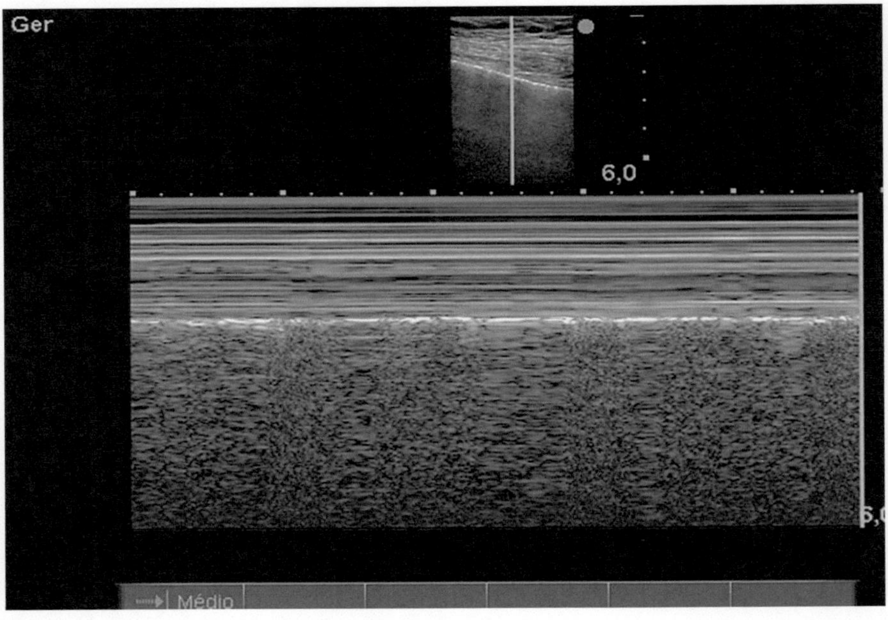

Fig. 10.1 Analysis of M-mode pleural slippage on ultrasound

corresponding to the junction of the parietal pleura, the visceral pleura, and the space between them, shows the A-lines when air is present in the lung field, signifying the reverberation of the pleural echo and indicating normal aeration of the lungs. The ribs create an acoustic shadow due to the reflection of the ultrasound waves when they hit the bone. As a result, a shadow called the rib acoustic shadow is visible below the rib. Between the two acoustic shadows of the ribs is the lung field where the pleural assessment is performed [6, 7]. The schematic representation of a normal lung field is shown in Fig. 10.2.

When the lung field is visualized in B-mode, the pleural line appears as a hyperechoic line; the same line can be visualized in M-mode along with respiratory motion. The absence of pleural sliding, which is promoted by air movement below the pleura, results in the generation of a distinct image in M-mode, referred to in the literature as a "barcode/stratosphere signal" (Fig. 10.3), indicating a lack of airflow in this specific area. Below the pleural line, an additional image pattern is observed that represents typical pleural motion in the lung field region, commonly known as the "beach sand sign" (Fig. 10.3B) [7].

After identifying the pleural line, a synchronous movement of inspiration and expiration is observed in correlation with the patient's respiratory cycle, where pleural sliding is observed. This sliding indicates that the surfaces of the parietal and visceral pleura are juxtaposed. Under normal circumstances, we observe the barcode sign above the pleura and the beach sand sign below the pleura in M-mode [6, 7]. Some image patterns can be identified in lung analysis and can identify dysfunction. Below, we describe the artifacts that are present in lung assessment.

A-lines

Repeating hyperechoic artifacts of the pleural line, they are identified below the pleural line and repeat at equal intervals. They are usually seen in healthy individuals. They represent normal aeration of the lungs and are generated by a physical

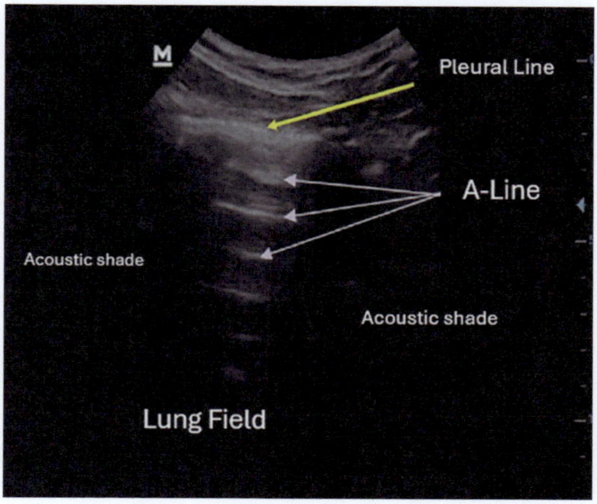

Fig. 10.2 Visualization of the lung field between two acoustic shadows of the ribs, identifying the pleural line (yellow arrow) and the A-lines (white arrows)

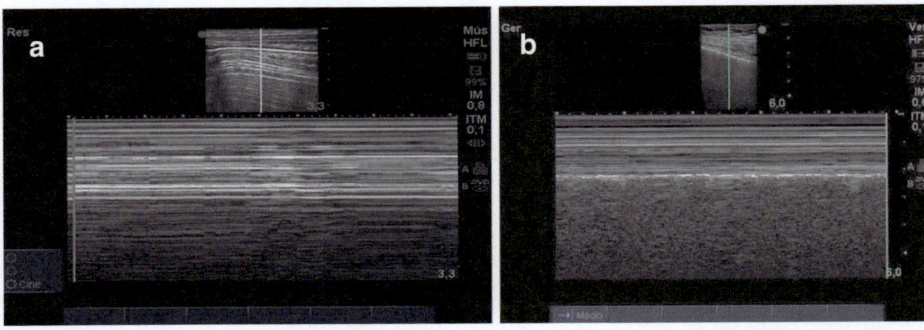

Fig. 10.3 (**a** and **b**) M-mode image of the barcode sign (**a**) and the beach sand sign (**b**)

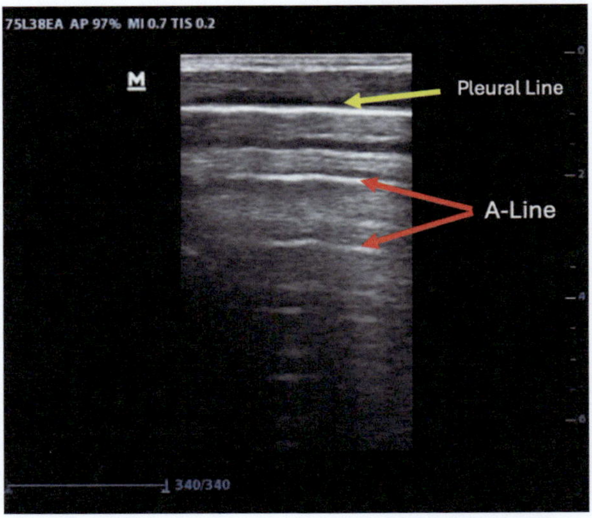

Fig. 10.4 Reverberation artifacts below the pleural line (yellow arrow), known as A-lines (red arrows)

phenomenon called pleural line reverberation, as shown in Fig. 10.4. When assessing the lung score, if pleural sliding and A-lines are seen in the assessed lung field, we score it as 0 [7, 8].

B-Lines

B-lines are categorized as B1-lines (distinct or separate) and B2-lines (merged or grouped), requiring different forms of identification when detected.

B1-lines are vertical lines that originate from the pleural line and extend toward the area of deepest visualization on the ultrasound screen (anteroposterior), resulting in a feature known as the "comet tail sign" (Fig. 10.5). The B1-line is produced by the mixing of air and fluid in the lung tissue and may represent thickening of the interlobular or intralobular septum. These B-lines move along the pleural line perpendicular to the pleura and erase the A-lines [6, 7]. When assessing the lung aeration score, if there are three or more B-lines in the assessed lung field, it is scored as 1 [8, 9].

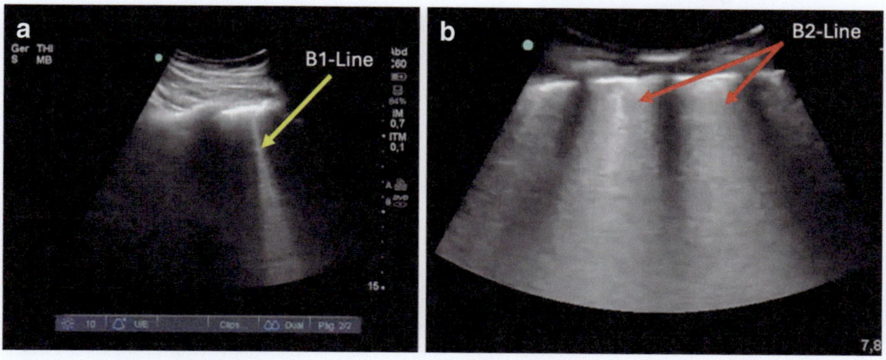

Figs. 10.5 (**a** and **b**) B-lines are categorized as B1-lines (distinct or separate—yellow arrow) and B2-lines (merged or grouped—red arrows) and require different forms of identification when detected

The B2-lines can be coalescent, i.e., grouped, if they are thicker than the B1-lines (greater than 3 mm) and form a kind of curtain on the ultrasound image, they also erase the A-lines [6, 7] (Fig. 10.5B). In this case, we can say that there is lung involvement in the interstitium and alveolus, which we call alveolar interstitial syndrome. This characteristic can accompany different pathologies and is represented on chest CT scans as "frosted glass," popularly known as "white lung," a pattern that became very well known during the pandemic because it was often seen in patients with COVID-19. The same pattern can be seen in patients with ARDS [6, 7]. In the evaluation of the lung aeration score, the evaluated lung field is scored as 2 [8, 9].

C-Lines

"Comet tail artifacts," also known as C-lines, are hyperechogenic lines seen subpleural, originating below the pleura in the context of a consolidated lung, with an absence of pleural line continuity (Fig. 10.6). These findings are indicative of lung consolidation processes that are usually seen in conditions such as pneumonia, for example, and result in a score of 3 on the Lung Aeration Score [8, 9].

Lung Consolidation

Lung consolidations are processes that cause the lung parenchyma to take on a liver-like appearance (hepatized lung). This occurs due to loss of aeration in the lung, resulting in lung collapse. This condition is usually infectious and replaces the normal air content with denser substances such as fluid, inflammatory cells, or exudates. Consolidations may be small and peripheral or larger and may present with dynamic air bronchograms, which appear as hyperechoic spots on ultrasound due to the presence of air in the bronchioles (Fig. 10.7). This condition results in complete loss of lung aeration. Therefore, if the assessed lung field is consolidated, it receives a score of 3 on the Lung Aeration Score [10].

Pulmonary Atelectasis

Atelectasis is the complete loss of aeration of part or all of the lung. A large pleural effusion can cause compressive atelectasis, while airway obstructions cause

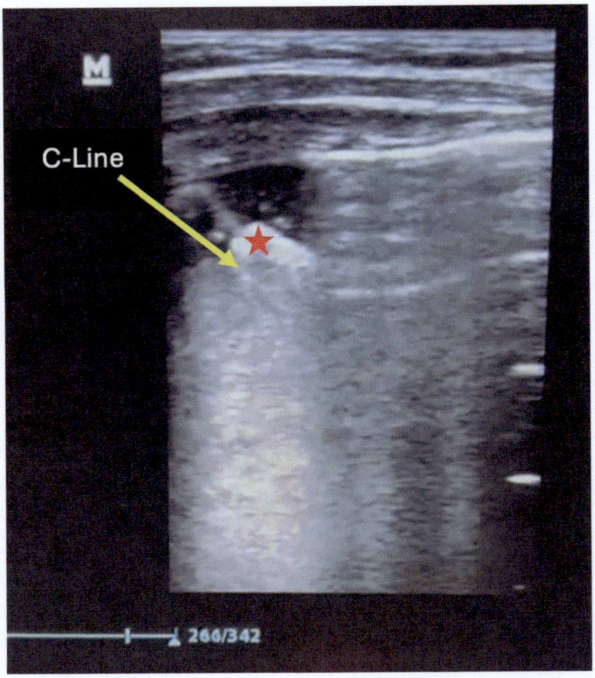

Fig. 10.6 C-lines are hyperechogenic lines seen subpleural (yellow arrow), originating below the pleural line in the context of a consolidated lung (red star)

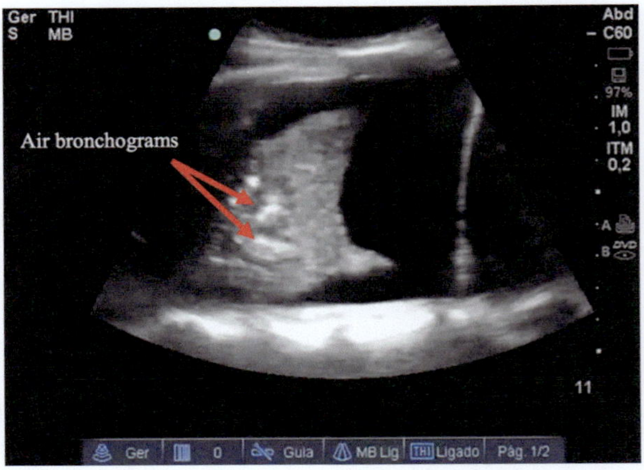

Fig. 10.7 Consolidations show dynamic air bronchograms, which on ultrasound appear as hyperechoic spots (red arrows) due to the presence of air in the bronchioles

obstructive atelectasis. They differ from consolidations in that they have static rather than dynamic air bronchograms, although a small proportion of atelectasis may have dynamic bronchograms. The lung tissue becomes hepatized and hypoechoic, indicating its collapse, as shown in Fig. 10.8. As with consolidations, if an atelectatic lung field is identified, it should be scored as 3 on the Lung Aeration Score, indicating a complete loss of aeration in that region [10].

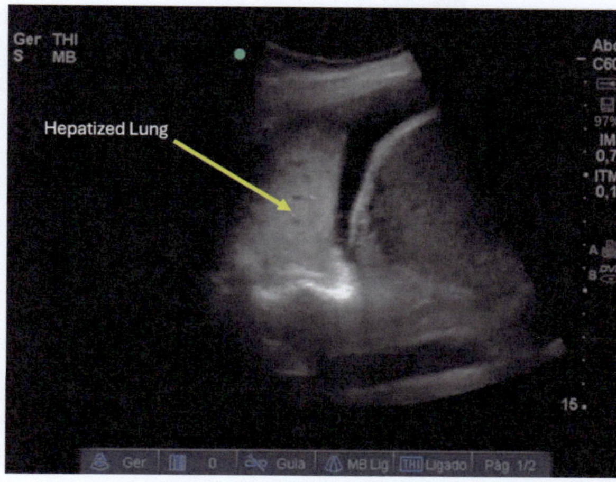

Fig. 10.8 The lung tissue becomes hepatized and hypoechoic (yellow arrow), indicating its collapse

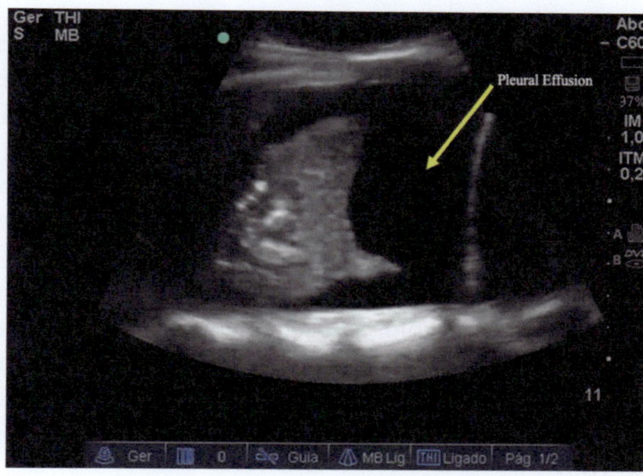

Fig. 10.9 Pleural effusion usually appears as an anechoic and homogeneous image

Pleural Effusion

Ultrasound has greater propagation through fluid media, making pleural effusion a pathologic condition that is readily identified with this assessment tool. Pleural effusion usually appears as an anechoic and homogeneous image if it is transudative, and in some cases as a hypoechoic and heterogeneous image, which is then referred to as a septate or trabeculated pleural effusion if it is exudative, as shown in Fig. 10.9.

Pneumothorax

Several criteria must be met to diagnose a pneumothorax. First, no pleural shift is observed during respiration because the gas in the pleural space prevents visualization of the shift of the underlying pleural line. Therefore, if no sliding is observed and it is out of sync with the phases of the patient's breathing, we should evaluate the following points. In this context, the physiological "beach sand sign" observed in M-mode is not seen and is replaced by the barcode sign above and below the pleural line (Fig. 10.10) [10].

The second criterion to look for is the absence of B-lines, because in pneumothorax we cannot see the pleural line, and because these lines emerge from the pleural line, they cannot be visualized. The third criterion is the presence of what we call the "pulmonary point," which is the transition between the normal aerated lung and the pneumothorax. The pulmonary point is pathognomonic for pneumothorax with a sensitivity of 66% and specificity of 100%, superior to radiography [10].

10.1.1 Protocols

In the ICU, pleuropulmonary assessment can be performed using two protocols, the BLUE (Beside Lung Ultrasound Emergency) protocol and the LUS (Lung Ultrasound Score) protocol, the latter of which has spawned several others with the same purpose but for different cases (LUSm, PLUE, CLUE, PINK, among others), as we will see below.

The BLUE protocol was developed specifically for rapid use in emergency situations involving patients with respiratory failure. The protocol involves the assessment of three different regions of the lung: the upper point, the lower point, and the lower lateral posterolateral point. To accurately perform this assessment, the patient should be placed in the supine position, and these designated areas of each hemithorax should be carefully examined with the examiner's hands placed on the patient's chest. The tops of the hands should be in contact with the clavicle (except for the thumbs) to ensure accurate location and delineation of the three standardized points. The upper BLUE point is located at the center of the upper hand, while the lower BLUE point is located at the center of the base of the palm. The lower lateral posterolateral point is determined by the intersection of a horizontal line drawn at the level of the lower BLUE point and a vertical line along the posterior axillary line [8, 10].

The BLUE protocol is designed to be performed in approximately 3 min to identify imaging patterns of lung structures such as normal, pulmonary edema, pneumonia, pulmonary embolism, pneumothorax, COPD, and asthma. It is a protocol that is widely used in emergency settings due to its efficacy in respiratory failure [8, 10].

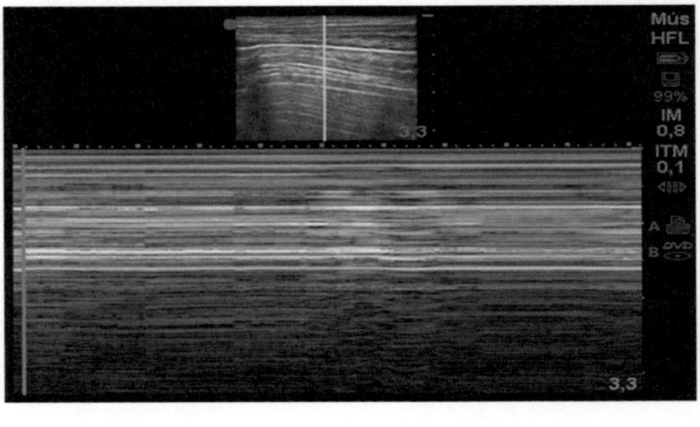

Fig. 10.10 (**a**) "Bar code sign" seen in the M-model of pneumothorax

Using this protocol, it is possible to profile patients when an association of signs is observed in a particular location and thus monitor the ventilatory weaning process. Any change in pulmonary ventilation that may interfere with the patient's progress toward weaning can be quickly and effectively identified using the BLUE protocol, which would prevent the patient from being extubated prematurely [11].

The second protocol is called the Lung Ultrasound Score (LUS) protocol. The LUS was derived from a study conducted by Soummer et al. [9], who evaluated the outcomes of patients undergoing mechanical ventilation following a pleuropulmonary ultrasound examination for ventilator weaning. Each of the 12 lung regions examined is evaluated based on its aeration, as shown in Fig. 10.11. A scoring system is proposed that assigns 0–3 points for each region (6 in each hemithorax), resulting in a total score of 0–36 points (Table 10.1) [9].

The use of the LUS protocol by healthcare professionals in the ICU seems to be of interest because this approach provides precise measurements of lung aeration levels, specifically related to lung diseases, so it can help to optimize the withdrawal of mechanical ventilation, facilitate the use of noninvasive ventilation, determine the need for bronchial hygiene, and evaluate in a quantitative way the positioning of the patient before and after the procedure.

The LUS protocol can also be performed in a focal manner (focal LUS). This is an analysis that eliminates the evaluation of the posterior regions bilaterally, so that a total of eight areas are evaluated, four in each hemithorax (Fig. 10.12). In this case, scores below 4–6 are associated with successful weaning from the ventilator [12]. Although this is a faster and more comprehensive analysis for patients who are unable to undergo further analysis, it must be remembered that the lack of analysis of dependent regions may lead to failure to identify dysfunction in these areas and compromise the diagnosis.

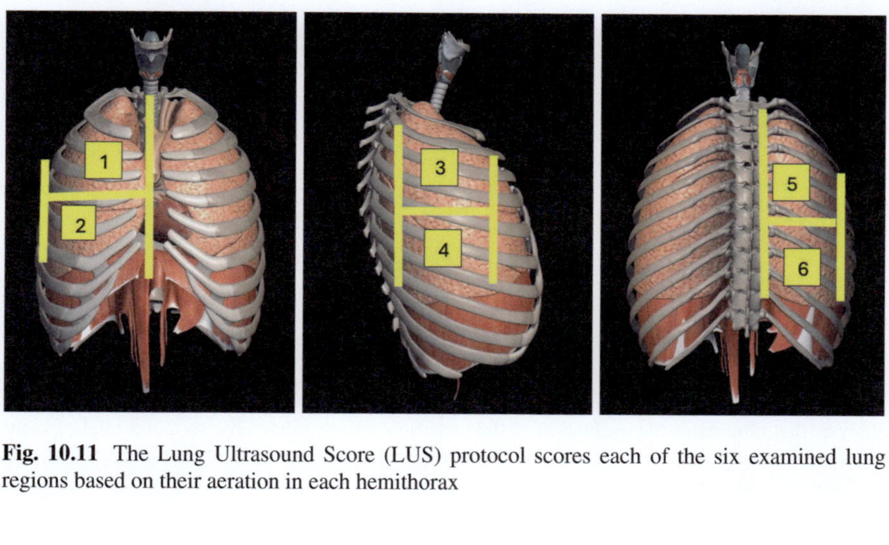

Fig. 10.11 The Lung Ultrasound Score (LUS) protocol scores each of the six examined lung regions based on their aeration in each hemithorax

Table 10.1 Modified Lung Ultrasound Score protocol (mLUSS)

Score system adopted distinguishes four patterns of lung aeration			
Profile A	**Presence of lines A and less than two isolated lines B**	0 point	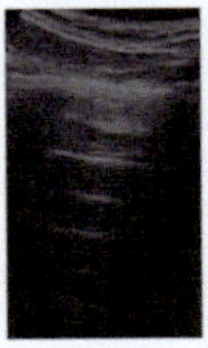
Profile B	**More than two lines B spaced and well defined**	1 point	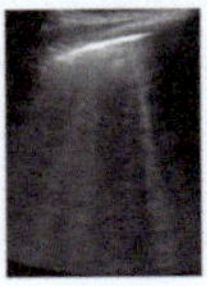
Profile B'	**Multiple coalescing lines B**	2 points	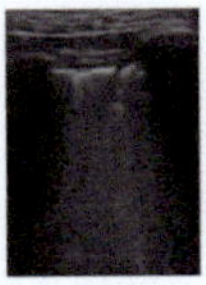
Profile C	**Presence of pulmonary consolidation**	3 points	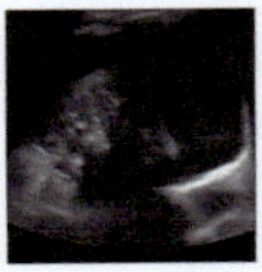

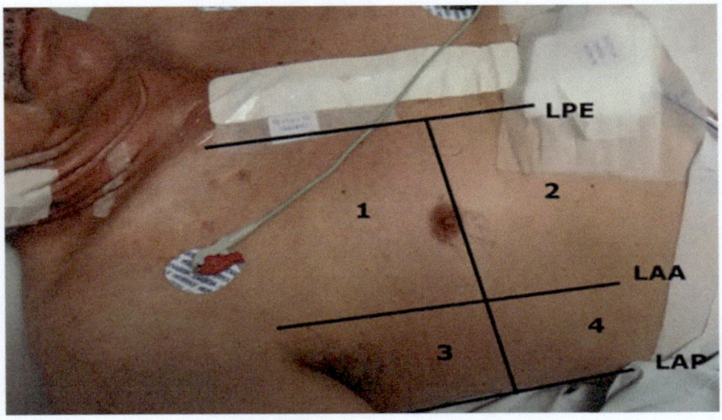

Fig. 10.12 The LUS protocol can also be performed in a focal manner (focal LUS). This is an analysis that eliminates the evaluation of the posterior regions bilaterally, so that a total of eight areas are evaluated, four in each hemithorax. *LPE* parasternal line, *LAA* anterior axillary line, and *LAP* posterior axillary line

The use of weaning protocols appears to reduce mechanical ventilation time and ICU length of stay compared to standard care. This reduction is due to the use of consistent and specific criteria to determine readiness for weaning and a targeted approach [13].

10.2 Diaphragmatic Ultrasound as a Tool for Predicting Weaning and Extubation Outcomes

As we have seen, remaining on a ventilator can increase patient morbidity and mortality. Ventilatory weaning depends on several factors and, most importantly, on effective supportive care. Therefore, identifying predictors of early weaning is a critical factor in the process of successfully weaning patients.

In this context, diaphragmatic analysis of these patients can help in the decision to wean by analyzing their dysfunction. By identifying diaphragm dysfunction, it is possible to monitor the patient and intervene early to reduce the complications associated with the length of stay on the mechanical ventilator [14].

Due to its complex structure and location, the diaphragm presents challenges in terms of direct assessment, especially in its entirety. Assessments of the diaphragm can take the form of static and/or dynamic examinations. Historically, assessments have relied heavily on radiographic methods, such as fluoroscopy, to measure the mobility of the diaphragm. Recent advances in diagnostics have shown that ultrasound has remarkable accuracy in examining lung artifacts and surrounding structures. Ultrasound of the diaphragm offers distinct advantages over alternative analytical approaches such as chest radiography, fluoroscopy, or tomography. This technique avoids radiation, is cost-effective, is noninvasive, and allows for immediate bedside application, complementing physical examination and clinical assessment with real-time dynamic muscle assessment [15, 16].

Alterations in diaphragmatic mobility are referred to as diaphragmatic dysfunction, which manifests as partial or complete loss of diaphragmatic contractility. Diaphragmatic dysfunction can also be manifested as paralysis or insufficiency and is categorized by the absence of one or both hemidiaphragms (Fig. 10.13). Most diaphragmatic changes are asymptomatic, and an abnormality in the position, shape, or configuration of the diaphragm may be discovered incidentally during a thoracic or abdominal examination performed for another clinical purpose [17, 18]. Thus, assessment of diaphragmatic mobility, thickness, muscle quality and strength, contractile velocity, and predictive indices can help guide decisions and progress in ventilator weaning [19].

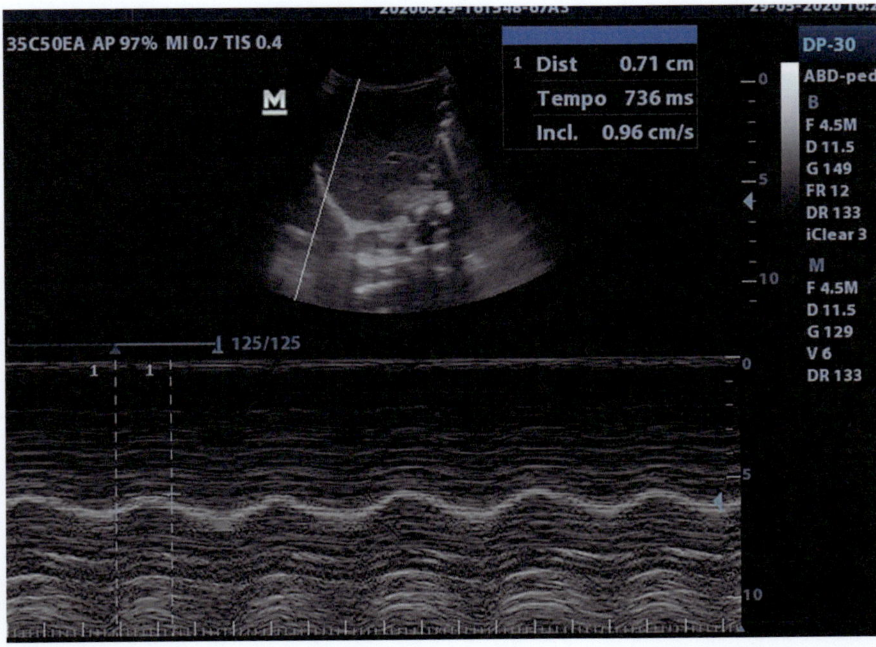

Fig. 10.13 Diaphragmatic mobility

10.2.1 Measuring Diaphragm Mobility

The measurement of descending diaphragmatic excursion (mobility), also known as diaphragmatic excursion (DE), is determined by the contraction velocity (DE/distance) / inspiratory time (cm/s) observed during the inspiratory ramp (Fig. 10.14). These ultrasound measurements are usually made with low-frequency transducers and greater depth to reach the tissue. The transducer used may be convex, curvilinear, or sectorial, and is positioned subcostal between the hemi-clavicular and axillary lines at an anterior and upward angle so that the ultrasound beam is perpendicular to the diaphragm. Patients may be supine, seated, or inclined at 30°–45° to facilitate observation of respiratory maneuvers at rest, during deep inspiration, and during sighing. Initially, B-mode is used to localize the muscle, followed by observation of its movement in M-mode ultrasound [20, 21].

Diaphragmatic mobility is positively correlated with inspiratory lung volumes, so we observed an increase in this measure during forced inspiration. When the patient is on mechanical ventilation, this measure may be affected, and the distinction between passive displacement due to ventilator driving pressures may not be clear [4]. Despite this, some studies to predict weaning from mechanical ventilation in ICU patients have found that DE has a sensitivity of 92% and a specificity of 100% with a cut-off greater than 1.1 cm [14].

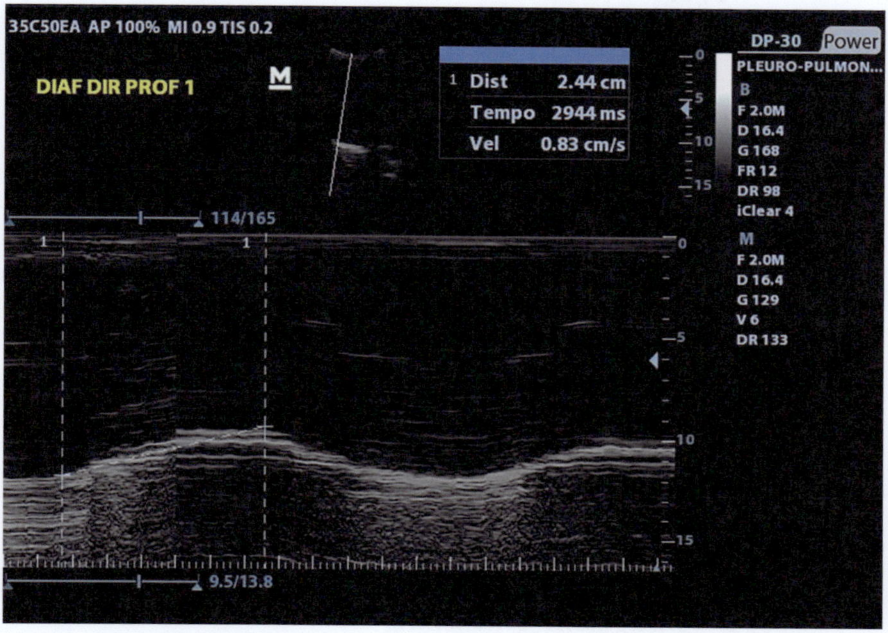

Fig. 10.14 The measurement of diaphragmatic excursion (DE) is determined by the contraction velocity (DE/distance)/inspiratory time (cm/s)

Reference values for diaphragmatic mobility have changed over the years and can vary depending on the type of analysis, the side analyzed, and the position. In the past, values of approximately 1.78 ± 0.58 cm at rest and 7.62 ± 1.44 at maximum inspiration have been observed in healthy individuals. Values greater than 1.0 cm in quiet breathing were considered normal for diaphragmatic mobility [21–23]. Currently, values of 2.32 ± 0.54 cm at rest and 5.54 ± 1.26 cm during deep breathing are observed, with values less than 1 cm characterizing diaphragmatic dysfunction [4]

Diaphragmatic motion changes in the supine, sitting, and standing positions and may show higher values, so it is important to determine positioning and technique for proper monitoring of patients. Values of 1.0–2.5 cm have been observed in healthy patients during quiet breathing bilaterally, with an average excursion of 3 cm and lower limits of 1.6 cm in females and 1.8 cm in males [24]. To predict successful extubation, values ≥1.0 cm are associated with success with a sensitivity of 69%–97.1% and a specificity of 62%–85%, DE < 1.0 cm can predict extubation failure with a lower sensitivity of 30%, but DE is generally lower in patients who fail extubation [25]. In elderly patients undergoing ventilator weaning, diaphragmatic mobility ≥1.3 cm was associated with better outcomes [26]. Diaphragmatic mobility appears to decrease with age, and mobility values of 0.9 cm in women and 1.0 cm in men during quiet breathing are within the normal range; during deep breathing, these values change to 3.7 in women and 4.7 in men over 65 years of age [27].

Pulmonary and diaphragmatic pathologies can cause alterations in diaphragmatic mobility and consequent impairment, as evidenced in individuals diagnosed with chronic obstructive pulmonary disease (COPD). In the COPD population, there appears to be a correlation between muscular dysfunction and pulmonary function decline, resulting in recorded measurements of approximately 1.58 ± 0.5 cm during quiet breathing periods and 4.58 ± 1.83 cm during deep inspiration in COPD patients classified in the moderate to severe spectrum. However, these findings have been controversial, with alternative studies reporting diaphragmatic mobility values of 3.62 ± 1.09 cm, 1.98 ± 0.75 cm according to Kang et al. [28], and 3.39 cm (20.8–51.6) according to Yamaguti et al. [29] in COPD patients during quiet breathing. In addition, changes in diaphragmatic mobility have been documented in cases of interstitial lung disease, with average measurements of approximately 4.5 ± 1.7 cm during quiet breathing and 7.6 ± 1.4 cm during deep breathing [30].

10.2.2 Thickness, Ratio, and Fraction of Diaphragmatic Thickening

Diaphragm thickness can be measured with the high-frequency rectilinear transducer in the diaphragmatic apposition zone, between the eighth and ninth intercostal spaces, and between the anterior axillary line and the midaxillary line. The B-mode is also used to locate the muscle and then follow its movement in the M-mode of the ultrasound; the thickness of the diaphragm can also be obtained in the B-mode. In both modes (B or M), thickness can be measured by the distance from the peritoneal line to the parietal pleura (hyperechoic lines) (Fig. 10.15) at rest, functional residual capacity (FRC), and total lung capacity (TLC) (Fig. 10.16A, B) [20, 21].

Diaphragm thickness measurements are used to identify diaphragm dysfunction by calculating the diaphragm thickness fraction (DTF): thickness at TLC (end of inspiration) − thickness at FRC (end of expiration) × 100 [20, 21].

Thickening fraction measurements appear to correlate with the assessment of respiratory effort using the Respiratory Effort Assessment Index (P01) and with the assessment of maximum inspiratory pressure (MPI), and thus may be an indicator of the need to discontinue ventilatory support. A thickening fraction between 15% and 30% during mechanical ventilation may be associated with stable thickness and a reduction in mechanical ventilation time, <20% are values associated with diaphragmatic dysfunction, and values >40% may indicate increased respiratory effort [31, 32].

Currently, DTF measurements above 29% in weaning patients indicate a high probability of success, without forgetting that the measurement can be influenced by the patient's condition, such as nutritional status, respiratory, cardiovascular, and

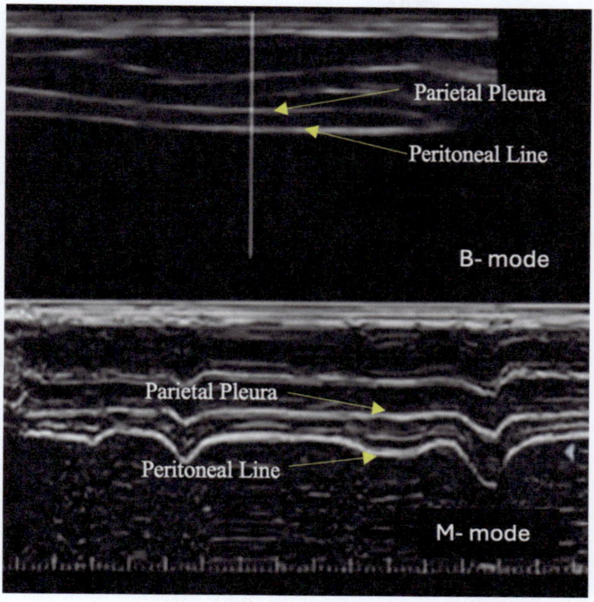

Fig. 10.15 Diaphragm thickness is measured by the distance from the peritoneal line to the parietal pleura in B-mode and M-mode

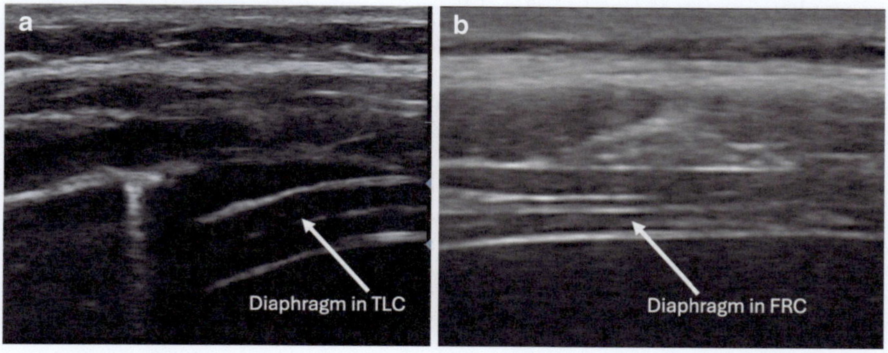

Fig. 10.16 (**a** and **b**) Diaphragm thickness measured in total lung capacity (TLC) (Fig. 10.16A) and functional residual capacity (FRC) (Fig. 10.16B)

psychological status [33]. Diaphragmatic dysfunction detected by DTF has values of less than 20%–30% [4]. In elderly patients undergoing ventilatory weaning, those who successfully extubated had a higher DTF than those who failed, and the cut-off for successful weaning was a DTF ≥30% [26].

Diaphragm thickness measurements may reflect the patient's ability to breathe unassisted and the risk of prolonged mechanical ventilation, length of ICU stay, and poor prognosis. These factors also reflect the potential impact of diaphragmatic myotrauma [31]. Prevention of diaphragmatic myotrauma during mechanical ventilation is a priority with the potential to significantly improve the prognosis of critically ill patients [32].

Techniques to assess diaphragmatic echo density provide information on muscle quality, and measurement of the thickening fraction can predict the outcome of weaning in a spontaneous breathing trial, reflecting diaphragmatic action; ultrasound can also help detect muscle weakness (HealthManagement.org).

Muscle strength can also be assessed using an analysis called thickening ratio, which corresponds to inspiratory thickening (total lung capacity—TLC) /expiratory thickening (functional residual capacity—FRC), with values >2.0 representing adequate muscle strength and values <2.0 representing muscle weakness [34, 35].

10.2.3 Diaphragmatic Index of Rapid Shallow Respiration (D-IRSS)

Prolonged dependence on the mechanical ventilator leads to diaphragmatic injury and worse outcomes. The Rapid Shallow Breathing Index (RSBI) is commonly used to analyze and guide weaning of critically ill patients. Using ultrasound, it is possible to perform the diaphragmatic rapid shallow breathing index (D-RSBI), which has a positive correlation with the RSBI, but with greater diagnostic accuracy [36].

The D-RSBI is equal to respiratory rate/diaphragmatic mobility and is expressed in breaths/min/mm. Values less than 1.7 for weaning patients and 1.9 for weaning COPD patients have been associated with successful weaning [37, 38]. Recently, a value of 1.24 ± 0.37 was found to be associated with successful weaning and 2.69 ± 0.98 with failure [36]. This index can also be expressed in breath/min/l, in which case values around 34.8 (23.7, 54.5) are associated with successful ventilatory weaning and values of 43.4 (33.1, 68.8) with failure [39].

10.2.4 Diaphragm Assessment Using Elastography

The immobilization time of critically ill patients exposed to mechanical ventilation can play a significant role in muscle structure and function, leading to weakness and, in more severe cases, paralysis. Techniques that allow assessment of muscle quality can assist in the weaning process of these patients [40].

Elastography allows the assessment of muscle elasticity and stiffness and tracks diaphragmatic muscle changes in the ICU. This analysis is based on the principle that each tissue has a specific elasticity, where ultrasound waves can measure this elasticity and/or stiffness in comparison to healthy tissue [40–42].

There are several forms of elastography assessment, including shear waves, transient waves, and acoustic radiation force, as well as the widely used compression or deformation technique. In this approach, real-time compression is performed by the ultrasound transducer to induce deformation, followed by an assessment of muscle quality before and after compression using a color-coded scale. The color schemes are predetermined on the ultrasound device, with red typically indicating more elastic tissue and blue representing firmer tissue [42, 43].

In the shear technique for diaphragm analysis, the higher the shear modulus, the greater the tissue stiffness. This physiological change in the diaphragmatic muscles may reflect damage such as fibrosis. Furthermore, this technique seems to correlate with the analysis of mean trans-diaphragmatic pressure, so it could be a technique to analyze diaphragmatic effort and help in the weaning process of critically ill patients [4].

10.2.5 Expiratory Muscles in the Weaning Process from Mechanical Ventilation

Ultrasound is useful in assessing the morphology, functionality, and performance of abdominal muscles in patients undergoing mechanical ventilation. Ultrasound assessment of abdominal muscle thickening in mechanically ventilated patients provides valuable information about abdominal muscle status, functionality, and weaning outcomes. Using a 10–15 MHz linear probe placed perpendicular to the abdominal wall with the patient in the supine position, it is quite possible to observe the expiratory muscles as hypoechoic layers surrounded by fascial sheaths. It is critical to apply minimal pressure with the probe to avoid distortion of the shape or thickness of the underlying muscles due to abdominal wall compression [19, 44].

The transducer is positioned in a transverse orientation approximately 2–3 cm above the umbilicus and 2–3 cm lateral to the midline to visualize the abdominal muscle. Maximum muscle thickness is obtained by moving the probe in a craniocaudal direction while maintaining it perpendicular to the skin. The semilunar line is first identified as a thick echogenic fascia that merges laterally with the rectus abdominis muscle and medially with the oblique muscles (Fig. 10.17). The external oblique, internal oblique, and transverse abdominal muscles can be identified as three parallel layers that are usually best visualized in the anterior axillary line, midway between the inferior border of the rib cage and the iliac crest. The reference values are 26.5 ± 8.0 (dominant side) and 26.0 ± 8.2 (nondominant side), men: 31.7 ± 6.3 and women: 20.0 ± 3.8 [19, 44].

The thickening fraction of the expiratory abdominal muscles (TFadb) can be quantified as the extent of the increase in thickness observed during expiration (TFadb = (end-expiratory thickness − end-inspiratory thickness) / end-inspiratory thickness × 100%) and may indicate the level of effort exerted by the expiratory muscles. Initial results suggest a reasonable relationship between TFadb and expiratory force production. It is important to note that the expiratory muscles have greater degrees of freedom compared to the diaphragm; active contraction of one muscle layer may directly influence the contraction and positioning of the adjacent layer, adding complexity to the interpretation of TFadb. Furthermore, the relationship between contraction, thickening, and pressure generation in abdominal muscles is

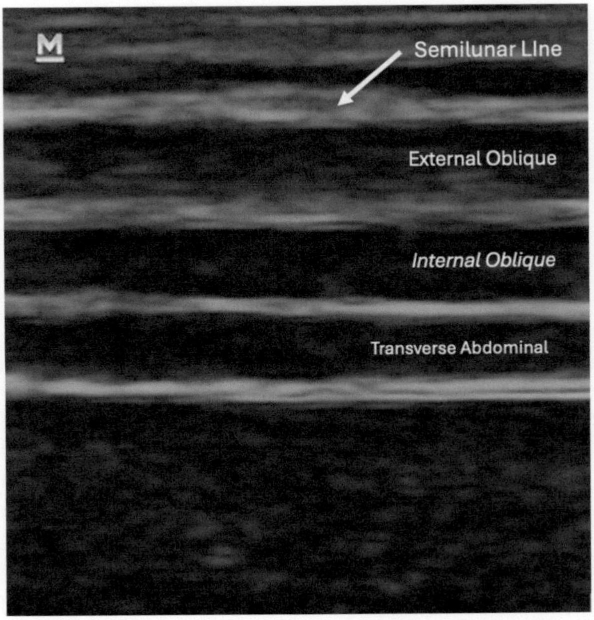

Fig. 10.17 The semilunar line is a thick echogenic fascia that merges laterally with the rectus abdominis muscle and medially with the oblique muscles. The external oblique, internal oblique, and transverse abdominal muscles can be identified as three parallel layers

complicated by their geometry during contraction. Subsequent research efforts should validate the relationship between expiratory muscle pressure and TFdb, along with its clinical significance [19, 44].

In healthy individuals, there is a positive correlation between the percentage of thickening of the internal oblique and rectus abdominis muscles and the pressure exerted during expiratory effort. In patients undergoing mechanical ventilation, it is possible to check muscle thickness and measure the thickening fraction of the abdominal muscles. This data can help in the process of weaning patients off the ventilator, as it shows an association between increased thickening in situations where the spontaneous ventilation test fails and during coughing, which is associated with an increased risk of reintubation or reconnection to the mechanical ventilator in these patients [44].

In the gradual process of ventilator weaning, ultrasound is an indispensable tool. This is a complicated process that must be accurately assessed to determine the point of continuity and progression. Analysis of factors such as lung aeration, areas of collapse, presence of fluid, and decreased diaphragm muscle strength and mobility is facilitated by the use of lung and diaphragm ultrasound. Both static and dynamic ultrasound measurements are possible, and over time, standards and protocols have been established for each pathologic condition. At the patient's bedside, ultrasound can now provide accurate, continuous assessment and monitoring, and quantification of physiologic changes. Early detection of the mechanisms causing ventilator weaning failure allows implementation of strategies to reduce failure and promote safe weaning.

References

1. Akella P, Voigt LP, Chawla S. To wean or not to wean: a practical patient focused guide to ventilator weaning. J Intensive Care Med. 2022;37:1417–25. https://doi.org/10.1177/08850666221095436.
2. Jaber S, De Jong A. Weaning from mechanical ventilation in intensive care units: a call for new international consensus guidelines. Lancet Respir Med. 2023;11:398–400. https://doi.org/10.1016/s2213-2600(22)00502-1.
3. Fadila M, Rajasurya V, Regunath H. Ventilator weaning. In: StatPearls [Internet]. Treasure Island: StatPearls Publishing; 2024.
4. Al-Husinat L, Jouryyeh B, Rawashdeh A, Robba C, Silva PL, Rocco PRM, Battaglini D. The role of ultrasonography in the process of weaning from mechanical ventilation in critically ill patients. Diagnostics. 2024;14:398. https://doi.org/10.3390/diagnostics14040398.
5. Zapata L, Blancas R, Conejo-Márquez I, García-De-Acilu M. Papel de la ecografía en la insuficiencia respiratoria aguda y en el weaning de la ventilación mecánica. Med Intensiva. 2023;47:529–42. https://doi.org/10.1016/j.medin.2023.03.009.
6. Leech M, Bissett B, Kot M, Ntoumenopoulos G. Lung ultrasound for critical care physiotherapists: a narrative review. Physiother Res Int. 2014;20:69–76. https://doi.org/10.1002/pri.1607.
7. Le Neindre A, Mongodi S, Philippart F, Bouhemad B. Thoracic ultrasound: Potential new tool for physiotherapists in respiratory management. A narrative review. J Crit Care. 2016;31(1):101–09. https://doi.org/10.1016/j.jcrc.2015.10.014.
8. Lichtenstein DA. Lung ultrasound in the critically ill. Ann Intensive Care. 2014;4:1. https://doi.org/10.1186/2110-5820-4-1.
9. Soummer A, Perbet S, Brisson H, Arbelot C, Constantin J-M, Lu Q, Rouby J-J, Lung Ultrasound Study Group. Ultrasound assessment of lung aeration loss during a successful weaning trial predicts post-extubation distress*. Crit Care Med. 2012;40(7):2064–72. https://doi.org/10.1097/ccm.0b013e31824e68ae.
10. McKiernan S, Chiarelli P, Warren-Forward H. Diagnostic ultrasound use in physiotherapy, emergency medicine, and anesthesiology. Radiography. 2010;16:154–9. https://doi.org/10.1016/j.radi.2009.12.004.
11. Lichtenstein DA. Lung ultrasound in the critically III. The BLUE protocol. 1st ed. Springer; 2016. https://doi.org/10.1007/978-3-319-15371-1.
12. Rocca E, Zanza C, Longhitano Y, Piccolella F, Romenskaya T, Racca F, Savioli G, Saviano A, Piccioni A, Mongodi S. Lung ultrasound in critical care and emergency medicine: clinical review. Adv Respir Med. 2023;91:203–23. https://doi.org/10.3390/arm91030017.
13. Blackwood B, Alderdice F, Burns K, et al. Use of weaning protocols for reducing duration of mechanical ventilation in critically ill adult patients: Cochrane systematic review and meta-analysis. BMJ Brit Med J. 2011;342:c7237. https://doi.org/10.1136/bmj.c7237.
14. Qian Z, Yang M, Li L, Chen Y. Ultrasound assessment of diaphragmatic dysfunction as a predictor of weaning outcome from mechanical ventilation: a systematic review and meta-analysis. BMJ Open. 2018;8:e021189. https://doi.org/10.1136/bmjopen-2017-021189.
15. Minami T, Manzoor K, McCool FD. Assessing diaphragm function in the chest wall and neuromuscular diseases. Clin Chest Med. 2018;39:335–44. https://doi.org/10.1016/j.ccm.2018.01.013.
16. Ricoy J, Rodríguez-Núñez N, Álvarez-Dobaño JM, Toubes ME, Riveiro V, Valdés L. Diaphragm Dysfunct Pulmonol. 2019;25:223–35. https://doi.org/10.1016/j.pulmoe.2018.10.008.
17. Kharma N. Dysfunction of the diaphragm. Curr Opin Pulm Med. 2013;1 https://doi.org/10.1097/mcp.0b013e3283621b49.
18. McCool FD, Manzoor K, Minami T. Disorders of the diaphragm. Clin Chest Med. 2018;39:345–60. https://doi.org/10.1016/j.ccm.2018.01.012.

19. Tuinman PR, Jonkman AH, Dres M, Shi ZH, Goligher EC, Goffi A, De Korte C, Demoule A, Heunks L. Respiratory muscle ultrasonography: methodology, basic and advanced principles and clinical applications in ICU and ED patients—a narrative review. Intensive Care Med. 2020;46:594–605. https://doi.org/10.1007/s00134-019-05892-8.
20. Cardenas LZ, Santana PV, Caruso P, De Carvalho CRR, De Albuquerque ALP. Diaphragmatic ultrasound correlates with inspiratory muscle strength and pulmonary function in healthy subjects. Ultrasound Med Biol. 2018;44:786–93. https://doi.org/10.1016/j.ultrasmedbio.2017.11.020.
21. Santana PV, Cardenas LZ, De Albuquerque ALP, De Carvalho CRR, Caruso P. Diaphragmatic ultrasound: a review of its methodological aspects and clinical uses. J Bras Pneumol. 2020;46:e20200064. https://doi.org/10.36416/1806-3756/e20200064.
22. Boussuges A, Gole Y, Blanc P. Diaphragmatic motion studied by M-mode ultrasonography. Chest. 2009;135:391–400. https://doi.org/10.1378/chest.08-1541.
23. Testa A, Soldati G, Giannuzzi R, Berardi S, Portale G, Silveri NG. Ultrasound M-mode assessment of diaphragmatic kinetics by anterior transverse scanning in healthy subjects. Ultrasound Med Biol. 2011;37:44–52. https://doi.org/10.1016/j.ultrasmedbio.2010.10.004.
24. Boussuges A, Rives S, Finance J, Brégeon F. Assessment of diaphragmatic function by ultrasonography: current approach and perspectives. World J Clin Cases. 2020;8:2408–24. https://doi.org/10.12998/wjcc.v8.i12.2408.
25. Marques MR, Pereira JM, Paiva JA, De Casasola-Sánchez GG, Tung-Chen Y. Ultrasonography to access diaphragm dysfunction and predict the success of mechanical ventilation weaning in critical care. J Ultrasound Med. 2023;43:223–36. https://doi.org/10.1002/jum.16363.
26. Li S, Chen Z, Yan W. Application of bedside ultrasound in predicting the outcome of weaning from mechanical ventilation in elderly patients. BMC Pulm Med. 2021;21 https://doi.org/10.1186/s12890-021-01605-4.
27. Siniscalchi C, Nouvenne A, Cerundolo N, et al. Diaphragm ultrasound in different clinical scenarios: a review with a focus on older patients. Geriatrics. 2024;9:70. https://doi.org/10.3390/geriatrics9030070.
28. Kang HW, Kim TO, Lee BR, Yu JY, Chi SY, Ban HJ, Oh IJ, Kim KS, Kwon YS, Kim YI, Kim YC, Lim SC. Influence of diaphragmatic mobility on hypercapnia in patients with chronic obstructive pulmonary disease. J Kor Med Sci. 2011;26:1209. https://doi.org/10.3346/jkms.2011.26.9.1209.
29. Yamaguti WP, Claudino RC, Neto AP, Chammas MC, Gomes AC, Salge JM, Moriya HT, Cukier A, Carvalho CR. Diaphragmatic breathing training program improves abdominal motion during natural breathing in patients with chronic obstructive pulmonary disease: a randomized controlled trial. Arch Phys Med Rehabil. 2012;93:571–7. https://doi.org/10.1016/j.apmr.2011.11.026.
30. Santana PV, Prina E, Albuquerque ALP, Carvalho CRR, Caruso P. Identifying decreased diaphragmatic mobility and diaphragm thickening in interstitial lung disease: the utility of ultrasound imaging. J Bras Pneumol. 2016;42:88–94. https://doi.org/10.1590/s1806-37562015000000266.
31. Goligher EC, Brochard LJ, Reid WD, Fan E, Saarela O, Slutsky AS, Kavanagh BP, Rubenfeld GD, Ferguson ND. Diaphragmatic myotrauma: a mediator of prolonged ventilation and poor patient outcomes in acute respiratory failure. Lancet Respir Med. 2019;7:90–8. https://doi.org/10.1016/s2213-2600(18)30366-7.
32. Schepens T, Dres M, Heunks L, Goligher EC. Diaphragm-protective mechanical ventilation. Curr Opin Crit Care Eval MEDLINE. 2019;25:77–85. https://doi.org/10.1097/mcc.0000000000000578.
33. Parada-Gereda HM, Tibaduiza AL, Rico-Mendoza A, Molano-Franco D, Nieto VH, Arias-Ortiz WA, Perez-Terán P, Masclans JR. Effectiveness of diaphragmatic ultrasound as a predictor of successful weaning from mechanical ventilation: a systematic review and meta-analysis. Crit Care. 2023;27 https://doi.org/10.1186/s13054-023-04430-9.

34. Schepens T, Fard S, Goligher EC. Assessing diaphragmatic function. Respir Care. 2020;65:807–19. https://doi.org/10.4187/respcare.07410.
35. Ueki J, De Bruin PF, Pride NB. In vivo assessment of diaphragm contraction by ultrasound in normal subjects. Thorax. 1995;50:1157–61. https://doi.org/10.1136/thx.50.11.1157.
36. Sen M, Kumar R, Chakrabarti S, Ish P, Gupta N, Gupta N, Shamil P. Prediction of weaning outcome from mechanical ventilation using diaphragmatic rapid shallow breathing index. Indian J Crit Care Med. 2022;26:1000–5. https://doi.org/10.5005/jp-journals-10071-24316.
37. Abbas A, Embarak S, Walaa M, Lutfy SM. Role of diaphragmatic rapid shallow breathing index in predicting weaning outcome in patients with acute exacerbation of COPD. Int J Chronic Obstruct Pulmon Dis. 2018;13:1655–61. https://doi.org/10.2147/copd.s161691.
38. Spadaro S, Grasso S, Mauri T, Corte FD, Alvisi V, Ragazzi R, Cricca V, Biondi G, Di Mussi R, Marangoni E, Volta CA. Can diaphragmatic ultrasonography performed during the T-tube trial predict weaning failure? The role of diaphragmatic rapid shallow breathing index. Crit Care. 2016;20 https://doi.org/10.1186/s13054-016-1479-y.
39. Xu X, Wu R, Zhang Y-J, Li H-W, He X-H, Wang S-M. Value of combination of heart, lung, and diaphragm ultrasound in predicting weaning outcome of mechanical ventilation. Med Sci Monit. 2020;26 https://doi.org/10.12659/msm.924885.
40. Dres M, Demoule A. Monitoring diaphragm function in the ICU. Curr Opin Crit Care. 2020;26(1):18–25. https://doi.org/10.1097/MCC.0000000000000682.
41. Drakonaki EE, Allen GM, Wilson DJ. Ultrasound elastography for musculoskeletal applications. Brit J Radiol. 2012;85:1435–45. https://doi.org/10.1259/bjr/93042867.
42. Li H, Bhatt M, Qu Z, Zhang S, Hartel MC, Khademhosseini A, Cloutier G. Deep learning in ultrasound elastography imaging: a review. Med Phys CD-ROM. 2022;49:5993–6018. https://doi.org/10.1002/mp.15856.
43. Klauser AS, Miyamoto H, Bellmann-Weiler R, Feuchtner GM, Wick MC, Jaschke WR. Sonoelastography: musculoskeletal applications. Radiology. 2014;272:622–33. https://doi.org/10.1148/radiol.14121765.
44. Schreiber AF, Sabatini U, Vorona S, et al. Measuring abdominal muscle function by abdominal muscle thickening on ultrasound: reproducibility, validity and normal range values. Ultrasound. 2019; https://doi.org/10.1183/13993003.congress-2019.oa5367.

Chapter 11
Weaning from Noninvasive Ventilation

Daniel Lago Borges, Antuani Rafael Baptistella, and Wan Cley Rabuske

11.1 Introduction

Noninvasive mechanical ventilation (NIV) is a widely recognized therapeutic option for managing various clinical conditions, including cardiogenic acute pulmonary edema (APE) and exacerbations of chronic obstructive pulmonary disease (COPD), with a strong evidence base supporting its use in these scenarios [1]. Despite its proven effectiveness, there are no standardized protocols for weaning patients from NIV. The weaning process is typically guided by the clinical judgment of the healthcare team, relying on signs of clinical improvement and complementary test results [2].

In 2008, British institutions proposed a protocol for NIV weaning, but it was not adopted as an official guideline and has not gained widespread use [3]. The absence of formal guidelines may be due to the relative ease of discontinuing and resuming NIV without significant adverse effects. However, this flexibility can lead to prolonged use of NIV, which may extend hospital stays, increase the risk of hospital-acquired infections, and raise overall costs [2].

On the other hand, premature weaning from NIV may worsen the patient's clinical condition, leading to a higher likelihood of intubation. The key challenge is determining the optimal time for weaning, balancing the risks associated with prolonged NIV use and those of early discontinuation [2].

D. L. Borges
Hospital Universitário of Maranhão Federal University (HUUFMA), São Luis, Maranhão, Brazil

A. R. Baptistella (✉) · W. C. Rabuske
Universidade do Oeste de Santa Catarina, Unoesc, Joaçaba, Brazil
e-mail: antuani.baptistella@unoesc.edu.br

A. R. Baptistella et al. (eds.), *Weaning from Mechanical Ventilation*,
https://doi.org/10.1007/978-3-032-01145-9_11

11.2 Identification of NIV Failure

Before considering weaning a patient from mechanical ventilation, the patient must be stable and tolerate NIV until the cause of the acute respiratory failure is controlled or resolved. Some physiological variables are associated with NIV failure and can be monitored to identify the patient's intolerance to noninvasive respiratory support.

Table 11.1 presents the physiological variables that indicate the increased risk of NIV failure [4].

An important tool for identifying NIV failure is the heart rate, acidosis, consciousness, oxygenation, and respiratory rate (HACOR) score. This score was proposed in 2017 by Duan et al. [5], and an updated HACOR score was published in 2022 [6], adding six variables to increase the accuracy of the score in predicting NIV failure after 1–2 h of noninvasive respiratory support. This update added the presence of pneumonia, cardiogenic pulmonary edema, pulmonary ARDS, immunosuppression, or septic shock and the SOFA score to the previously published score (Table 11.2).

According to the updated HACOR score results, 1–2 h of noninvasive respiratory support is estimated to reduce the risk of NIV failure (Table 11.3).

Assessing the risk of NIV failure may be an initial strategy for screening patients for weaning from NIV once the cause of acute respiratory failure (ARF) is controlled or resolved.

Table 11.1 Physiologic variables associated with NIV failure

Variable	Description
PaO_2/FiO_2	$PaO_2/FiO_2 < 200$ at 1 h after NIV → increased risk of intubation $PaO_2/FiO_2 < 150$ → increased risk of death (as compared with up-front strategy of invasive mechanical ventilation)
Tidal volume	VT >9–9.5 ml/kg of PBW 1 h after NIV → increased risk of intubation and death
Respiratory rate	Low or decreasing RR → greater likelihood of NIV success
Simplified Acute Physiology Score II	Higher scores → higher likelihood of failure (without a threshold defined in the literature)
HACOR score	Threshold of >5 at 1 h after initiation of NIV → the NIV failure rate was 87.1%
Point-of-care lung ultrasound score	The total lung ultrasound score was significantly higher in patients with Covid-19 who had NIV failure

Adapted from Munshi et al. [4]
VT tidal volume, *PBW* predicted body weight, *RR* respiratory rate

Table 11.2 Updated HACOR score

Variables	Category	Assigned points
Heart rate (bpm)	≤120	0
	≥121	1
pH	≥7.35	0
	7.30–7.34	2
	7.25–7.29	3
	<7.25	4
GCS	15	0
	13–14	2
	11–12	5
	≤10	10
PaO_2/FiO_2	≥201	0
	176–200	2
	151–175	3
	126–150	4
	101–125	5
	≤100	6
Respiratory rate (bpm)	≤30	0
	31–35	1
	36–40	2
	41–45	3
	≥ 46	4
Additional variables		
Presence of pneumonia	+2.5	
Cardiogenic pulmonary edema	−4	
Pulmonary ARDS	+3	
Immunosuppression	+1.5	
Septic shock	+2.5	
SOFA score	+0.5 × SOFA	

Adapted from Duan et al. [6]

Table 11.3 Rate of NIV failure

Updated HACOR score	Rate of NIV failure
≤7	12.4%
7.5–10.5	38.2%
11–14	67.1%
>14	83.7%

Updated HACOR score
Adapted from Duan et al. [6]

11.3 Criteria for Starting Weaning from NIV

Patients may be screened daily for the clinical criteria to be met before the weaning attempt. The main criteria for considering it are as follows [7]:

- Cause of ARF controlled or resolved
- Arterial pH $\geq$ 7.30
- Fraction of inspired oxygen (FiO_2) $\leq$ 0.5
- Arterial partial pressure of oxygen (PaO_2) > 60 mmHg
- PaO_2/FiO_2 ratio > 150
- Arterial oxygen saturation (SaO_2) $\geq$ 92%
- Respiratory rate (RR) between 8 and 30 breaths per minute
- Systolic blood pressure (SBP) between 90 and 180 mmHg without vasopressors
- Body temperature between 36 and 38 °C
- Heart rate (HR) between 50 and 120 bpm
- Glasgow Coma Scale (GCS) score $\geq$ 13

More liberal weaning criteria can promote earlier discontinuation of NIV, leading to a reduced incidence of complications, shorter NIV duration, and decreased hospital stay. Conversely, stricter criteria tend to result in higher weaning success rates, akin to the approach used in extubation [8].

If patients pass the baseline screening criteria, they can be discontinued from NIV onto nasal/Venturi oxygen at the minimal level (maximum of 5 L/min) to achieve the same oxygenation targets of NIV [9].

11.4 General Care During Weaning from NIV

Some factors that cause discomfort in the patient and compromise weaning. They are:

Interface Potential source of pain and claustrophobia leading to discontinuation of NIV and consequently orotracheal intubation. Choosing the best interface also depends on the fastening and sealing system, as they play an important role in minimizing leaks and consequently patient-ventilator asynchronies. In addition, leaks increase noise, especially when NIV is delivered through face masks.

Ventilator Settings and Asynchrony Inadequate ventilator settings can lead to asynchrony between the patient's demand and the ventilator's supply. Pressure support levels that are too low or too high lead to patient discomfort, while air leaks promote the dispersion of inspired airflow and are the main causes of auto-triggering, putting the patient at risk of volutrauma.

Humidification Inadequate humidification during NIV is associated with discomfort in the upper airway mucosa and dehydration of bronchial secretions. Adequate humidification can be achieved actively or with a heat and moisture exchanger (HME). It should be borne in mind that using the HME increases the dead space and resistance to flow in the ventilation circuit, thus increasing the patient's respiratory load. Patients in the acute phase of respiratory failure, especially hypercapnic patients, benefit from the active humidification system or the absence of HME. However, if NIV needs to be maintained for a longer period and $PaCO_2$ values are lower than at the start of therapy, it is suggested that HME be installed to improve patient comfort.

Position The patient's position is important for the comfort and efficiency of NIV. A semi-sitting position (45°) was associated with lower respiratory efforts and intrinsic PEEP, in addition to being considered more comfortable by patients who were weaning from MV [10].

11.5 NIV Weaning Strategies

Weaning from invasive mechanical ventilation has been widely studied, but weaning from NIV still lacks standardization of the safest and most effective way to discontinue ventilatory support. NIV should be discontinued as soon as the cause of respiratory failure has been resolved or controlled, but premature discontinuation of ventilatory support can result in a worsening of the patient's clinical condition.

A study comparing physician-guided weaning versus protocol-guided weaning showed a reduction in the duration of NIV (4.4 ± 2.5 days vs. 2.6 ± 1.5 days, $p < 0.001$) and the length of ICU stay (8.1 ± 5.5 days vs. 5.8 ± 2.7 days, $p = 0.02$) when weaning was protocol-guided [7].

There are three main reported types of protocols to wean patients from NIV:

- Immediate weaning: When patient is disconnected from the NIV as they meet the weaning criteria [11].
- Stepwise pressure reduction: Inspiratory positive airway pressure (IPAP) and expiratory positive airway pressure (EPAP) are reduced by 2–4 cm of H_2O every 4–6 h [12, 13].
- Stepwise duration reduction: Each day, the patient spends more time without the NIV, e.g., first day, for every 3 h, 1 h without NIV, second day, for every 3 h, 2 h without NIV and third day patient receives only supplemental O_2 [12, 13].

A comparison of the three NIV weaning strategies employed for the patients in the immediate withdrawal group showed that 76.6% were successful in weaning, in the gradual reduction of pressure support group, 90% were successful, while in the gradual reduction of time group 86.6% of patients were successful in weaning, however, no statistically significant difference was observed between the groups [14].

Different studies have compared immediate weaning with stepwise weaning. Lun et al. [11] did not observe any difference in the weaning outcome between these two strategies. Sellares et al. conducted a clinical trial involving 120 patients with COPD in which they compared abrupt versus gradual NIV discontinuation (use for three additional nights) and found no difference in the outcomes: new episode of respiratory failure, long-term NIV dependence, length of hospital stay and readmission, or hospital survival at 6 months. However, the abrupt discontinuation group had a shorter ICU stay (4 (2–6) versus 5 (4–7) days, $p = 0.036$), showing that NIV can be discontinued immediately in COPD patients once the episode has resolved and the patients tolerate unassisted breathing [15].

In another study, Purohit et al. compared abrupt discontinuation with gradual weaning of NIV duration and observed a similar weaning success rate (80% vs 90%, $p = 0.472$), but a significantly shorter total duration of NIV use (38.97 ± 17 h vs 64.3 ± 7.74 h; $p < 0.0001$) and length of hospital stay (5.8 ± 1.6 days vs 7.7 ± 0.61 days; $p < 0.0001$) in the abrupt discontinuation group, concluding that this would be a safe method [16].,

Patients with COPD may experience hypoventilation and elevated $PaCO_2$ during sleep, which is why gradual weaning of the duration of NIV is recommended. The duration of daytime NIV should be reduced daily once the cause of respiratory failure has been resolved, maintaining therapy at night, avoiding exacerbations of COPD [14]. On the other hand, patients with a greater number of comorbidities, who may not tolerate a protocol based on gradual time reduction, may benefit from a protocol of gradual pressure reduction, and it is possible to monitor signs of tolerance in the face of decreased patient care [9, 14].

Comparing the stepwise duration reduction with the stepwise pressure reduction, NIV duration during weaning was significantly lower for patients undergoing weaning by pressure reduction [17]. Studies showed no difference in the weaning outcome between these two types of weaning protocol [12, 13, 17].

Studies evaluating predictors of successful weaning from NIV are rare. A study conducted with 85 patients with acute exacerbation of COPD, the rapid shallow breathing index (RSBI), maximum inspiratory pressure, and maximum expiratory pressure were significantly different between success and failure group, and the RSBI predicted the NIV weaning success with an AUCROC of 0.804, suggesting that this index can be useful for selecting patients that can be successfully weaned from the NIV [18].

11.6 NIV Weaning Protocols

Weaning guided by protocol has better outcomes than weaning guided by clinical opinion. However, unlike invasive MV, discontinuing and returning to noninvasive therapy does not present direct risks to the patient, but interruption or maintenance, when not properly indicated, is related to worse outcomes for the patient.

The first step of the weaning protocol is to establish the criteria to wean the patient from the NIV. The resolution or control of the cause of the ARF that leads the patient to NIV and stabilization of clinical signs are essential criteria to proceed the weaning.

There is no consensus on the best NIV weaning protocol. Once the cause of respiratory failure has been resolved, *immediate weaning*, *stepwise pressure reduction*, or *stepwise duration reduction* have high weaning success rates, and there is no important difference between them.

The heterogeneity and low sample size of the studies are a limitation in reaching a consensus on the best method. However, when there is not a high number of comorbidities associated with respiratory failure and the condition is resolved in a short time, NIV can be discontinued immediately, reducing the number of days spent in the ICU and hospital. When there is an unfavorable clinical condition, more precise monitoring and the use of a protocol for gradual weaning are necessary.

Hypercapnic patients or those at risk of hypoventilation can benefit from the strategy of stepwise duration reduction, since NIV is only withdrawn at night on the third day. The stepwise pressure reduction is equally effective for weaning and enables precise control of the relationship between the support offered by the ventilator and the patient's clinical responses to the decrease in ventilatory support [19].

In addition to the possibility of immediate weaning, we present the following two possibilities of gradual weaning (Figs. 11.1 and 11.2).

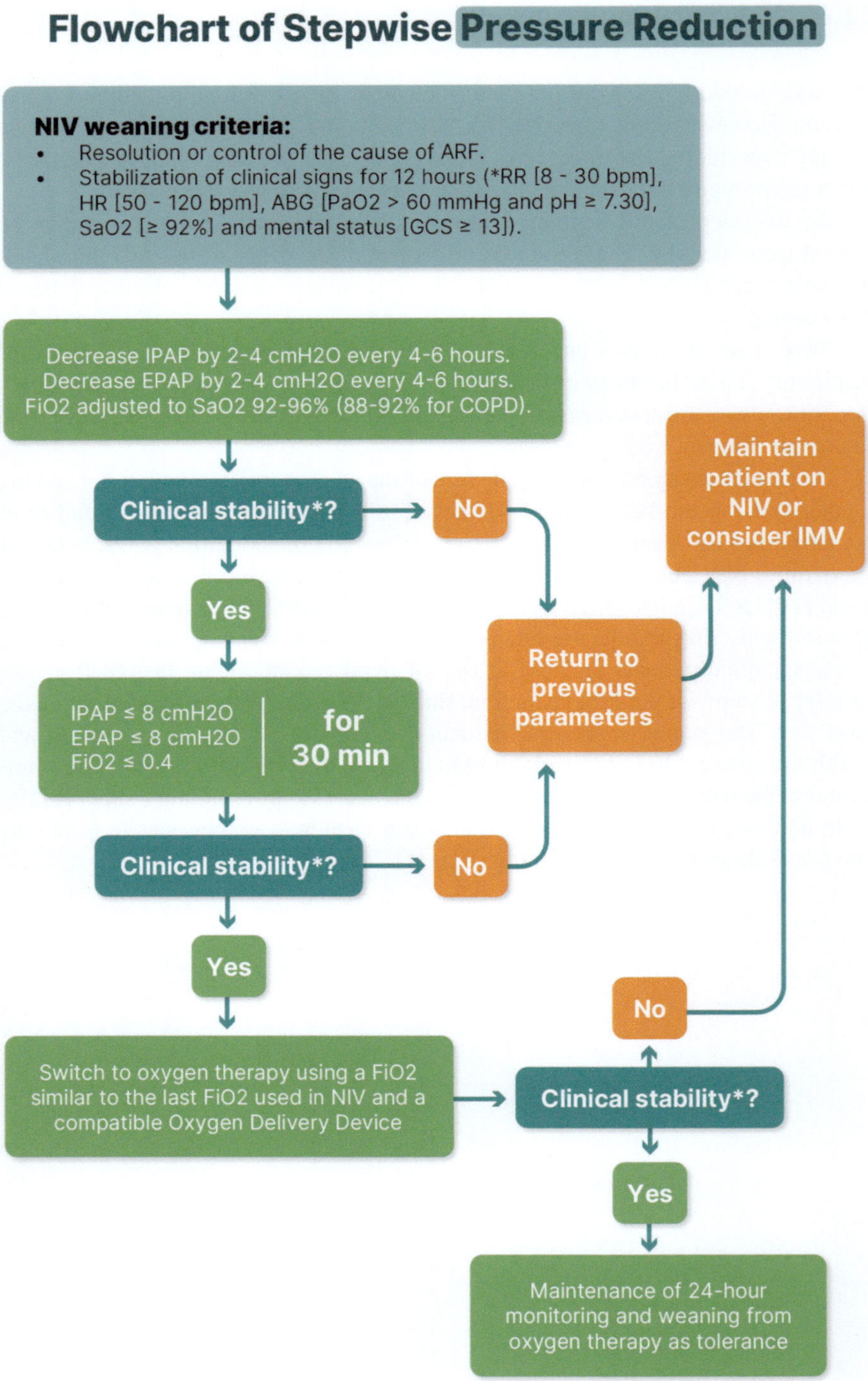

Fig. 11.1 Flowchart of stepwise pressure reduction. *RR* respiratory rate, *HR* heart rate, *ABG* arterial blood gases. (Refs. [8, 13, 20, 21])

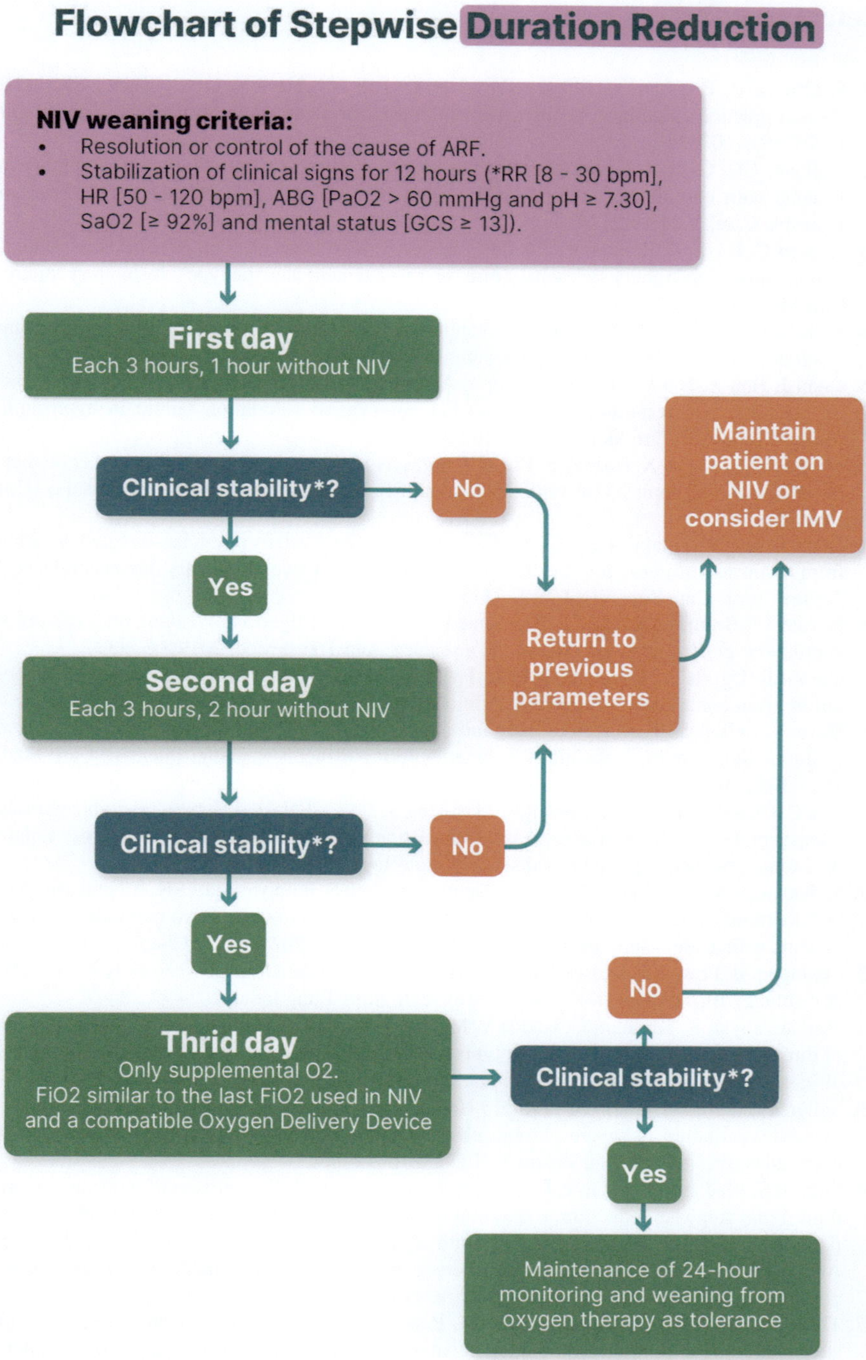

Fig. 11.2 Flowchart of stepwise pressure reduction. *RR* respiratory rate, *HR* heart rate, *ABG* arterial blood gases. (Refs. [8, 13, 20, 21])

References

1. Rochwerg B, Brochard L, Elliott MW, Hess D, Hill NS, Nava S, et al. Official ERS/ATS clinical practice guidelines: noninvasive ventilation for acute respiratory failure. Eur Respir J. 2017;50:1602426.
2. Khilnani GC, Galle AD, Hadda V, Sharma SK. Non-invasive ventilation after extubation in patients with chronic obstructive airways disease: a randomised controlled trial. Anaesth Intensive Care. 2011;39:217–23.
3. Roberts C, Brown J, Reinhardt A, Kaul S, Scales K, Mikelsons C, et al. Non-invasive ventilation in chronic obstructive pulmonary disease: management of acute type 2 respiratory failure. Clin Med. 2008;8:517–21.
4. Munshi L, Mancebo J, Brochard LJ. Noninvasive respiratory support for adults with acute respiratory failure. Hardin CC, organizador. N Engl J Med. 2022;387:1688–98.
5. Duan J, Han X, Bai L, Zhou L, Huang S. Assessment of heart rate, acidosis, consciousness, oxygenation, and respiratory rate to predict noninvasive ventilation failure in hypoxemic patients. Intensive Care Med. 2017;43:192–9.
6. Duan J, Chen L, Liu X, Bozbay S, Liu Y, Wang K, et al. An updated HACOR score for predicting the failure of noninvasive ventilation: a multicenter prospective observational study. Crit Care. 2022;26:196.
7. Duan J, Tang X, Huang S, Jia J, Guo S. Protocol-directed versus physician-directed weaning from noninvasive ventilation: the impact in chronic obstructive pulmonary disease patients. J Trauma Acute Care Surg. 2012;72:1271–5.
8. Navalesi P, Bruni A, Garofalo E, Biamonte E, Longhini F, Frigerio P. Weaning off mechanical ventilation: much less an art, but not yet a science. Ann Transl Med. 2019;7:S353.
9. Özsancak Uğurlu A, Ergan B. How do I wean a patient with acute hypercapnic respiratory failure from noninvasive ventilation? Pulmonology. 2023;29:144–50.
10. Deye N, Lellouche F, Maggiore SM, Taillé S, Demoule A, L'Her E, et al. The semi-seated position slightly reduces the effort to breathe during difficult weaning. Intensive Care Med. 2013;39:85–92.
11. Lun C, Chan VL, Leung W, Cheung APS, Cheng S, Tsui MSN, et al. A pilot randomized study comparing two methods of non-invasive ventilation withdrawal after acute respiratory failure in chronic obstructive pulmonary disease. Respirology. 2013;18:814–9.
12. Sadanandan AM, George S, Mohamed Nambipunnilath S, Puthiyaveettil SK. A comparison of two weaning strategies for non-invasive ventilation in chronic obstructive pulmonary disease patients with acute respiratory failure. Ir J Med Sci (1971). 2024;193:2419–25.
13. Thampan SJ, Prasath A, Moses J, Kisku KH, Sagar P, Ravichandran K. Wean early leave early: Apt strategy for weaning from non-invasive ventilation. Lung India. 2024;41:284–7.
14. Venkatnarayan K, Khilnani G, Hadda V, Madan K, Mohan A, Pandey R, et al. A comparison of three strategies for withdrawal of noninvasive ventilation in chronic obstructive pulmonary disease with acute respiratory failure: randomized trial. Lung India. 2020;37:3.
15. Sellares J, Ferrer M, Anton A, Loureiro H, Bencosme C, Alonso R, et al. Discontinuing noninvasive ventilation in severe chronic obstructive pulmonary disease exacerbations: a randomised controlled trial. Eur Respir J. 2017;50:1601448.
16. Purohit S, Madan M, Kumar R, Kaushik R, Ish P, Aj M, et al. Comparison of immediate withdrawal and stepwise reduction in duration of non-invasive ventilation in chronic obstructive pulmonary disease patients presenting with acute hypercapnic respiratory failure. Monaldi Arch Chest Dis [Internet]. 2023. Recuperado de: https://www.monaldi-archives.org/index.php/macd/article/view/2755. [citado 12 de novembro de 2024];
17. Thampan SJ, Varughese PG, Varghese M, Prasath A, Sagar P. Comparison of two weaning strategies from non-invasive ventilation in patients with acute acidotic hypercapnic respiratory failure – a RCT. Sleep Breath Disord [Internet]. Eur Resp Soc. 2023:97. Recuperado de: http://publications.ersnet.org/lookup/doi/10.1183/23120541.sleepandbreathing-2023.97. [citado 22 de outubro de 2024]

18. Yu J, Lee M-R, Chen C-T, Lin Y-T, How C-K. Predictors of successful weaning from noninvasive ventilation in patients with acute exacerbation of chronic obstructive pulmonary disease: a single-center retrospective cohort study. Lung. 2021;199:457–66.
19. Damas C, Andrade C, Araújo JP, Almeida J, Bettencourt P. Weaning from non-invasive positive pressure ventilation: experience with progressive periods of withdraw. Rev Port Pneumol. 2008;14:49–53.
20. Chay S, Gonzalez I. Clinical guidelines for non-invasive ventilation in acute respiratory failure. South Tees Hospitals; 2014.
21. Grieco DL, Menga LS, Cesarano M, Rosà T, Spadaro S, Bitondo MM, et al. Effect of helmet noninvasive ventilation vs high-flow nasal oxygen on days free of respiratory support in patients with COVID-19 and moderate to severe hypoxemic respiratory failure: the HENIVOT randomized clinical trial. JAMA. 2021;325:1731.

Chapter 12
Weaning-Induced Cardiac Failure

Saint-Clair Bernardes Neto

12.1 Introduction

Invasive mechanical ventilation (MV) is an advanced life support treatment commonly used for critically ill patients admitted to an intensive care unit (ICU). Its benefits are multiple and consistent with the primary goal of these units: to preserve life. However, prolonged use of MV is associated with several complications, including increased morbidity and mortality.

For this reason, critically ill patients on MV should be weaned from the ventilator as early as possible, depending on their clinical conditions [1]. This weaning process must be performed with great care, as the weaning failure rate can be as high as 26%–42% [2].

Considering that the cardiovascular system is responsible for capturing and transporting oxygen from the respiratory system to the body, as well as conducting carbon dioxide captured in the tissues for later elimination through ventilation, it is possible to understand that the proper functioning of the heart and lungs, which work in an interconnected manner, constitutes a continuous and complex mechanism [3].

The relationship between these organs and their respective systems is so close that a change in the functioning of one can directly affect the other [4].

Weaning from MV is an extremely delicate process and has been compared to a cardiovascular stress test [5]. The delicacy of this process stems from the transition from positive intrathoracic pressure to spontaneous breathing with negative intrathoracic pressure. This transition promotes hemodynamic and respiratory changes that culminate in adverse conditions for the cardiac system, primarily with increased

S.-C. Bernardes Neto (✉)
Faculdade de Ciências da Saúde (FACISA), Universidade Federal do Rio Grande do Norte (UFRN), Natal, Brazil

A. R. Baptistella et al. (eds.), *Weaning from Mechanical Ventilation*,
https://doi.org/10.1007/978-3-032-01145-9_12

left ventricular filling pressure and subsequent weaning-induced pulmonary edema (WiPO) [6–8].

12.2 Pathophysiology of Cardiac Dysfunction in the Post-Extubation Period

Cardiac dysfunction after extubation is relatively common and needs to be thoroughly understood from a pathophysiological point of view to determine the most appropriate treatment strategies.

The transition of a patient from invasive mechanical ventilation (MV) to spontaneous ventilation can be difficult for many, as spontaneous breathing itself involves greater oxygen consumption, diversion of blood flow to the muscles, and increased carbon dioxide production. Therefore, a higher cardiac output is required, while variations in lung volumes during spontaneous breathing can lead to hemodynamic effects [9, 10].

The close relationship between the heart and the respiratory system is fundamental to understanding the pathophysiology of cardiac dysfunction after extubation and removal from invasive MV. One theory that explains this relationship is that the organs are connected by blood vessels and are located within the same compartment: the thoracic cage. Since this cage is considered rigid, it can be imagined that the heart, with its atrial and ventricular cavities, experiences frequent and constant pressure changes while being held within a compartment that also undergoes pressure changes [9, 11, 12].

Both mechanical and spontaneous ventilation promote variations in intrathoracic pressure, leading to different effects on cardiac function [3, 11]. In a more general analysis, we can say that spontaneous ventilation, through the contraction of the inspiratory muscles, promotes a reduction in intrapleural pressure during the inspiratory phase (Fig. 12.1). Conversely, positive pressure MV is responsible for increasing intrathoracic pressure. These variations affect venous return and the blood ejection capacity of the left ventricle [10, 13].

On the left side of the heart, blood ejection is performed by the left ventricle (LV) and is determined by the difference between arterial pressure and intrathoracic pressure. As a result, the LV encounters resistance in the arterial vasculature, and the pressure required for ejection is also increased by the heightened work of breathing caused, for example, by weaning from mechanical ventilation (MV) (by reducing intrathoracic pressure). The LV overload due to the increased afterload described above may promote the induction of heart failure as well as pulmonary edema [4, 9, 11, 12].

Considering the right side of the heart, the reduction in intrapleural pressure is responsible for the decrease in ventricular pressure, increasing venous return and right ventricular (RV) preload. The increased volume of blood entering the RV during spontaneous inspiration is also responsible for the dilation of the right

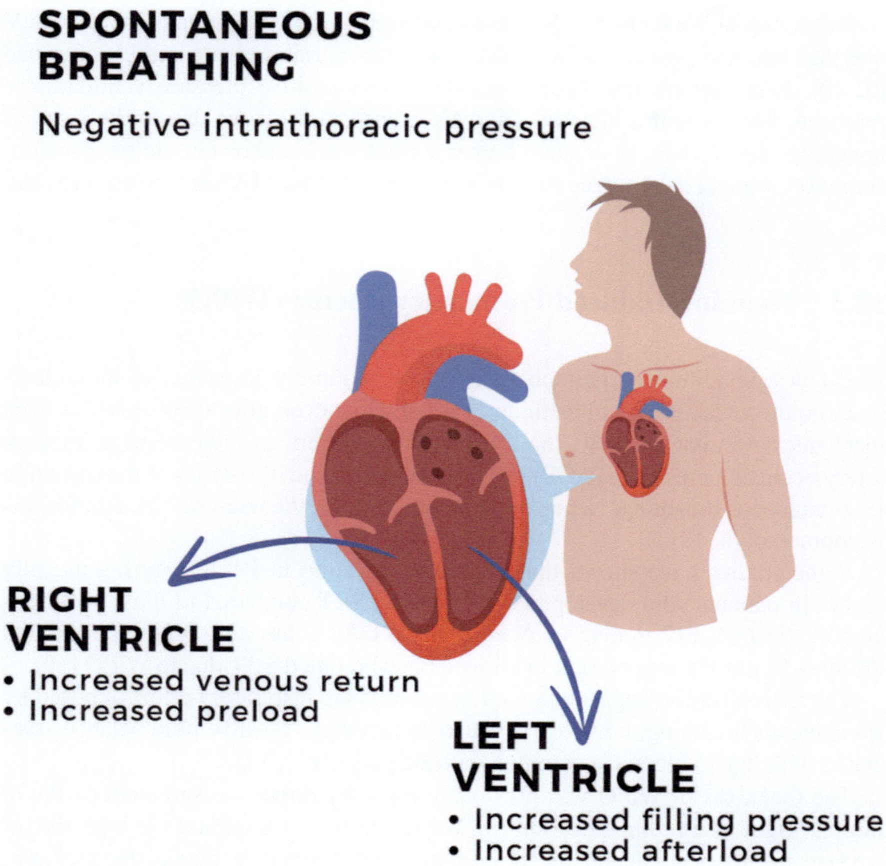

Fig. 12.1 Effect of spontaneous breathing pressure variations in the right and left ventricles

ventricular chamber and the consequent deviation of the intraventricular septum toward the LV, reducing its ability to expand and receive blood volume [4, 9, 11–13].

During MV, the left heart is less affected in terms of contractility because the increase in intrathoracic pressure promotes a decrease in venous return to the RV, an increase in pulmonary vascular resistance to RV ejection, and a decrease in systemic vascular resistance to LV ejection [4]. However, in the reverse situation of spontaneous ventilation, as previously described, there is greater damage to LV function.

Adjusting PEEP to inappropriately high levels during MV can promote compression and/or collapse of the alveolar vessels, significantly altering pulmonary vascular resistance. High levels of PEEP promote compression of extra-alveolar vessels due to alveolar hyperdistension. Conversely, when PEEP is set too low, alveolar collapse and the collapse of intra-alveolar vessels occur, in addition to increasing the stimulus for hypoxic vasoconstriction. Both situations lead to increased pulmonary vascular resistance [4, 14].

Nevertheless, we know that MV itself can mask the development of increased LV overload because positive pressure decreases transmural pressure and LV afterload [9, 10]. It is important to understand that when positive pressure ventilation is removed, venous return increases, and LV afterload also rises due to the work of breathing. These changes demand higher cardiac work and/or muscle oxygen consumption, which could induce cardiac ischemia and reduce LV compliance [15, 16].

12.3 Weaning-Induced Pulmonary Edema (WiPO)

WiPO is a condition of pulmonary edema that rapidly increases in individuals undergoing a spontaneous breathing trial (SBT) or even after disconnection from mechanical ventilation (MV) [6, 17]. In this condition, an increase in pulmonary artery occlusion pressure (PAOP) can be observed within 5–10 min of the transition to spontaneous breathing. Negative pleural pressure is the main mechanism for this phenomenon [6, 18].

Some studies have shown that the mean elevation in PAOP was significantly higher in patients who developed WiPO during SBT compared to those with successful trials (Δ ±17 mmHg vs Δ ±4 mmHg) [18]. It has also been reported that PAOP > 18 mmHg was present in all patients who failed SBT due to WiPO [19].

The reason for the negative pleural pressure is the inspiratory effort imposed by spontaneous breathing; however, it is also known that a positive fluid balance associated with hypervolemia is common in these patients [7, 17].

The diagnosis of WiPO was previously made by direct measurement of PAOP through right heart catheterization [6], but its invasive nature and the high risk of adverse events necessitated the development of alternative diagnostic methods. Nowadays, the use of bedside echocardiography plays a crucial role, as it can be employed for diagnosis as well as for managing respiratory failure due to WiPO. It can also be utilized for early identification of WiPO prior to the initiation of SBT in mechanically ventilated patients at high risk for WiPO development [20, 21].

The use of echocardiography in clinical practice can be combined with ultrasound assessment of the lungs and respiratory muscles. This combination allows for a more thorough and detailed evaluation of the respiratory impairment presented by patients with WiPO [20, 22–24].

The specificity of diagnosis by echocardiography, when applied to patients at high risk of developing WiPO, is achieved by detecting excessive fluid balance and elevated LV filling pressure. Another important method to assess fluid accumulation and the cardiological system's response to such a situation can be performed using a bedside clinical test called passive leg raising, which consists of moving the patient from a semi-reclining position to a supine position with the legs elevated at 45°. This maneuver favors venous return while simultaneously measuring cardiac function (for example, with echocardiography itself). The maneuver can increase venous return blood volume by approximately 300 ml, and an increase in cardiac output of 10% or more indicates responsiveness to fluid infusion. A smaller increase or no increase may indicate a propensity for WiPO [7, 17, 25, 26].

12.4 Risk Factors for Cardiac Dysfunction After Mechanical Ventilation

When weaning critically ill patients from mechanical ventilation, it is crucial to identify patients at increased risk of developing pulmonary edema during the process. The risk of weaning failure is approximately two times higher in this subgroup [17, 27] and may be the leading cause of weaning failure in patients with heart and lung disease [8, 15].

Several conditions have been described as risk factors for the development of WiPO, such as advanced age (>65 years), chronic obstructive pulmonary disease (COPD), chronic heart failure, and obesity [7, 8, 10, 15–17, 27].

Left heart failure with prior impairment of left ventricular (LV) systolic function is a significant risk factor for the development of WiPO. Greater negativity of intrathoracic pressure imposes additional overload on the ventricle, leading to pulmonary edema due to retrograde pressures and exacerbating heart failure [10, 16]. This change is less frequent in individuals without left ventricular impairment, as the muscle's contractile capacity remains robust in the presence of afterload variations [9].

In patients with COPD, specific WiPO features should be considered, particularly due to the increased work of breathing resulting from airflow obstruction and myocardial compression due to hyperinflation, which leads to greater negative pressure [6, 15]. Additionally, ventricular septal deviation occurs due to right ventricular (RV) dilation resulting from increased venous return [6].

12.5 Weaning in Patients at Risk for Cardiac Dysfunction Post-Mechanical Ventilation

Weaning from mechanical ventilation (MV) is a challenge for healthcare professionals in an ICU, regardless of the patient type, as its failure is associated with prolonged MV, extended ICU stays, and other complications. Given that the patients described above are at high risk for developing WiPO, we must exercise even greater caution [28]. Careful assessment is crucial when performing the spontaneous breathing trial (SBT).

The decision to wean a patient from mechanical ventilation is primarily made after a successful SBT. It is important to emphasize that, in clinical practice, SBT can be performed both by disconnecting the ventilator completely and allowing for spontaneous breathing with an artificial airway still in place. In such cases, oxygen support may be provided as needed, a process known as T-tube SBT. Alternatively, the patient may remain on the mechanical ventilator with reduced pressure support ventilation (PSV) settings, which simulates the work of breathing that will be required after support is withdrawn.

A systematic review analyzing physiological parameters related to work of breathing has described that SBT performed in a T-tube provides work of breathing that closely resembles that of spontaneous ventilation after cessation of MV [29]. Another systematic review evaluating the predictability of weaning success or failure found no significant difference between these methods [30].

For patients at risk for WiPO, there is an ongoing search for more specific testing. Cabello et al. [31] found that the failure rate of SBT in patients with left heart failure or COPD was significantly higher when performed in a T-tube (79%) compared to PSV + PEEP (21%) or PSV without PEEP (43%), particularly in patients who were difficult to wean—defined as those who had already failed at least one SBT and had been on MV for more than 3 days.

Another reflection of the ability of T-tube SBT to accurately detect the risk of developing WiPO is that when this test is performed, there is a more significant increase in pulmonary artery occlusion pressure (PAOP), reaching values greater than 18 mmHg in patients with heart disease or COPD [31].

Therefore, due to the specificity of these patients and the likely ability of T-tube SBT to detect changes in ventricular filling pressure, patients at high risk of WiPO should undergo a T-tube spontaneous breathing test prior to extubation [32, 33].

Performing mechanical ventilation prior to weaning is essential to minimize major changes and the effects of MV on the patient's cardiac function [9]. A strategy that utilizes reduced tidal volumes, minimizes hyperinflation, and employs low PEEP levels can help prevent myocardial overload. Continuous monitoring and ventilatory adjustments that avoid increased ventilatory effort are also beneficial in reducing the risk of WiPO during the weaning process.

For patients who inevitably experience respiratory changes due to pulmonary edema induced by weaning, treatment should address the primary pathophysiological mechanisms of the condition: fluid accumulation and myocardial dysfunction. The use of diuretics to reduce fluid overload and circulating volume within the cardiovascular system is the most recommended approach [6, 15, 16].

A practical method for monitoring and achieving negative fluid balance in volume management is through the measurement of circulating BNP levels. Elevated BNP levels indicate cardiac overload and a higher likelihood of weaning failure. One study found that BNP-guided volume management facilitates a more negative fluid balance, allows for the safe use of increased diuretics, and reduces mechanical ventilation duration in patients with left heart failure [34].

If patients at high subjective risk for WiPO are identified, they should be monitored with echocardiography at the beginning of the weaning process to accurately detect signs of WiPO risk. After making any necessary treatment adjustments based on this information, a repeat echocardiogram should be conducted at the start of the SBT to fine-tune treatment, followed by another at the end of the test for comparison with baseline values.

References

1. Girard TD, Alhazzani W, Kress JP, Ouellette DR, Schmidt GA, Truwit JD, et al. An official American Thoracic Society/American College of Chest Physicians clinical practice guideline: liberation from mechanical ventilation in critically ill adults. Rehabilitation protocols, ventilator liberation protocols, and Cuf leak tests. Am J Respir Crit Care Med. 2017;195:120–33.
2. Boles J-M, Bion J, Connors A, Herridge M, Marsh B, Melot C, Pearl R, Silverman H, Stanchina M, Vieillard-Baron A, Welte T. Weaning from mechanical ventilation. Eur Respir J. 2007;29:1033–56.
3. Verhoeff K, Mitchell JR. Cardiopulmonary physiology: why the heart and lungs are inextricably linked. Adv Physiol Educ. 2017;41(3):348–53.
4. Alviar CL, Miller PE, McAreavey D, Katz JN, Lee B, Moriyama B, Soble J, van Diepen S, Solomon MA, Morrow DA. ACC critical care cardiology working group. Positive pressure ventilation in the cardiac intensive care unit. J Am Coll Cardiol. 2018;72(13):1532–53.
5. Pinsky M. Breathing as exercise: the cardiovascular response to weaning from mechanical ventilation. Intensive Care Med. 2000;26:1164–6.
6. Lemaire F, Teboul JL, Cinotti L, Giotto G, Abrouk F, Steg G, et al. Acute left ventricular dysfunction during unsuccessful weaning from mechanical ventilation. Anesthesiology. 1988;69:171–9.
7. Liu J, Shen F, Teboul JL, Anguel N, Beurton A, Bezaz N, et al. Cardiac dysfunction induced by weaning from mechanical ventilation: incidence, risk factors, and effects of fluid removal. Crit Care. 2016;20:369.
8. Teboul JL, Monnet X, Richard C. Weaning failure of cardiac origin: recent advances. Crit Care. 2010;14:211.
9. Mahmood SS, Pinsky MR. Heart-lung interactions during mechanical ventilation: the basics. Ann Transl Med. 2018;6(18):349.
10. Pinsky MR. Cardiopulmonary interactions: physiologic basis and clinical applications. Ann Am Thorac Soc. 2018;15(Suppl 1):S45–8.
11. Avila MB. Interação cardiopulmonar durante a ventilação mecânica. In: PROFISIO. Programa de atualização em fisioterapia em terapia intensiva adulto. Ciclo 12. Módulo 3. Editora Secad Artmed, 2022.
12. Grübler MR, Wigger O, Berger D, Blöchlinger S. Basic concepts of heart-lung interactions during mechanical ventilation. Swiss Med Wkly. 2017;147:w14491.
13. Pinsky MR. Heart-lung interactions. Curr Opin Crit Care. 2007;13(5):528–31.
14. Barbas CSV, Bueno MAS, Amato MBP, Hoelz C, Rodrigues JM. Interação cardiopulmonar durante a ventilação mecânica. Rev Soc Cardiol Estado de São Paulo. 1998;8(3):406–19.
15. Perren A, Brochard L. Managing the apparent and hidden difficulties of weaning from mechanical ventilation. Intensive Care Med. 2013;39:1885–95.
16. Teboul JL. Weaning-induced cardiac dysfunction: where are we today? Intensive Care Med. 2014;40:1069–79.
17. Goudelin M, Champy P, Amiel JB, Evrard B, Fedou AL, Daix T, et al. Left ventricular overloading identified by critical care echocardiography is key in weaning-induced pulmonary edema. Intensive Care Med. 2020;46:1371–81.
18. Teboul JL, Abrouk F, Lemaire F. Right ventricular function in COPD patients during weaning from mechanical ventilation. Intensive Care Med. 1988;14:483–5.
19. Jubran A, Mathru M, Dries M, Tobin MJ. Continuous recordings of mixed venous oxygen saturation during weaning from mechanical ventilation and the ramifications thereof. Am J Respir Crit Care Med. 1998;158:1763–9.
20. Mayo P, Volpicelli G, Lerolle N, Schreiber A, Doelken P, Vieillard-Baron A. Ultrasonography evaluation during the weaning process: the heart, the diaphragm, the pleura and the lung. Intensive Care Med. 2016;42:1107–17.
21. Vignon P, Repessé X, Vieillard-Baron A, Maury E. Critical care ultrasonography in acute respiratory failure. Crit Care. 2016;20:228.

22. Bataille B, Riu B, Moussot PE, Mari A, Brunel E. Integrated use of bedside lung ultrasound and echocardiography in acute respiratory failure: a prospective observational study in ICU. Chest. 2014;146:1586–93.
23. Llamas-Alvarez AM, Tenza-Lozano EM, Latour-Perez J. Diaphragm and lung ultrasound to predict weaning outcome: systematic review and meta-analysis. Chest. 2017;2017(152):1140–50.
24. Tuinman PR, Jonkman AH, Dres M, Shi ZH, Goligher EC, Goffi A, et al. Respiratory muscle ultrasonography: methodology, basic and advanced principles and clinical applications in ICU and ed patients. A narrative review. Intensive Care Med. 2020;46:594–605.
25. Dres M, Teboul J-L, Anguel N, Guerin L, Richard C, Monnet X. Passive leg raising performed before a spontaneous breathing trial predicts weaning-induced cardiac dysfunction. Intensive Care Med. 2015;41:487–94.
26. Monnet X, Teboul JL. Passive leg raising: five rules, not a drop of fluid! Crit Care. 2015;19(18):18.
27. Thille AW, Muller G, Gacouin A, Coudroy R, Decavèle M, Sonneville R, et al. Effect of postextubation high-flow nasal oxygen with noninvasive ventilation vs highflow nasal oxygen alone on reintubation among patients at high risk of extubation failure: a randomized clinical trial. JAMA. 2019;322:1465–75.
28. Epstein SK, Ciubotaru RL, Wong JB. Effect of failed extubation on the outcome of mechanical ventilation. Chest. 1997;112:186–92.
29. Sklar MC, Burns K, Rittayamai N, Lanys A, Rauseo M, Chen L, et al. Effort to breathe with various spontaneous breathing trial techniques. A physiologic meta-analysis. Am J Resp Crit Care Med. 2017;195:1477–85.
30. Burns KEA, Soliman I, Adhikari NKJ, Zwein A, Wong JTY, Gomez-Builes C, et al. Trials directly comparing alternative spontaneous breathing trial techniques: a systematic review and meta-analysis. Crit Care. 2017;21(1):127.
31. Cabello B, Thille AW, Roche-Campo F, Brochard L, Gomez FJ, Mancebo J. Physiological comparison of three spontaneous breathing trials in difficult-to-wean patients. Intensive Care Med. 2010;36:1171–9.
32. Fructos-Vivar F, Esteban A. Our paper 20 years later: how has withdrawal from mechanical ventilation changed? Intensive Care Med. 2014;40:1449–59.
33. Kuhn BT, Bradley LA, Dempsey TM, Puro AC, Adams JY. Management of mechanical ventilation in decompensated heart failure. J Cardiovasc Dev Dis. 2016;3:33.
34. Mekontso-Dessap A, Roche-Campo F, Kouatchet A, Tomicic V, Beduneau G, Sonneville R, et al. Natriuretic peptide-driven fluid management during ventilator weaning: a randomized controlled trial. Am J Resp Crit Care Med. 2012;186:1256–63.

Chapter 13
Pathophysiology and Management of Weaning and Extubation Failure

Amanda Pereira Cruz, Nathane Santanna Felix, and Pedro Leme Silva

13.1 What Is Extubation Failure, and Why Is the Weaning Process from Mechanical Ventilation Important?

Weaning from mechanical ventilation (MV), which consists of transition from positive pressure ventilation to spontaneous ventilation, lasts for approximately 40% of the duration of MV and may be one of the most complex issues during MV management [1]. Weaning failure substantially worsens the clinical status of critically ill patients, and it may occur in 20% of high-risk patients (old patients and those with chronic heart, lung, or kidney diseases) [1–4].

The terms “extubation” and “MV weaning” need to be defined. The term extubation refers to the removal of an advanced airway, and it involves factors related only to the airway or the route for invasive ventilatory support. MV weaning describes the gradual removal of positive airway pressure toward completely spontaneous ventilation. In general, and for the sake of simplicity, we refer to extubation as the final step in MV weaning.

The definition of extubation failure is more complex and varies among authors. According to Boles et al. [5], extubation failure is defined as failure of the

A. P. Cruz
Laboratory of Pulmonary Investigation, Institute of Biophysics Carlos Chagas Filho, Federal University of Rio de Janeiro, Rio de Janeiro, Brazil

Gloria D’Or Hospital, D’Or Institute for Research and Education, Rio de Janeiro, Brazil

N. S. Felix
Gloria D’Or Hospital, D’Or Institute for Research and Education, Rio de Janeiro, Brazil

P. L. Silva (✉)
Laboratory of Pulmonary Investigation, Institute of Biophysics Carlos Chagas Filho, Federal University of Rio de Janeiro, Rio de Janeiro, Brazil
e-mail: pedroleme@biof.ufrj.br

A. R. Baptistella et al. (eds.), *Weaning from Mechanical Ventilation*,
https://doi.org/10.1007/978-3-032-01145-9_13

spontaneous breathing test (SBT) or the need for re-intubation within 48 h after extubation. In 2017, a task force within the WIND (Weaning according to a New Definition) study and the REVA (Réseau Européen de Recherche en Ventilation Artificielle) network [2] described successful weaning or separation as extubation without death or re-intubation within the next 7 days, whether post-extubation non-invasive ventilation was used or not, or discharge from the intensive care unit (ICU) without invasive MV (see Chap. 2 for more information).

Regardless of the definition, there is agreement that extubation failure and consequent re-intubation increase MV time, the risk of healthcare-related infections, particularly ventilator-associated pneumonia, and mortality [4].

13.2 Pathophysiology of Extubation Failure

The decision to intubate and initiate MV generally occurs in relation to respiratory failure or not. Respiratory failure, by definition, is characterized by impaired lung function and is the primary cause of intubation with pneumonia or exacerbation of chronic lung diseases. Extubation failure can be related to the primary reason for intubation, likely related to respiratory failure.

When respiratory distress is secondary to an underlying cause, it may or may not have an impact on lung function. Some examples are sepsis, delirium, a heart condition, or acute/chronic kidney failure [6]. It may also be related to impairment of the upper airways. Examples include cases of severe bronchospasms in asthma exacerbations or the inability to protect the upper airways due to neurologic impairment.

Thus, the pathophysiology of extubation failure can be directly associated with the primary reason for respiratory distress. The most common mechanism is generally an imbalance between the force-generating capacity of the respiratory muscles and the load they must face once MV is discontinued. However, failure can occur without respiratory distress, referred to as an unrelated cause of respiratory failure [4].

13.3 Risk Factors for Extubation Failure

The main risk factors for weaning and extubation failures are (1) factors related to the airway, such as upper airway obstruction or difficulty in protecting the upper airway and (2) factors unrelated to the upper airways, such as conditions that lead to changes in gas exchange, respiratory muscle pump disorders, and extrapulmonary causes [3].

13.3.1 Airway-Related Extubation Failure

Extubation failure due to airway failure is associated with loss of defense capabilities or patency of the upper and/or lower airway and can be understood as an inability to breathe without a tracheal tube [7].

13.3.1.1 Superior Airway Obstruction

- Laryngospasm
- Tracheal stenosis
- Tracheomalacia
- Hypersecretion

The main causes of upper airway obstruction or increased upper airway resistance are the presence of an endotracheal tube, tracheal injury such as tracheal stenosis, tracheomalacia, or granulation tissue formation. Flexible bronchoscopy can help with an accurate diagnosis.

Laryngospasm is one of the most common causes of extubation failure. There are few options to prevent this condition, but steroids should be used at least 4 h before extubation in patients who fail a cuff leak test [8].

13.3.1.2 Lack of Airway Protection

- Decreased level of consciousness (neurologic cause)
- Swallowing disability
- Hypersecretion

13.3.2 Non-airway-Related Extubation Failure

13.3.2.1 Gas Exchange Alterations

Some conditions can interfere with gas exchange and make weaning more difficult. Previous lung diseases such as fibrosis and chronic obstructive pulmonary disease (COPD) are involved in impairment of gas exchange. When planning to wean, metabolic disturbance (such as alkalosis) and anemia should be considered and corrected to improve gas exchange.

13.3.2.2 Muscle Pump Insufficiency

Several factors related to critical illness can lead to dysfunction of diaphragmatic muscles. First, the underlying disease can promote a state of increased inflammation and a catabolic state. Distributive shock, mainly septic shock, plays a fundamental role in muscle proteolysis and consequent loss of muscle strength in both peripheral and respiratory muscles. Furthermore, other conditions can generate muscle dysfunction such as hyperglycemia, multiple organ dysfunction, and the use of sedatives and neuromuscular blocks that promote prolonged immobility in bed [9, 10].

Diaphragmatic dysfunction can be induced by MV (DDIMV). DDIMV can be directly associated with weaning and extubation failure. There are several pathophysiologic mechanisms for DDIMV; however, the main mechanisms rely on an imbalance between MV support and patient demand [10].

Insufficient or absent diaphragmatic activity, whether due to sedation or neuromuscular blockade, or even due to MV over-assistance, can lead to muscle atrophy. Over-assistance can be defined as excessive support of MV, whether by pressure, volume, or flow, in response to the patient's demand. This condition prevents the individual from achieving a minimally effective muscle contraction to avoid or minimize the loss of muscle fibers due to disuse. It has been demonstrated that just 18 h of diaphragmatic inactivity can lead to loss of diaphragmatic muscle fibers [11].

On the other hand, excessive diaphragmatic activity induced by under-assistance (i.e., when MV does not fully meet the patient's demand) can lead to muscle injury due to a concentric load, in addition to lung injury due to increased dynamic pulmonary stress. The latter is of particular interest because excessive diaphragmatic load can generate increases in transpulmonary pressure generated by the patient, also known as self-inflicted lung injury (P-SILI).

Goligher et al. [10] demonstrated that lower and upper extremes of diaphragmatic effort, assessed via the fraction of diaphragmatic thickness fraction by ultrasonography, can be a predictor of prolonged MV. The lower and upper extremes of diaphragmatic effort were associated with longer duration of weaning from MV and longer ICU length of stay, in addition to a greater risk of in-hospital complications. In contrast, the authors observed that patients who had adequate diaphragmatic thickness (which was close to breathing at rest) after the first 3 days off MV required less time on MV.

Other variables associated with MV can have a negative influence on the weaning and extubation process, such as positive end-expiratory pressure (PEEP) and even oxygen therapy. PEEP is essential to restore functional residual capacity due to losses caused by sedation and anesthesia during the ICU stay. However, inadequate adjustment can promote diaphragmatic and pulmonary damage, allied to respiratory muscle weakness and greater patient-ventilator asynchrony. Furthermore, excessive or insufficient supply of oxygen therapy during MV may induce tissue damage, promote a pro-oxidative reaction (in cases of excessive supply), or cause injury to tissues and organs due to hypoxia (in cases of insufficient supply).

The pathophysiology of over-assistance and under-assistance in relation to MV parameters is presented in Tables 13.1 and 13.2.

Table 13.1 The pathophysiology of over-assistance and under-assistance

Over-assistance		Under-assistance	
Excessive support	Diaphragm atrophy (reduction in cross-sectional area)	Insufficient support	Concentric diaphragm injury (excessive load)
	Insufficient diaphragm activity (respiratory weakness)		Excessive diaphragm activity
Ventilator-induced lung injury (VILI)	VILI (volutrauma or atelectrauma)	Patient self-inflicted lung injury (P-SILI)	Increase in stress and strain
			Increase in pulmonary transcapillary pressure; pulmonary edema
			Ventilation heterogeneity (pendelluft)
Asynchrony	Ineffective triggering	Asynchrony	Double triggering with breath stacked
	Delayed cycling		Premature cycling (eccentric diaphragm load)
	Excessive flow		Insufficient flow
	Reverse triggering		
Excessive positive end-expiratory pressure (PEEP)	Longitudinal diaphragm atrophy	Insufficient PEEP	Expiratory braking (diaphragmatic reflex due to alveolar instability at end expiration)
	Caudal displacement of the diaphragm appositional zone (reduction in force generation)		
	Diaphragm injury due to overstretch		
Excessive FiO_2	Hyperoxia	Insufficient FiO_2	Hypoxia

Over-assistance, excessive delivery of ventilation parameters. Excessive inspiratory support (pressure, volume, or flow) exceeds the patient's demand, which leads to insufficient diaphragmatic activity and induces diaphragmatic muscle atrophy. The cross-sectional area reduces and, consequently, the force generated decreases. Excessive PEEP can induce diaphragm shortening. This leads to greater mechanical maneuvering of the muscle, which loses its ability to generate force (according to the stretch-tension relationship). A consequence of this particular atrophy is that when PEEP is removed (weaning and extubation), there is a greater risk of a rebound effect with pulmonary edema and diaphragmatic injury due to over-stretch. Over-assistance can cause excessive flow asynchronies (increase in peak inspiratory flow [overshooting], which can be harmful to circulation) and late cycling (when the patient tries to start exhaling, but the mechanical ventilation (MV) does not allow the expiratory valve to open). Excessive adjustment of ventilatory parameters can generate current volumes or pressures above safety values, which may evolve to VILI. Under-assistance can also cause asynchronies. The asynchrony of insufficient flow and premature cycling (the MV interrupts the patient's inspiration by opening the expiratory valve and closing the inspiratory valve) causes eccentric diaphragmatic injury. When the patient is causing a muscle contraction, which in the case of the diaphragm leads to fiber shortening, the MV promotes a fiber stretching mechanism by inducing expiration, leading to eccentric contraction. Diaphragmatic contraction leads to large oscillations in transpulmonary pressure (due to an intense decrease in pleural pressure), which triggers harmful mechanisms related to P-SILI, causing greater lung stress and strain, greater pulmonary transcapillary pressure (promoting sequestration of liquid from the pulmonary capillaries to the alveolar area), greater heterogeneity in the distribution of ventilation (promoting pendelluft, a mechanism of air displacement from nondependent areas to dependent lung areas), and greater regional strain. Excess oxygen leads to hyperoxia, which contributes to the production of reactive oxygen species, inflammation, and risk of absorption atelectasis. Insufficient oxygen settings can lead to hypoxemia, which triggers the brain controllers of respiration followed by increased ventilatory drive. Organic dysfunction can also occur due to tissue hypoxia

Table 13.2 Main indexes, tests, and scores for evaluating extubation success and failure

	Acquisition mode	Respiratory outcomes	Other outcomes	Disadvantages	References
Main predictive integrative index, tests, and scores					
IWI	IWI = [(Cst,rs × SaO_2) (RR/VT ratio)]	≥25 predict weaning success		Patients need to be in controlled ventilation modes Arterial blood gas analysis is needed	[12]
RSBI	RR/VT (liters) in 1 min	<105 predict extubation success			[13]
RISC score	Underweight (body mass index, <18.5 kg/m^2)–1 GCS score prior to CPAP mode ≥ 10–1 MAP <10 after SBT start within 15 min <10–1 Fluid balance 24 h prior to extubation ≥1500 ml–2 Total ventilation days ≥5–3	>4 predict extubation failure within 72 h		A modest value to determine extubation failure (sensitivity of 0.80 and a specificity of 0.54 with AUC of 0.67)	[14]
Peak flow	Measurement done with an external flowmeter or a ventilator Voluntary peak flow—under the investigator stimulus Involuntary peak flow—injection of 3 ml of normal saline or with a suction catheter	>60 L/min		Variability of techniques and instruments makes different cutoffs	[15]
Cuff leak test	Qualitative measurement—deflection of cuff is followed by the detection of air leak sound through the trachea Quantitative measurement—difference between the expired tidal volume with the cuff inflated and with the cuff deflated	≤110 ml or 12% of air leak indicates high risk of extubation failure	The higher the leak, the lower the likelihood that post-extubation stridor will occur	The low sensitivity suggests that a negative test cannot completely exclude post-extubation airway obstruction and that patients still need to be closely monitored post-extubation	[16]

MV ventilation measures					
$P_{0.1}$	Expiratory pause of 0.1 s	≤ −4 indicates higher risk of weaning failure	Independently associated with a higher 90-day mortality and duration of MV	Lack of MV with the $P_{0.1}$ analysis	[17–19]
Pocc	Expiratory pause of 4 s	< −10 can predict a relapse of respiratory failure in MV patients		Lack of MV with expiratory pause in PS Risk of superimposed effort	[18]
$P_{0.1}$ + Pocc		Pocc ≤ − 15 + $P_{0.1}$ ≤ − 4 is associated with a higher risk of relapse of respiratory failure in MV patients			[18]
Diaphragm ultrasound				Moderate interprofessional variability Requires greater professional expertise	

(continued)

Table 13.2 (continued)

	Acquisition mode	Respiratory outcomes	Other outcomes	Disadvantages	References
Tdi	Measured from the center of the pleural line to the center of the peritoneal line, at the end of expiration (Tdi-exp) and then at the end of inspiration (Tdi-insp) in B- and M-modes	≥30% predict weaning success >10% decrease and >10% increase predict weaning failure	Higher risk of remaining on MV for at least 3 weeks Fewer ventilator-free days at day 60 Prolonged duration of MV Prolonged ICU admission Higher risk of reintubation Higher risk of reintubation		[10, 20]
FE (diaphragmatic thickness fraction)	FE = [(Tdi − insp) − (Tdi − exp) / Tdi − exp] × 100	<15% higher duration of MV Between 15% and 30% is associated with the shortest duration of MV <20% predict weaning failure			[3, 10]

DE (diaphragmatic excursion)	Measures the distance that the diaphragm can move during the respiratory cycle	≥10 mm predicts extubation success <10 mm predicts extubation failure <14 mm predicts weaning failure		The assessment during assisted-controlled mode may be overestimated due to the additional presence of pressure applied by the MV in addition to muscle contraction	[20–22]
Posterior lung ultrasound score	LUS assigns 0 points to A lines or < 2 separate B lines plus regular sliding; 1 point with lines B ≥ 3 or spaced focal points plus regular sliding; 2 points with coalescing B lines; and 3 points to pulmonary consolidations with a score ranging from 0 (normal lungs) to 36 (worst case scenario). LUS evaluation has been subsequently integrated with the following four additional parameters: Presence of pleural effusion (cm) (value 0 absent, value 1 present) Presence of pericardial effusions (cm) (value 0 absent, value 1 present) Measurement of the IVC respiratory variation (<0–33%) (value 0 absent, value 1 present) Diaphragm excursion (cm). This last parameter was measured during normal breathing (in O_2 therapy or before non-invasive ventilation, NIV), in M-mode through a right subcostal scan. An excursion >2 ± 0.5 cm was considered as normal (value 0, absent) while the value below as abnormal (value 1, present)	Higher posterior lung US scores are associated with extubation failure			[23]

(continued)

Table 13.2 (continued)

	Acquisition mode	Respiratory outcomes	Other outcomes	Disadvantages	References
EIT				High-cost assessment instrument, requiring an expert professional May be influenced by cardiac artifacts More validation studies are needed	
GI	The sum of the absolute differences between the median value of tidal variation and every pixel value divided by the sum of all impedance values for normalization $GI = \frac{\sum_{x,y\,lung}\left[DI_{xy} - \text{Median}\left(DI_{lung}\right)\right]}{\sum_{x,y\,lung} DI_{xy}}$	Higher GI index (up to 24 h before and after extubation) is associated with SBT failure	Higher values of GI before the start of the SBT on pressure support ventilation in patients failing the SBT		[24]
ΔEELI	The average end-expiratory global impedance values in 10 consecutive breaths	Lower EELI (up to 24 h before and after extubation) is associated with SBT failure			[25, 26]
ΔEELI/VT	The difference of EELI with the tidal volume of five subsequent breathing cycles at the last 1 min before SBT and calculated the average tidal volume (VT)	0.89 in SBT-15 min predicts weaning successful			[24]

$\lvert\Delta(CW–CL)\rvert$	Calculated compliance win (CW) and compliance loss (CL), expressed as a percentage, from the EIT recordings. Compliance change percentage variation ($\lvert\Delta(CW\text{-}CL)\rvert$) was defined as the difference between CW and CL regarding SBT at 5, 15, and 30 min compared to SBT at 0 min	**7.7** in SBT-5 min predicts weaning failure			[24]

Legend: Main predictive integrative index, tests, and scores involve the most traditional predictive instruments of extubation failure or success

IWI = integrative weaning index; RSBI = rapid and shallow breathing index; RISC score = re-intubation summation calculation; MV ventilation measures uses values provided by the VM. P0,1 = airway occlusion pressure in the first 100 ms of inspiration; Pocc = occlusion pressure at the end of expiration. Diaphragm ultrasound provides ultrasound measurements of the diaphragm. Tdi = diaphragmatic thickness; excursion represents the diaphragmatic contraction plus the pressure applied by the ventilator; FE = diaphragmatic thickness fraction. Reflect variation in thickness of the diaphragm during a respiratory effort; DE = diaphragmatic excursion; EIT = electrical impedance tomography; tomographic images evaluated during the respiratory cycle, which provide measurements of pulmonary ventilation distribution. GI = global inhomogeneity index; ΔEELI = end-expiratory lung volume. ΔEELI represents the variation in end-expiratory lung impedance during the SBT. The decrease in ΔEELI suggested that there may be part of the alveoli collapsed or the VT decreased; ΔEELI/VT = relationship between an end-expiratory lung volume and tidal volume; $\lvert\Delta(CW\text{-}CL)\rvert$ = change in compliance change percentage variation. Especially in the early time of SBT, the value of $\lvert\Delta(CW\text{-}CL)\rvert$ with the failure group was more obvious. It may be related to excessive or weak spontaneous breathing. Excessive spontaneous breathing can easily lead to ventilator fatigue and self-induced lung damage, while weak spontaneous breathing may lead to carbon dioxide retention; both excessive and weak spontaneous breathing lead to failed ventilator weaning

13.3.3 Extrapulmonary Causes

In addition to causes of weaning failure related to the respiratory system and gas exchange, extrapulmonary causes must be considered in critically ill patients [27, 28].

Delirium is a common psycho-organic disorder in critically ill patients, and it is associated with a higher risk of prolonged MV and reduced probability of successful extubation [29]. Tools to detect delirium in the ICU have been validated and should be used for early detection. Depression, anxiety, and sleep disturbances are also causes of weaning failure.

Weaning-induced pulmonary edema is caused by transition from a positive pressure to negative pressure ventilation, which creates overloading conditions for the heart. COPD, cardiopathy, and obesity were found to be independent risk factors for weaning-induced pulmonary edema. Treatment includes the removal of fluid to change the result of a passive leg raising test from negative to positive. A positive accumulated fluid balance may be a factor indicative of extubation failure, because pulmonary edema may be difficult to control with the removal of positive pressure ventilation.

Nutritional status also can affect the success of weaning. A low or high body mass index is a risk factor for weaning failure. Malnutrition is common in critically ill patients. Ideally, energetic needs should be determined by indirect calorimetry to prevent under- or over-feeding. As well as a low body mass index, conditions that are related to muscle weakness, such as pre-existing neuromuscular disorders, and advanced age, were also found to be strongly associated with weaning failure in patients who survived their stay in hospital. Metabolic disorders that could interfere with muscle contraction, such as hypophosphatemia, hypomagnesemia, hypokalemia, and hypocalcemia, should be corrected to promote a better weaning process.

Peripheral neuromuscular abnormalities should also be considered in patients who fail the spontaneous breath test. Primary causes of muscle weakness, such as Guillain-Barré syndrome, myasthenia gravis, and motor neuron disease, can interfere with ventilation weaning. However, most cases of neuromuscular dysfunction that complicate weaning result from muscle weakness acquired in the ICU. Critical illness polyneuropathy may affect the diaphragm to some degree, which makes the process of weaning more difficult. Several risk factors for the development of neuromuscular complications in the ICU have been reported, including sepsis, inflammation, age, and prolonged use of neuromuscular blocking agents [30]. The risk factors for extubation failure are summarized in Fig. 13.1.

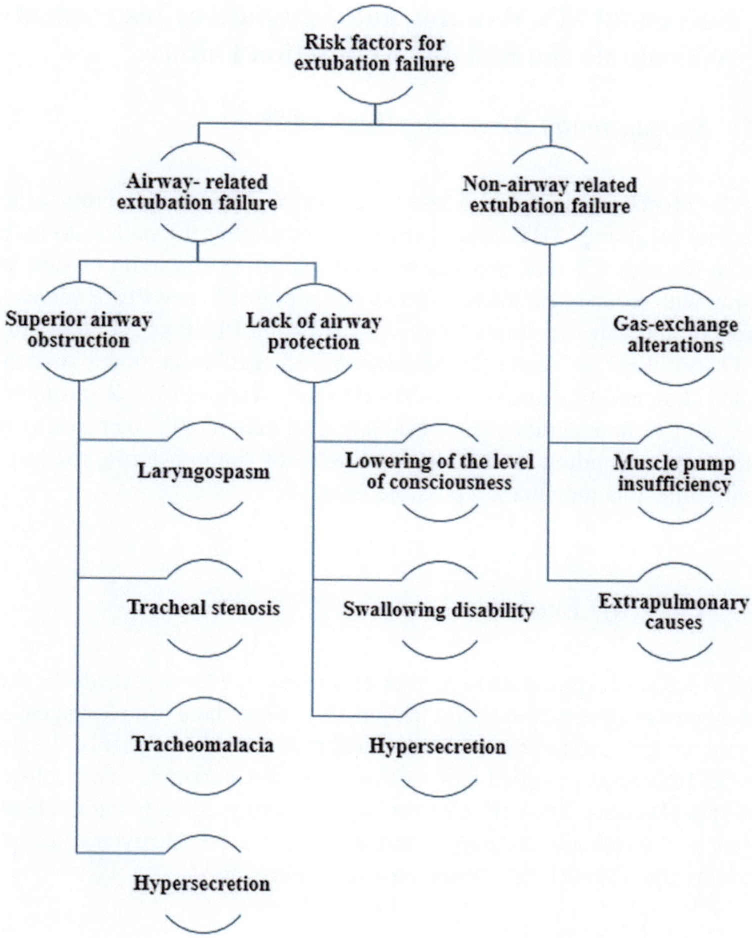

Fig. 13.1 The risk factors for extubation failure may be due to (A) airways, such as superior airway obstruction, the main causes of which are (1) laryngospasm, defined as spasm of the tracheal muscles (may be accompanied by edema); this obstruction can be caused by the presence of the orotracheal tube, considered as a foreign object, associated with pressure stimuli from the cuff, which may lead to local ischemia, in addition to the patient's inherent predisposition; (2) tracheal stenosis, i.e., the formation of collagen tissue due to repetitive injuries leading to a reduction in the diameter of the airway; (3) tracheomalacia, which is also a condition of tissue alteration, but with tracheal laxity and instability during breathing. (B) Lack of airway protection. The main causes are (1) reduced level of consciousness, generally due to neurologic issues such as trauma, sedation, hypoactive delirium, tumor, or brain injury. The Glasgow Coma Scale score ≤ 8 is regularly used to define the need for re-intubation due to the risk of bronchoaspiration; (2) inability to swallow, when the patient partially or completely loses the ability to swallow; (3) hypersecretion due to excessive production of secretion, related to both obstruction and a lack of airway protection. In general, the assessment can be made by identifying tongue mobility, swallowing ability, and coughing (peak expiratory flow). Extubation factors not related to the airways evolve with (1) alteration of gas exchange, such as metabolic acidosis, which can stimulate the neurologic center of ventilation, leading to tachypnea and metabolic alkalosis, leading to depression of the respiratory drive; (2) insufficiency of the respiratory muscle pump, related to weakness or diaphragmatic injury; (3) extrapulmonary causes, which can be understood as any other cause not related to the respiratory system

13.4 Successful MV Weaning and Extubation: Instruments to Evaluate the Risk for Extubation Failure

13.4.1 *Spontaneous Breathing Test*

SBT is the most commonly used test to assess an individual's ability to tolerate spontaneous breathing. SBT usually involves connecting the patient to an orotracheal tube through a T-tube and macro nebulization, or through pressure support ventilation with reduced parameters (pressure support [PS] and PEEP values are not standardized and can vary from PS of 7 cmH_2O and PEEP of 5 cmH_2O to PS of 0 cmH_2O and PEEP of 5 cmH_2O). More advanced ventilation modes such as automatic tube compensation are also described in the literature [31]. Regardless of the protocol, SBT is an essential test for evaluating an individual's tolerance to extubation. However, depending on the minimum level of support during the test or the evaluation time, this may mask a possible failure.

13.4.2 *The Cuff Leak Test*

The cuff leak test was proposed to predict the presence of laryngeal edema and post-extubation airway obstruction [16]. Theoretically, when there is no laryngeal edema, there is an air leak around the tube after deflating the balloon cuff of the endotracheal tube. In contrast, a failed cuff leak test suggests potential airway obstruction from laryngeal edema. The cuff leak test has excellent specificity but moderate sensitivity for post-extubation airway obstruction. That means that even with a positive test, patients should be closely observed after extubation.

13.4.3 *MV Ventilation Measurements ($P_{0,1}$ and $\Delta Pocc$)*

Monitoring the respiratory drive and effort can be useful in assessing the timing of SBT and extubation. For example, progressive increases in esophageal pressure oscillations during SBT can be observed in cases of weaning failure [13]. However, this is rarely done in clinical practice due to the need for a catheter to measure esophageal pressure (to assess diaphragmatic effort) or diaphragmatic electrical activity (EAdi) (to assess the ventilatory drive). Both require time, availability of equipment, and experienced staff [17]. On the other hand, several noninvasive measurements provided by MV are being widely developed and validated in the literature to meet this demand quickly, safely, effectively, and practically.

Recent studies demonstrate that expiratory occlusion measurements have good correlation with the extremes of respiratory effort and drive and with excessive extremes of dynamic pulmonary stress. Thus, occlusion measurements may help to monitor and maintain protective ventilation even in spontaneous ventilation [32, 33]. In addition, the risk of developing ventilator-induced diaphragm dysfunction during spontaneous breathing may be minimized [10].

Occlusion pressure at the end of expiration (**Δ**Pocc) has been described recently; its absolute value or its mathematical derivative, muscle pressure (Pmus), can be used to assess respiratory effort. In addition, **Δ**Pocc can be used to estimate dynamic transpulmonary pressure (Ptp, din). Accordingly, Bertoni et al. [32] showed that Pmus, derived from **Δ**Pocc > 15 cmH_2O, showed good accuracy for excessive values of respiratory effort.

The measurement of occlusion pressure in the first 100 ms at the beginning of inspiration ($P_{0.1}$) helps to infer respiratory drive and effort, so that extreme values may be related to worse outcomes [19]. Moreover, Telias et al. [17] demonstrated that $P_{0.1}$ values >1 and <−3.5 cmH_2O showed good sensitivity and specificity for detecting low and high respiratory effort, respectively.

The validation of noninvasive measurements helps to identify over-assistance and under-assistance in spontaneous MV. Esnault et al. [18] showed that excessive $P_{0.1}$ and ΔPocc values are associated with a high risk of weaning failure in patients with COVID-19. $P_{0.1}$ values <−4 cmH_2O and **Δ**Pocc < −15 cmH_2O were associated with a new episode of respiratory failure during the weaning process. De Vries et al. [33] carried out a secondary analysis of two previous studies and observed that $P_{0.1}$ and **Δ**Pocc had excellent accuracy in detecting low and high respiratory effort. Furthermore, by using respective mathematical derivatives, both provided good accuracy for detecting high dynamic pulmonary stress. Recently, Le Marec et al. [19] identified a higher prevalence of dyspnea in patients with high $P_{0.1}$, which was an independent risk factor for longer MV time and 90-day mortality. Furthermore, when the patient had $P_{0.1}$ values <−3.5 cmH_2O at ICU admission, survival was lower at 90 days. These results reinforce the need for further studies to analyze the influence of respiratory effort in critically ill patients on their weaning process from MV.

13.4.4 Impedance Electrical Tomography

Impedance electrical tomography (EIT) is a noninvasive bedside tool that provides real-time images of the ventilation. Around 16–32 electrodes are positioned around the chest, applying low alternating current between pairs of electrodes, which results in a reconstructed image of a given moment of breathing [34]. In general, EIT allows visualization of regional collapse and over-distention in ventilation distribution, unlike many monitoring techniques and resources, where the variables can only provide a global view of ventilation in a static (or quasi-static) mode of the respiratory system.

Considering the importance of monitoring ventilation distribution during spontaneous breathing, EIT can provide more precise monitoring during weaning from MV and has the potential to be a predictor of extubation success or failure. In addition, it may allow rapid identification of possible mechanisms of P-SILI, such as a heterogeneous distribution of ventilation and pendelluft. It may also indicate possible under-assistance of ventilation and a greater risk of factors associated with non-airway-related extubation failure, such as the primary cause of endotracheal intubation and initiation of MV, dysfunction of the respiratory muscle pump, and gas exchange disorders [35]. Wisse et al. [35] evaluated the SBT process. The authors adapted the patient to a continuous positive airway pressure of 2 cmH_2O, no PS, and FiO_2 adjusted to SpO_2 between 92% and 94% for 30 min. Overall, there was a reduction in ΔEELI (end-expiratory lung impedance) during SBT. Furthermore, the group who failed the SBT showed an increase in the heterogeneity index (gradient index [GI]) at the beginning and the end of the 30 min of SBT compared with the group with a successful SBT.

Considering that the ΔEELI is the variation in impedance at the end of expiration in the lungs while the GI allows the heterogeneity of ventilation within the lung to be quantified, both give an idea of the distribution of ventilation. Thus, those patients who failed the SBT had greater lung de-recruitment and lack of homogeneity during the process. One point to be evaluated is the short SBT time (30 min), which contrasts with the previous literature (120 min). The authors explained that a long time period may predispose to EIT artifacts and noises due to patient and belt movements and reapplication of contact agent on the EIT belt [35].

Joussellin et al. [23] compared the regional ventilation distribution by EIT in patients before and after extubation. The authors noted that patients who progressed to extubation failure had a greater loss of lung aeration after extubation. Although discreet, their results showed that both the increase in GI and regional ventilation delay may indicate that extubation failure is associated with inhomogeneous ventilation distribution. Furthermore, the authors suggested that, at the end of SBT, these changes were associated with a decrease in tidal volume and lung compliance, likely reflecting a situation of respiratory muscle weakness at the time of weaning.

Regardless of how ventilatory assistance is assessed at the bedside, it is commonly understood that its extremes, whether over-assistance or under-assistance, are related to a greater risk of extubation failure. This can be due to possible diaphragmatic dysfunction as a result of disuse and atrophy, or likely lung and diaphragm injuries induced by the patient's extreme effort.

13.5 Conclusions

The timing of MV removal can be an extremely demanding challenge for clinicians. Failure to wean from MV and extubation has a significant negative impact on the patient, with an increased risk of morbidity and mortality. The causes related to failure are diverse and may involve airway, non-airway factors and extrapulmonary causes, especially when the patient is subjected to over- or under-assistance during MV.

Prevention of this event is essential and can be done through multifactorial assessment, such as early identification of patients with higher non-modifiable risk factors such as advanced age and the presence of comorbidities such as heart failure and COPD. Other factors include the clinical status of the patient, such as the prevention and treatment of delirium, metabolic disorders, and water balance. Furthermore, some resources can be used, such as some measurements predicted by MV and advanced instruments such as diaphragmatic ultrasonography and bioimpedance tomography.

The spectrum of causes of extubation failure should be identified and treated promptly. Systematic protocols should be used to evaluate risk factors, prepare and correctly apply the SBT, and assess post-extubation care with rapid re-intubation in cases of failure. More studies are needed to evaluate the effects of systematic protocols.

References

1. Pham T, Heunks L, Bellani G, et al. Weaning from mechanical ventilation in intensive care units across 50 countries (WEAN SAFE): a multicentre, prospective, observational cohort study. Lancet Respir Med. 2023;11:465–76. https://doi.org/10.1016/S2213-2600(22)00449-0.
2. Béduneau G, Pham T, Schortgen F, et al. Epidemiology of weaning outcome according to a new definition. The WIND study. Am J Respir Crit Care Med. 2017;195:772–83. https://doi.org/10.1164/rccm.201602-0320OC.
3. Jung B, Vaschetto R, Jaber S. Ten tips to optimize weaning and extubation success in the critically ill. Intensive Care Med. 2020;46:2461. https://doi.org/10.1007/s00134-020-06300-2.
4. Thille AW, Richard J-CM, Brochard L. The decision to extubate in the intensive care unit. Am J Respir Crit Care Med. 2013;187:1294–302. https://doi.org/10.1164/rccm.201208-1523CI.
5. Boles J-M, Bion J, Connors A, et al. Weaning from mechanical ventilation. Eur Respir J. 2007;29:1033–56. https://doi.org/10.1183/09031936.00010206.
6. Heunks LM, Van den Hoeven JG. Clinical review: the ABC of weaning failure – a structured approach. Crit Care. 2010;14(6):245. https://doi.org/10.1186/cc9296.
7. Jaber S, Quintard H, Cinotti R, et al. Risk factors and outcomes for airway failure versus non-airway failure in the intensive care unit: a multicenter observational study of 1514 extubation procedures. Crit Care. 2018;22:236. https://doi.org/10.1186/s13054-018-2150-6.
8. Fan E, Zakhary B, Amaral A, et al. Liberation from mechanical ventilation in critically ill adults. An official ATS/ACCP clinical practice guideline. Ann Am Thorac Soc. 2017;14:441–3. https://doi.org/10.1513/AnnalsATS.201612-993CME.
9. Bureau C, Van Hollebeke M, Dres M. Managing respiratory muscle weakness during weaning from invasive ventilation. Eur Respir Rev. 2023;32:220205. https://doi.org/10.1183/16000617.0205-2022.
10. Goligher EC, Dres M, Fan E, et al. Mechanical ventilation-induced diaphragm atrophy strongly impacts clinical outcomes. Am J Respir Crit Care Med. 2018;197:204–13. https://doi.org/10.1164/rccm.201703-0536OC.
11. Levine S, Nguyen T, Taylor N, et al. Rapid disuse atrophy of diaphragm fibers in mechanically ventilated humans. N Engl J Med. 2008;358:1327–35. https://doi.org/10.1056/NEJMoa070447.
12. Nemer SN, Barbas CSV, Caldeira JB, et al. A new integrative weaning index of discontinuation from mechanical ventilation. Crit Care. 2009;13:R152. https://doi.org/10.1186/cc8051.
13. Jubran A, Grant BJB, Laghi F, et al. Weaning prediction. Am J Respir Crit Care Med. 2005;171:1252–9. https://doi.org/10.1164/rccm.200503-356OC.

14. Bansal V, Smischney NJ, Kashyap R, et al. Reintubation summation calculation: a predictive score for extubation failure in critically ill patients. Front Med. 2022;8:789440. https://doi.org/10.3389/fmed.2021.789440.
15. Duan J, Zhang X, Song J. Predictive power of extubation failure diagnosed by cough strength: a systematic review and meta-analysis. Crit Care. 2021;25:357. https://doi.org/10.1186/s13054-021-03781-5.
16. Kuriyama A, Jackson JL, Kamei J. Performance of the cuff leak test in adults in predicting post-extubation airway complications: a systematic review and meta-analysis. Crit Care. 2020;24:640. https://doi.org/10.1186/s13054-020-03358-8.
17. Telias I, Junhasavasdikul D, Rittayamai N, et al. Airway occlusion pressure as an estimate of respiratory drive and inspiratory effort during assisted ventilation. Am J Respir Crit Care Med. 2020;201:1086–98. https://doi.org/10.1164/rccm.201907-1425OC.
18. Esnault P, Cardinale M, Hraiech S, et al. High respiratory drive and excessive respiratory efforts predict relapse of respiratory failure in critically ill patients with COVID-19. Am J Respir Crit Care Med. 2020;202:1173–8. https://doi.org/10.1164/rccm.202005-1582LE.
19. Le Marec J, Hajage D, Decavèle M, et al. High airway occlusion pressure is associated with dyspnea and increased mortality in critically ill mechanically ventilated patients. Am J Respir Crit Care Med. 2024;210:201–10. https://doi.org/10.1164/rccm.202308-1358OC.
20. Qian Z, Yang M, Li L, Chen Y. Ultrasound assessment of diaphragmatic dysfunction as a predictor of weaning outcome from mechanical ventilation: a systematic review and meta-analysis. BMJ Open. 2018;8:e021189. https://doi.org/10.1136/bmjopen-2017-021189.
21. Spadaro S, Grasso S, Mauri T, et al. Can diaphragmatic ultrasonography performed during the T-tube trial predict weaning failure? The role of diaphragmatic rapid shallow breathing index. Crit Care. 2016;20:305. https://doi.org/10.1186/s13054-016-1479-y.
22. Palkar A, Mayo P, Singh K, et al. Serial diaphragm ultrasonography to predict successful discontinuation of mechanical ventilation. Lung. 2018;196:363–8. https://doi.org/10.1007/s00408-018-0106-x.
23. Joussellin V, Bonny V, Spadaro S, et al. Lung aeration estimated by chest electrical impedance tomography and lung ultrasound during extubation. Ann Intensive Care. 2023;13:91. https://doi.org/10.1186/s13613-023-01180-3.
24. Li J, Zeng F, Yang F, et al. Electrical impedance tomography predicts weaning success in adult patients with delayed upper abdominal surgery: a single-center retrospective study. Front Med (Lausanne). 2021;8:748493. https://doi.org/10.3389/fmed.2021.748493.
25. Longhini F, Maugeri J, Andreoni C, et al. Electrical impedance tomography during spontaneous breathing trials and after extubation in critically ill patients at high risk for extubation failure: a multicenter observational study. Ann Intensive Care. 2019;9:88. https://doi.org/10.1186/s13613-019-0565-0.
26. Lima JNG, Fontes MS, Szmuszkowicz T, et al. Electrical impedance tomography monitoring during spontaneous breathing trial: physiological description and potential clinical utility. Acta Anaesthesiol Scand. 2019;63:1019–27. https://doi.org/10.1111/aas.13383.
27. Akella P, Voigt LP, Chawla S. To wean or not to wean: a practical patient focused guide to ventilator weaning. J Intensive Care Med. 2022;37:1417–25. https://doi.org/10.1177/08850666221095436.
28. Liu J, Shen F, Teboul J-L, et al. Cardiac dysfunction induced by weaning from mechanical ventilation: incidence, risk factors, and effects of fluid removal. Crit Care. 2016;20:369. https://doi.org/10.1186/s13054-016-1533-9.
29. Doorduin J, van der Hoeven JG, Heunks LMA. The differential diagnosis for failure to wean from mechanical ventilation. Curr Opin Anaesthesiol. 2016;29:150–7. https://doi.org/10.1097/ACO.0000000000000297.
30. Hermans G, Van den Berghe G. Clinical review: intensive care unit acquired weakness. Crit Care. 2015;19:274. https://doi.org/10.1186/s13054-015-0993-7.
31. Guérin C, Terzi N, Mezidi M, et al. Low-pressure support vs automatic tube compensation during spontaneous breathing trial for weaning. Ann Intensive Care. 2019;9:137. https://doi.org/10.1186/s13613-019-0611-y.

32. Bertoni M, Telias I, Urner M, et al. A novel non-invasive method to detect excessively high respiratory effort and dynamic transpulmonary driving pressure during mechanical ventilation. Crit Care. 2019;23:346. https://doi.org/10.1186/s13054-019-2617-0.
33. de Vries HJ, Tuinman PR, Jonkman AH, et al. Performance of noninvasive airway occlusion maneuvers to assess lung stress and diaphragm effort in mechanically ventilated critically ill patients. Anesthesiology. 2023;138:274–88. https://doi.org/10.1097/ALN.0000000000004467.
34. Heines SJH, Becher TH, van der Horst ICC, Bergmans DCJJ. Clinical applicability of electrical impedance tomography in patient-tailored ventilation: a narrative review. Tomography. 2023;9:1903–32. https://doi.org/10.3390/tomography9050150.
35. Wisse JJ, Goos TG, Jonkman AH, et al. Electrical impedance tomography as a monitoring tool during weaning from mechanical ventilation: an observational study during the spontaneous breathing trial. Respir Res. 2024;25:179. https://doi.org/10.1186/s12931-024-02801-6.

Chapter 14
Intensive Care Unit-Acquired Weakness (ICU-AW) and Weaning

Daniel Lago Borges, Mayara Gabrielle Barbosa Borges, and Stefany Alves Furtado

14.1 Introduction

Muscular dysfunction that develops during severe illness, commonly known as intensive care unit-acquired weakness (ICU-AW), significantly influences various clinical outcomes, including weaning from mechanical ventilation (MV), duration of ICU and hospital stays, physical functioning, and mortality [1, 2]. In the initial week of an ICU stay, muscle mass can decrease by around 2%–4% daily [3, 4].

ICU-AW represents a frequent complication of critical illnesses with a multifaceted origin, impacting both limb and respiratory muscles [5]. Patients with multiple organ failure typically experience a more marked reduction in limb muscle mass [3], whereas fast declines in diaphragm muscle strength and thickness are linked to sepsis [6] and decreased diaphragm contractile activity [4].

Efforts to prevent or manage ICU-AW are limited and primarily concentrate on addressing or mitigating factors known to be associated with ICU-AW, such as hyperglycemia, catabolism, sepsis, use of neuromuscular blocking agents (NMBA), and corticosteroids [3]. Moreover, immobility and lack of physical activity significantly contribute to muscle wasting [7]. Therefore, reversing muscle inactivity holds promise for preventing, reversing, or improving muscle degradation [8].

D. L. Borges · M. G. B. Borges (✉)
University Hospital of Federal University of Maranhão, São Luís, Maranhão, Brazil

S. A. Furtado
Health Department of the State of Pernambuco, Garanhuns, Pernambuco, Brazil

A. R. Baptistella et al. (eds.), *Weaning from Mechanical Ventilation*,
https://doi.org/10.1007/978-3-032-01145-9_14

14.2 Pathophysiology of ICU-AW

ICU-AW is a common issue in critically ill patients, with the implication that this neuromuscular dysfunction lacks a plausible etiology beyond critical illness and its treatments. Additionally, the literature also highlights a spectrum of disability, where the degree of disability is linked to differences in pre-morbid functional status, the burden of comorbid illness, and the nature and duration of critical illness. The cellular signaling networks and molecular mechanisms that regulate the development and persistence of ICU-AW are not fully understood but appear to be complex [9].

ICU-AW is largely related to damage caused by the systemic inflammatory response syndrome (SIRS), which affects the morphology and physiology of skeletal muscles and their conduction system. Axonal depolarization occurs due to microvascular changes, leading to hypoperfusion of small nerve capillaries and reduced oxygen delivery (DO_2), resulting in the accumulation of acidic metabolites, such as endotoxins and pro-inflammatory agents released during sepsis or SIRS [10].

The reduction in muscle function and weakness primarily results from an imbalance between muscle protein synthesis and lysis, leading to significant muscle loss and maintaining a catabolic state [11].

Several factors were examined for their association with myopathy: molecular factors, such as interleukin-6 (IL-6), C-reactive protein (CRP), and insulin-like growth factor binding protein 1 (IGFBP-1); serum osmolarity; drugs (norepinephrine, dobutamine, hydrocortisone, aminoglycosides, analgesics, sedatives, and NMBA); and multisystem factors, assessed by Simplified Acute Physiology Scores (SAPS-2) and Sequential Organ Failure Assessment (SOFA) [11].

The role of IL-6 and other cytokines in muscle dysfunction is still unclear. However, IL-6 is also associated with proteolysis and myosin loss. Among patients with chronic inflammatory conditions/diseases, serum IL-6 is related to muscle loss and dysfunction. In ICU patients, IL-6 may not be related to disease severity but can be predictive of mortality [12].

Corticosteroid treatment has been associated with the development of ICU-AW, particularly in mechanically ventilated patients. Although corticosteroids attenuate systemic inflammation and improve hypoxemia, they induce catabolic effects on skeletal muscles. Additionally, treatment with NMBA may be associated with muscle weakness because it causes complete muscle disuse, which can contribute to ICU-AW [11].

The frequent association between myopathy and neuropathy has led to the central theory that critical illness polyneuropathy (CIP) and critical illness myopathy (CIM) are not isolated events but integral parts of the process leading to multiple organ dysfunction syndrome (MODS) in critically ill patients. In this context, neurogenic and myogenic changes of varying severity and progression over time would be linked [13].

CIP is characterized by a symmetric distal sensorimotor axonal alteration that affects the respiratory and limb muscles, as well as sensory and autonomic nerves.

Proposed causes for muscle destruction include chemokine-induced muscle autophagy, muscle membrane inexcitability, acquisition of channelopathies or direct toxicity, and effects of ICU care, including corticosteroids or NMBA. It is increasingly recognized that muscle atrophy, CIM, and CIP are not necessarily distinct entities but likely constitute an overlapping spectrum triggered by an acute inflammatory response, often occurring simultaneously [9].

There are multifaceted factors leading to skeletal muscle atrophy in critically ill patients, including prolonged bed rest, catabolic signaling (including pro-inflammation and insulin resistance), and malnutrition through low caloric and protein intake. Insufficient caloric intake generally compromises proteins, leading to reduced protein synthesis [14].

To compensate for the increased protein needs of the body during critical illnesses, skeletal muscle degradation is increased to provide amino acids for the synthesis of other proteins that may be necessary for immune function, for example, resulting in muscle atrophy. On the other hand, bed rest, regardless of illness, can result in muscle loss. Reduced blood flow is related to decreased amino acid delivery to skeletal muscle. Given the extent of bed rest combined with accelerated catabolic processes in a critically ill patient, reduced delivery of amino acids to skeletal muscle would likely contribute extensively to muscle loss [15].

14.3 Diagnosis of ICU-AW

14.3.1 Evaluation of Peripheral Muscle Strength

The diagnosis of ICU-AW is clinical, involving the manual evaluation of peripheral muscle strength or using handgrip dynamometry (HGD). ICU-AW symmetrically affects all limbs, impacting proximal muscles more than distal ones. Deep tendon reflexes may be reduced or unchanged; respiratory muscles are variably affected, while facial and extraocular muscles generally remain intact. These characteristics, along with their onset after "exposure to critical illness" and ICU admission, distinguish ICU-AW from other neuromuscular disorders that instead lead to ICU admission [16].

For the evaluation of muscle strength aimed at diagnosing ICU-AW, patients must be adequately awake and cooperative. In the classic study by De Jonghe and colleagues [17], after 7 days of MV, patients were screened daily for muscle strength evaluation based on their responses to the following five commands: "Open (close) your eyes," "Look at me," "Open your mouth and stick out your tongue," "Nod your head," and "Raise your eyebrows when I count to 5." The appropriate time for assessment was considered the first day the patient responded to at least three of these commands in two consecutive evaluations within a 6-h interval.

The total score of the Medical Research Council sum score (MRCss) is considered the gold standard for diagnosing ICU-AW. For this assessment, the MRC scale is applied to six muscle groups bilaterally, scoring from 0 to 5 for each tested movement (Table 14.1). ICU-AW is diagnosed when the sum score is 48 or less. MRCss less than 36 identifies a more severe form of ICU-AW; however, even a mild reduction in limb muscle strength with an MRCss of less than 55 is associated with increased long-term morbidity and mortality [16].

HGD is a simple and repeatable test that assesses the strength of the dominant hand in cooperative patients. Dominant HGD values below 11 kg in men and 7 kg in women strongly suggest the diagnosis of ICU-AW and can be used for rapid detection, which should be confirmed with MRCss. Handgrip strength is also independently associated with poor in-hospital prognosis and can serve as a simple test to identify ICU-AW [11].

14.3.2 Electrophysiological Tests and Muscle Biopsy

Conducting neurophysiological tests or muscle biopsies in critically ill patients remains challenging. The presence of tissue edema and electrical interference theoretically reduces the accuracy of nerve conduction studies (NCS) in ICU patients, although the extent to which these concerns affect the diagnosis is unknown [18].

Electrophysiological testing of peripheral nerves and muscles can reveal neuromuscular electrical abnormalities before weakness occurs and is essential not only for differentiating CIP from CIM but also for distinguishing them from other acute neuromuscular disorders. Among NCS, the simplified peroneal nerve test (PENT) can detect a reduction in the amplitude of the common peroneal nerve compound muscle action potential (CMAP) and has been validated in two multicenter studies as a screening method to identify CIM or CIP with 100% sensitivity and high specificity of 85.2%. Stimulation occurs through an active electrode placed on the belly of the extensor digitorum brevis muscle, and the recording electrode is placed on its distal tendon. In the presence of polyneuropathy or myopathy, CMAP amplitude is reduced [18].

Table 14.1 MRC Scale and movements tested for the MRC sum score

MRC	Description
0	No visible contraction
1	Visible contraction, but no limb movement
2	Active movement, but not against gravity
3	Active movement against gravity
4	Active movement against gravity and resistance
5	Active movement against full resistance
Upper limbs	**Lower limbs**
Shoulder abduction Elbow flexion Wrist extension	Hip flexion Knee extension Ankle dorsiflexion

To differentiate between CIP and CIM, other characteristics should be evaluated. For example, a sensory nerve action potential (SNAP) can be recorded in the sural or median nerve, and a decreased amplitude of both CMAP and SNAP indicates polyneuropathy, as it signifies injury to both motor and sensory nerves. Conversely, a delayed muscle contraction with a normal SNAP suggests myopathy [18].

Altered electrical excitability of nerves and muscles is associated with increased long-term mortality, independent of muscle weakness. The PENT remains the best test to diagnose CIP and/or CIM in all uncooperative patients [19].

Muscle biopsy may be necessary in these cases to clarify the pathological diagnosis and provide additional prognostic information. For example, muscle necrosis usually indicates a poor prognosis, while myopathy with myosin filament loss is associated with better functional recovery. A biopsy of the motor nerve from the gracilis muscle can be considered for research purposes or complex differential diagnoses. Coagulopathy, lack of trained pathologists for interpretation, cost, and patient refusal due to pain limit the utility of routine muscle biopsy [18].

14.3.3 Ultrasonography

Ultrasonography (USG) of the limbs' nerves and muscles is a noninvasive bedside technique that can be used for daily monitoring of muscle changes.

Although the predictive validity of USG has not yet been fully evaluated, it has been sensitive in identifying changes in muscle density, such as a daily reduction of 1.6%–6% in the quadriceps muscle density. Puthucheary and colleagues described that patients with multiple organ dysfunction experienced muscle mass loss throughout their ICU stay, with an average reduction of 17% in the cross-sectional area of the quadriceps by the tenth day of ICU stay. This study concluded that the loss was greater in the group with more than one organ dysfunction and that there is rapid and early degradation within the first week of critical illness [3].

In quantitative evaluation, a modality that can differentiate muscle tissue from fibrous tissue and intramuscular fat is used, utilizing a feature of the ultrasound device called echogenicity. In quantitative evaluation, the following modalities can be used: cross-sectional area, muscle thickness, and pennation angle [20]. Reductions of 20% in muscle thickness, 10% in cross-sectional area, 5% in pennation angle, and an increase in echogenicity of at least 8% seem reasonable indicators of ICU-AW, although this technique has not been standardized and no clear threshold has been determined yet [11].

Diaphragmatic ultrasonography complements the evaluation of ICU-acquired diaphragmatic weakness (DW) since this condition accompanies ICU-AW. It is still unclear whether these are two distinct entities or parts of the same syndrome. DW translates into a reduced ability of the diaphragm to generate pressure, a decrease in diaphragm thickness, and a reduced thickening fraction after the initiation of MV. Diaphragm excursion on muscular ultrasonography less than 11 mm during normal breathing and a diaphragm thickening fraction on muscular ultrasonography less than 20% are indicative [21].

14.4 Impact of ICU-AW on Weaning

ICU-AW has been diagnosed in up to 67% of patients with prolonged ventilation and appears to be both the cause and consequence of extended MV. In fact, respiratory muscle weakness due to CIP or CIM impairs weaning from MV, while the risk of developing ICU-AW increases with the duration of MV exposure [19].

Critically ill patients frequently receive sedatives while in the ICU, especially on MV. Deep sedation and paralysis lead to more severe muscle weakness, likely due to the concomitant immobility these drugs cause. However, the burden of muscle loss and weakness during critical illness is not limited to limb muscles. The diaphragm is also affected by muscle loss and weakness, leading to prolonged MV, impacting on ventilator liberation [11].

Over the last decade, clinical efforts and research have focused almost entirely on ICU-acquired limb muscle weakness, with little emphasis on the diaphragm. This may be due to a lack of knowledge about the effects of critical illness on respiratory muscles or the limited availability of tools to assess and monitor diaphragm function in ICU patients. However, several recent studies have shown that severe ICU-acquired diaphragmatic weakness develops in a large percentage of patients on MV in the ICU [22].

When DW is found in mechanically ventilated patients, it is crucial to first exclude the presence of easily treatable endocrine and electrolyte disorders such as hypophosphatemia, hypomagnesemia, and hypocalcemia. Severe diaphragmatic dysfunction can occur in hypothyroidism, and sometimes the primary manifestation of this disease can be respiratory failure due to respiratory muscle weakness. Prolonged hyperglycemia, severe malnutrition, untreated severe renal failure, the use of NMBA, and sustained administration of high-dose corticosteroids can all contribute to reduced muscle strength in a subset of mechanically ventilated ICU patients [22].

Most DW in ICU patients, however, is not a consequence of easily treatable conditions. In many cases, diaphragmatic dysfunction is believed to occur primarily as a consequence of MV itself (ventilator-induced diaphragmatic dysfunction [VIDD]). There is also strong evidence that other processes besides VIDD, including sepsis and other systemic infections, are responsible for many cases of ICU-acquired diaphragmatic weakness [22].

Limb and respiratory muscle weakness have been identified as independent predictors of prolonged MV need. Limb muscle weakness at the time of extubation has been independently associated with higher rates of extubation failure in clinical patients. Among predominantly surgical patients with limb muscle weakness, 80% also exhibited diaphragmatic dysfunction. Extubation failed in 50% of these cases, with reintubation required within 72 h, and 50% of these patients died in the ICU [9].

Controlled MV with complete unloading of the diaphragm causes significant atrophy of diaphragm myofibers within a few hours. Conversely, excessive diaphragm loading is associated with high levels of inspiratory effort, increased inflammation, edema, and injury to diaphragm myofibers. While disuse atrophy and muscle fiber injuries are likely linked, they represent two distinct insults to the diaphragm, with the latter appearing to be a more immediate phenomenon. The associations do not necessarily reflect causality. Weak patients were less likely to achieve early weaning from MV, early ICU discharge, and early hospital discharge than non-weak patients [9].

14.5 Prevention Strategies for ICU-AW

Search for prevention strategies for ICU-AW is crucial to mitigate the deleterious effects of this condition, promote functional recovery, and improve patients' quality of life after hospital discharge. For this reason, a mnemonic was created using the word "FRAQUEZA" (weakness in Portuguese) to provide step-by-step guidance to avoid the detrimental effects of ICU-AW [20]. Here we present an adapted version of this mnemonic using the word "WEAKNESS" (Table 14.2).

In this chapter, each of these strategies will be systematically addressed in detail.

14.5.1 Weapons for Screening and Diagnosing Functionality

Functional evaluation is fundamental for diagnosing ICU-AW. In this context, three main pillars should be considered: muscle mass, muscle strength, and mobility.

The loss of muscle mass is a critical factor in the development of ICU-AW. Among the various methods to assess it, USG stands out. This evaluation method offers

Table 14.2 Bundle of strategies to prevent ICU-acquired weakness (ICU-AW) [20]

Weapons for screening and diagnosing functionality
Examination of nutritional risk and periodic reassessment
Adapted protein and energy adequacy
Keep muscle quantity and quality
Nuanced use of sedatives, opioids, and neuromuscular blockers
Exercises and early mobility
Scope of control and glycemic variability
Seamless mechanical ventilation from start to finish

several advantages: it is portable, radiation-free, low-cost, and highly reproducible both inter-evaluator and intra-evaluator [23].

Muscle strength can be assessed through HGD or MRC-ss. Although HGD directly measures only hand strength, it can extrapolate the assessment to a global dimension. It provides reference values according to age and gender [24] and through anthropometric measurements [25].

Lastly, mobility can be evaluated using scales such as the ICU Mobility Scale (IMS), with scores ranging from 0 to 10, as shown in Table 14.3 [26].

Thus, following this triad (lean mass, strength, and mobility), a functional evaluation can be conducted, allowing for the development of an effective multidisciplinary therapeutic plan.

14.5.2 Examination of Nutritional Risk and Periodic Reassessment

Nutritional planning in combating ICU-AW involves a structured approach that includes nutritional screening, assessment, and periodic reassessment. This strategy aims to establish a care pathway to identify and treat malnutrition and its early signs, using nutritional evaluation as a guide for individual decisions. Maintaining this care pathway is crucial as nutritional risk is a significant indicator of malnutrition, necessitating an early and planned approach for high-risk patients [14, 27].

Nutritional screening should be performed on all patients upon hospital admission to identify those who are malnourished or at risk of malnutrition, and to predict clinical outcomes and complications in a noninvasive and cost-effective manner [28, 29]. Patients at high nutritional risk exhibit greater loss of lean mass,

Table 14.3 ICU Mobility Scale [26]

0	Nothing (lying in bed)
1	Sitting in bed, exercising in bed
2	Passively moved to chair (no standing)
3	Sitting on the edge of the bed
4	Standing
5	Transferring from bed to chair
6	Marching on spot (at bedside)
7	Walking with the assistance of two or more people
8	Walking with the assistance of one person
9	Walking independently with a gait aid
10	Walking independently without a gait aid

highlighting the importance of screening tools such as the NRS 2002 and the NUTRIC score, especially in ICUs [28–30].

Nutritional assessment complements screening and follows defined protocols, such as the Subjective Global Assessment and the GLIM method [31, 32]. Periodic reassessment of nutritional status during hospitalization is essential due to variations in clinical condition and dietary intake [27]. An efficient screening system significantly contributes to nutritional diagnosis and the implementation of necessary interventions within a treatment and rehabilitation plan [14].

14.5.3 Adapted Protein and Energy Adequacy

Individualizing nutritional therapy with an emphasis on energy and protein provision, varying according to the treatment phase and the patient's metabolic condition, is fundamental [20]. This approach should be implemented gradually over 3–4 days of admission to avoid refeeding syndrome and inhibition of autophagy [33–36].

Moreover, preventing cumulative energy deficits during ICU stay is crucial. An accumulated deficit of 1000 kcal approximately doubles the risk of ICU-AW and malnutrition at ICU discharge [37]. Despite recommendations for the use of indirect calorimetry to assess energy needs, its availability is limited, leading to the use of predictive equations as a viable alternative [30, 38, 39].

14.5.4 Keep Muscle Quantity and Quality

The reduction of muscle mass, with a prevalence ranging from 20% to 70% among ICU admissions, is a complex clinical challenge associated with adverse outcomes, such as prolonged hospital stay and MV [15, 40]. The cause is multifactorial, including prolonged bed rest, intense catabolic response, and insulin resistance, necessitating comprehensive interventions that address both physical and nutritional rehabilitation [20, 34].

Accurately assessing lean mass loss and muscle strength in critically ill patients is challenging, mainly due to fluid retention and the ability to cooperate. Practically, for cooperative patients, functional tests are recommended, which can be confirmed with imaging exams. For patients with cognitive impairment (sedation, delirium, etc.), non-volitional strategies should be used, such as computed tomography at the L3 level, ultrasonography of the quadriceps femoris, and phase angle assessment through bioelectrical impedance analysis [20].

14.5.5 Nuanced Use of Sedatives, Opioids, and Neuromuscular Blockers

ICU patients undergoing MV often require heightened sedation due to factors like inflammation, respiratory drive, and potential neurological issues [41, 42]. Optimal sedation levels are determined based on individual clinical conditions, assessed through scales like Ramsay or Richmond Sedation-Agitation Scale (RASS), and sophisticated monitoring tools as bispectral index [43–45].

Current sedation and analgesia guidelines prioritize lighter sedation to avoid adverse events, prolonged ICU stays, and economic burdens [46]. Adherence to protocol-driven guidelines, aided by tools such as sedation scales and pain assessments, enhances precision and cost-effectiveness in sedation management [47, 48].

Preference is given to maintaining patients at superficial sedation levels (RASS −1 to 0), while deeper sedation (RASS −4 to −5) is warranted for severe conditions like acute respiratory distress syndrome (ARDS) or when neuromuscular blockade is needed. Common sedatives include benzodiazepines or propofol, with cautious consideration of their effects on patient cognition and the risk of complications like propofol infusion syndrome [49, 50]. Neuromuscular blockade, employed for hypoxemia management and ventilation support, requires careful administration to balance benefits and risks, particularly in ARDS scenarios [51].

14.5.6 Exercises and Early Mobility

Early mobilization is a logical intervention to improve muscle strength and function in ICU patients, proven effective and safe in preventing ICU-AW with minimal adverse events [52, 53].

Early mobilization involves various activities such as exercises, rolling in bed, sitting, standing, and walking, tailored to each patient's condition [54]. A recent meta-analysis demonstrated its effectiveness in preventing ICU-AW, reducing ICU and hospital length of stay, and enhancing functionality. However, some patients may not immediately engage in mobilization due to acute clinical conditions, necessitating alternative interventions like cycle ergometry or electrical stimulation [55].

Electrical stimulation implemented early in ICU care has shown promise in preventing ICU-AW and improving quality of life by enhancing muscle strength and shortening ventilation and hospital stays [56].

Integration of early mobilization into ICU care requires a multidisciplinary approach involving various healthcare professionals to ensure patient safety and program success. Therefore, the combination of early mobilization and protein supplementation emerges as a key strategy in treating lean mass loss in critically ill patients, highlighting the necessity of integrated approaches in ICU rehabilitation programs [57].

14.5.7 Scope of Control and Glycemic Variability

Glycemic control in critically ill patients, referred to as dysglycemia, encompasses hyperglycemia, hypoglycemia, and glycemic variability, posing a significant challenge in clinical management [58].

Hyperglycemia, often seen as an adaptive response to systemic inflammation, is prevalent among critically ill patients and correlates with adverse outcomes such as increased mortality, prolonged hospital stays, and impaired wound healing [59, 60].

In diabetic patients, sarcopenia, characterized by muscle mass decline, may result from insulin deficiency, which plays a vital role in stimulating muscle growth and protein synthesis [61].

Current guidelines from the American Association of Clinical Endocrinologists (AACE) and the American Diabetes Association (ADA) recommend initiating continuous insulin therapy when blood glucose levels exceed 180 mg/dL in critically ill patients, aiming for glycemic control between 140 and 180 mg/dL. Prompt treatment of hypoglycemia is crucial to prevent worsening clinical conditions, and protocol-driven approaches are advocated by organizations like the Surviving Sepsis Campaign (SSC) for severe sepsis cases [62].

Monitoring blood glucose levels every 1–2 h until stabilization, followed by transitioning to every 4 h, helps manage glycemic levels effectively, with caution advised when interpreting point-of-care capillary blood tests to avoid overestimating serum glucose values [63].

This integrated approach underscores the importance of glycemic control in optimizing clinical outcomes for critically ill patients, necessitating multidisciplinary collaboration and adherence to evidence-based guidelines for effective management of dysglycemia in the ICU setting [20].

14.5.8 Seamless Mechanical Ventilation from Start to Finish

The management of acute respiratory failure (ARF) presents various challenges and requires tailored support strategies depending on the underlying cause and severity. Oxygen supplementation is the primary intervention for hypoxemic ARF, starting from nasal cannulas and escalating to devices like non-rebreather masks for higher fraction of inspired oxygen (FiO_2) levels [64–66].

When ventilation fails, noninvasive ventilation options such as continuous positive airway pressure (CPAP) or bi-level positive airway pressure (BiPAP) may be considered, with close monitoring of parameters like tidal volume and pressure to ensure patient comfort and efficacy [65–67].

In cases where invasive ventilatory support is necessary, lung-protective ventilation strategies must be initiated immediately post-intubation. This involves maintaining optimal tidal volumes, positive end-expiratory pressure (PEEP) levels, and FiO_2 concentrations to prevent further lung injury. Monitoring for patient-ventilator asynchrony is crucial during ventilation to mitigate adverse outcomes and respiratory muscle dysfunction [65–70].

Sedo-analgesia and, at times, muscle paralysis may be employed during invasive ventilation to ensure patient comfort and optimize ventilator synchrony. Prompt assessment for weaning readiness is essential, with daily evaluations to gradually reduce ventilator support and initiate spontaneous breathing trials. Post-extubation support varies depending on patient characteristics and ARF etiology, emphasizing the importance of tailored care to minimize the risk of extubation failure and optimize patient outcomes [65–67].

14.6 Rehabilitation in the ICU and Weaning

The recovery of respiratory and peripheral musculature is crucial for the weaning process from MV. However, the enhancement of cognitive function, cardiac status, hemodynamic and nutrition, and, not least, mental health and motivation play pivotal roles in the success of this process [71].

In the presence of ICU-AW, the implementation of an early, well-structured, protocol-based physical activity intervention can lead to better outcomes in intensive care unit patients. However, current research on prevention strategies for ICU-AW is limited and lacks robust evidence [9].

In recent systematic reviews and meta-analyses [72, 73], the following rehabilitation treatments for patients undergoing weaning from MV have been considered:

- Positioning and progressive mobilization, including assisted, active, or resisted exercises, balance training, transfers, orthostatism, stationary walking, ambulation, and cycle ergometry
- Neuromuscular electrical stimulation
- Inspiratory muscle training

14.6.1 Positioning and Progressive Mobilization

A progressive rehabilitation program consisting of six intensity levels, from positioning and rotational therapy to walking close to the bedside (Table 14.4) lasting 3–4 days, was able to reduce MV time and time to extubation by an average of 2 days, while also increasing the diaphragmatic thickening fraction [74].

A quality improvement program to introduce early and progressive mobilization on the outcomes of patients with MV was associated with shortened MV durations and ICU stays. A multidisciplinary team—a critical care nurse, nursing assistant, respiratory therapist, physical therapist, and even family—was set up to initiate the early mobilization program within 72 h of MV. The protocol was divided into four

Table 14.4 Protocol for positioning and progressive mobilization in mechanically ventilated patients [74]

Level	Activity
0	Turning over once every 2 h for unconscious patients with unstable vital signs
1–2	In addition to turning over, maintaining joint range of motion to prevent muscle atrophy and placing normal limb position for conscious patients who could sit up for at least 20 min, 3 times a day
3	Similar to level 2, but sitting on the edge of the bed for patients who could perform upper-limb antigravity training
4	Similar to level 3, but standing up or sitting in a chair for at least 20 min a day for patients who could perform lower-limb antigravity training
5	Patients actively moved from the bed and walked bedside

levels and was provided twice daily, 5d/wk during the 30-min family visiting time, and, if possible, cooperating with family [75]:

- Level I, passive extremities movement for unconscious patients
- Level II, active extremities movement and interaction with the physical therapist for conscious patients who can respond to simple commands in a sitting position on the bed
- Level III, similar to level II, but sitting on the edge of the bed for patient's biceps strength of >3/5 on the MRC scale
- Level IV, similar to level II, but the patient had actively moved from the bed to a chair beside the bed for patient's quadriceps strength of >3/5

In another study, the effects of two different protocols were evaluated compared to conventional treatment (involving passive and active range of motion exercises). The first protocol included passive and active range of motion (ROM), sitting position for a minimum of 20 min, sitting on the edge of the bed, and active transfer to a chair for a minimum of 20 min. In the second protocol, exercises with elastic bands were added (diagonal pull, shoulder flexion, flyer, and reverse flyer postures—3 × 10 repetitions, 1 × day, 5 × week) [76].

The authors observed a significant reduction in ventilation duration in patients from both intervention protocols (12.82 ± 5.69, 5.78 ± 2.74, and 6.52 ± 4.40 days; $p < 0.05$), as well as greater gains in peripheral muscle strength assessed by hand grip and in the level of physical activity [76].

14.6.2 Neuromuscular Electrical Stimulation (NMES)

The implementation of an abdominal NMES protocol (30 min, twice per day, 5 days per week) alongside standard care allowed an improvement in ventilation duration and ICU length of stay, which were shorter compared to the control group. Nevertheless, no significant differences were noted in terms of muscle thickness in the rectus abdominis, diaphragm, or combined lateral abdominal muscles [77].

A systematic review and meta-analysis [73] incorporating studies utilizing NMES alone or combined with exercises as an intervention did not demonstrate a significant benefit for ventilator weaning.

Curiously, another recent systematic review and meta-analysis indicates that NMES combined with physical therapy (PT) significantly improved the extubation success rate against standard ICU care and NMES alone and showed a better ranking over PT or NMES alone in improving clinical outcomes such as ICU length of stay, MV duration, extubation success rate, and mortality in critically ill patients undergoing MV [78].

14.6.3 Inspiratory Muscle Training (IMT)

Respiratory muscle dysfunction is present in 80% of mechanically ventilated patients with ICU-AW. Inadequate ventilatory drive, increased work of breathing, and respiratory muscle weakness are probable factors contributing to weaning failure [79].

A daily intermittent inspiratory loading comprising six to eight contractions repeated in three to four sets at moderate to high intensity was deemed safe and enhanced inspiratory muscle strength and weaning success in patients encountering difficulties in weaning [80].

Several studies attempted to assess the impact of IMT on MV weaning. A protocol of IMT twice daily, 7 days a week, 5 min per session, with a load of 30% of the maximum inspiratory pressure increasing daily by 10%, led to a substantial increase in maximal inspiratory pressure (MIP) and a reduction in weaning duration by 1.7 days [81].

Another IMT protocol increased the success rate of weaning from MV and MIP. In this research, participants completed four sets of 6–10 breaths daily, with 2 min of rest with mechanical ventilator support between each set, 5 days a week, utilizing a threshold inspiratory muscle training device (pressure load ranging between 4 and 20 cmH_2O). The device was adjusted to the maximum pressure setting achievable by the subject during inspiration consistently and was advanced daily based on tolerance [82].

The use of an inspiratory muscle training regimen involving an electronic resistive loading device demonstrated significant muscle strength improvement and notable positive effects on two critical clinical outcomes: ICU survival rates and successful weaning [83, 84]. The inspiratory load protocol entailed applying an inspiratory load for 60 breaths in 2 sets of 30 breaths each, with a rest interval of 2–3 min between sets. Each set consisted of three subsets of 10 breaths each. Within every subset of 10 breaths, the load initiation was set at half of the target (defined as 40% of the MIP) and gradually increased until reaching the target load. The final five breaths of each subset were performed under the target load [84].

References

1. Hermans G, Van Mechelen H, Clerckx B, Vanhullebusch T, Mesotten D, Wilmer A, et al. Acute outcomes and 1-year mortality of intensive care unit-acquired weakness. A cohort study and propensity-matched analysis. Am J Respir Crit Care Med. 2014;190:410–20.
2. Wieske L, Dettling-Ihnenfeldt DS, Verhamme C, Nollet F, van Schaik IN, Schultz MJ, et al. Impact of ICU-acquired weakness on post-ICU physical functioning: a follow-up study. Crit Care. 2015;19:196.
3. Puthucheary ZA, Rawal J, McPhail M, Connolly B, Ratnayake G, Chan P, et al. Acute skeletal muscle wasting in critical illness. JAMA. 2013;310:1591–600.
4. Goligher EC, Fan E, Herridge MS, Murray A, Vorona S, Brace D, et al. Evolution of diaphragm thickness during mechanical ventilation. Impact of inspiratory effort. Am J Respir Crit Care Med. 2015;192:1080–8.
5. Friedrich O, Reid MB, Van den Berghe G, Vanhorebeek I, Hermans G, Rich MM, et al. The sick and the weak: neuropathies/myopathies in the critically ill. Physiol Rev. 2015;95:1025–109.
6. De Jonghe B, Bastuji-Garin S, Durand M-C, Malissin I, Rodrigues P, Cerf C, et al. Respiratory weakness is associated with limb weakness and delayed weaning in critical illness. Crit Care Med. 2007;35:2007–15.
7. Llano-Diez M, Renaud G, Andersson M, Marrero HG, Cacciani N, Engquist H, et al. Mechanisms underlying ICU muscle wasting and effects of passive mechanical loading. Crit Care. 2012;16:R209.
8. Gosselink R, Langer D. Recovery from ICU-acquired weakness; do not forget the respiratory muscles! Thorax. 2016;71(9):779.
9. Vanhorebeek I, Latronico N, Van den Berghe G. ICU-acquired weakness. Intensive Care Med. 2020;46:637–53.
10. Godoy MDP, Costa HLLS, Silva Neto AE, Serejo ALC, Souza LC, Kalil MR, et al. Muscular weakness acquired in ICU (ICU-AW): effects of systemic neuromuscular electrical stimulation. Rev Bras Neurol. 2015;51(4):110–3.
11. Boelens YFN, Melchers M, van Zanten ARH. Poor physical recovery after critical illness: incidence, features, risk factors, pathophysiology, and evidence-based therapies. Curr Opin Crit Care. 2022;28:409–16.
12. Winkelman C. The role of inflammation in ICU-acquired weakness. Crit Care. 2010;14:186.
13. Dos Santos CC, Batt J. ICU-acquired weakness: mechanisms of disability. Curr Opin Crit Care. 2012;18:509–17.
14. Ceniccola GD, Holanda TP, Pequeno RSF, Mendonça VS, Oliveira ABM, Carvalho LSF, et al. Relevance of AND-ASPEN criteria of malnutrition to predict hospital mortality in critically ill patients: a prospective study. J Crit Care. 2018;44:398–403.
15. Parry SM, Chapple LS, Mourtzakis M. Exploring the potential effectiveness of combining optimal nutrition with electrical stimulation to maintain muscle health in critical illness: a narrative review. Nutr Clin Practice. 2018;33(6):772–89.
16. Le Stanga V, Nicola Latronicoc N, Dresa M, Bertoni M. Critical illness-associated limb and diaphragmatic weakness. Curr Opin Crit Care. 2024;30:121–30.
17. De Jonghe B, Sharshar T, Lefaucheur JP, Authier FJ, Durand-Zaleski I, Boussarsar M, et al. Paresis acquired in the intensive care unit, a prospective multicenter study. JAMA. 2002;288:2859.
18. Jolley SE, Bunnell AE, Hough CL. ICU-acquired weakness. Chest. 2016;150(5):1129–40.
19. Attwell C, Sauterel L, Jöhr J, Piquilloud L, Kuntzer T, Diserens K. Early detection of ICU-acquired weakness in septic shock patients ventilated longer than 72 h. BMC Pulm Med. 2022;22:466.
20. Machado JC, Castro MG, Giacomassi IWS, Giorelli GV, Isola AM, Silva JM Jr, et al. Bundles do combate à fraqueza adquirida na unidade de terapia intensiva. BRASPEN J. 2021;36(2):131–44.

21. Piva S, Fagoni N, Latronico N. Intensive care unit–acquired weakness: unanswered questions and targets for future research. F1000Res. 2019;8:508.
22. Supinski GS, Morris PE, Dhar S, Callahan LA. Diaphragm dysfunction in critical illness. Chest. 2018;153(4):1040–51.
23. Toledo DO, Silva DCLE, Santos DMD, Freitas BJ, Dib R, Cordioli RL, et al. Bedside ultrasound is a practical measurement tool for assessing muscle mass. Rev Bras Ter Intensiva. 2017;29(4):476–80.
24. Caporrino FA, Faloppa F, Santos JBG, Réssio C, Soares FHC, Nakachima LR, Segre NG. Estudo populacional da força de preensão palmar com dinamômetro Jamar ®. Rev Bras Ortop. 1998;33(2)
25. Lopes J, Grams ST, Silva EF, Medeiros LA, Brito CMMB, Yamaguti WP. Reference equations for handgrip strength: normative values in young adult and middle-aged subjects. Clin Nutr. 2018 Jun;37(3):914–8.
26. Hodgson CL, Bailey M, Bellomo R, Berney S, Buhr H, Denehy L, et al. A binational multicenter pilot feasibility randomized controlled trial of early goal-directed mobilization in the ICU. Crit Care Med. 2016;44:1145–52. https://doi.org/10.1097/CCM.0000000000001643.
27. Field LB, Hand RK. Differentiating malnutrition screening and assessment: a nutrition care process perspective. J Acad Nutr Diet. 2015;115(5):824–8.
28. Kondrup J, Rasmussen HH, Hamberg O, Stanga Z, Ad Hoc ESPEN Working Group. Nutritional risk screening (NRS 2002): a new method based on an analysis of controlled clinical trials. Clin Nutr. 2003;22(3):321–36.
29. Heyland DK, Dhaliwal R, Jiang X, Day AG. Identifying critically ill patients who benefit the most from nutrition therapy: the development and initial validation of a novel risk assessment tool. Crit Care. 2011;15(6):R268.
30. Castro MG, Ribeiro PC, Souza IAO, Cunha HFR, Silva MHN, Rocha EEM, et al. Diretriz brasileira de terapia nutricional no paciente grave. BRASPEN J. 2018;33(Supl 1):2–36.
31. Detsky AS, McLaughlin JR, Baker JP, Johnston N, Whittaker S, Mendelson RA, et al. What is subjective global assessment of nutritional status? JPEN J Parenter Enteral Nutr. 1987;11(1):8–13.
32. Cederholm T, Jensen GL, Correia MITD, Gonzalez MC, Fukushima R, Higashiguchi T, et al. GLIM Core Leadership Committee, GLIM Working Group. GLIM criteria for the diagnosis of malnutrition: a consensus report from the global clinical nutrition community. J Cachexia Sarcopenia Muscle. 2019;10(1):207–17.
33. van Zanten ARH, De Waele E, Wischmeyer PE. Nutrition therapy and critical illness: practical guidance for the ICU, post-ICU, and long-term convalescence phases. Crit Care. 2019;23(1):368.
34. Wischmeyer PE, Molinger J, Haines K. Point-counterpoint: indirect calorimetry is essential for optimal nutrition therapy in the intensive care unit. Nutr Clin Pract. 2021;36(2):275–81.
35. McClave SA, Omer E. Point-counterpoint: indirect calorimetry is not necessary for optimal nutrition therapy in critical illness. Nutr Clin Pract. 2021;36(2):268–74.
36. Whittle J, Molinger J, MacLeod D, Haines K, Wischmeyer PE, LEEP-COVID Study Group. Persistent hypermetabolism and longitudinal energy expenditure in critically ill patients with COVID-19. Crit Care. 2020;24(1):581.
37. Fetterplace K, Beach LJ, MacIsaac C, Presneill J, Edbrooke L, Parry SM, et al. Associations between nutritional energy delivery, bioimpedance spectroscopy and functional outcomes in survivors of critical illness. J Hum Nutr Diet. 2019;32(6):702–12.
38. Singer P, Blaser AR, Berger MM, Alhazzani W, Calder PC, Casaer MP, et al. ESPEN guideline on clinical nutrition in the intensive care unit. Clin Nutr. 2019;38(1):48–79.
39. McClave SA, Martindale RG, Vanek VW, McCarthy M, Roberts P, Taylor B, A.S.P.E.N. Board of Directors, American College of Critical Care Medicine, Society of Critical Care Medicine, et al. Guidelines for the provision and assessment of nutrition support therapy in the adult critically ill patient: Society of Critical Care Medicine (SCCM) and American Society for Parenteral and Enteral Nutrition (A.S.P.E.N.). J Parenter Enter Nutr. 2009;33(3):277–316.

40. Toledo DO, Freitas BJ, Dib R, Pfeilsticker FJDA, Santos DM, Gomes BC, et al. Peripheral muscular ultrasound as outcome assessment tool in critically ill patients on mechanical ventilation: an observational cohort study. Clin Nutr ESPEN. 2021;43:408–14.
41. Ammar MA, Sacha GL, Welch SC, Bass SN, Kane-Gill SL, Duggal A, et al. Sedation, analgesia, and paralysis in COVID-19 patients in the setting of drug shortages. J Intensive Care Med. 2021;36(2):157–74.
42. Hanidziar D, Bittner EA. Sedation of mechanically ventilated COVID-19 patients: challenges and special considerations. Anesth Analg. 2020;131(1):e40–1.
43. Namigar T, Serap K, Esra AT, Özgül O, Can ÖA, Aysel A, et al. The correlation among the Ramsay sedation scale, Richmond agitation sedation scale and Riker sedation agitation scale during midazolam-remifentanil sedation. Rev Bras Anestesiol. 2017;67(4):347–54.
44. Pop MK, Dervay KR, Dansby M, Jones C. Evaluation of Richmond agitation sedation scale (RASS) in mechanically ventilated in the emergency department. Adv Emerg Nurs J. 2018;40(2):131–7.
45. Rüsch D, Arndt C, Eberhart L, Tappert S, Nageldick D, Wulf H. Bispectral index to guide induction of anesthesia: a randomized controlled study. BMC Anesthesiol. 2018;18(1):66.
46. Terada Y, Inoue S, Konda M, Egawa J, Ueda J, Kirita T, et al. Effects of deep sedation under mechanical ventilation on cognitive outcome in patients undergoing surgery for oral and maxillofacial cancer and microvascular reconstruction. Med Intensiva (Engl Ed). 2019;43(1):3–9.
47. Olson MD, Saw J, Visscher SL, Balakrishnan K. Cost comparison and safety of emergency department conscious sedation for the removal of ear foreign bodies. Int J Pediatr Otorhinolaryngol. 2018;110:140–3.
48. Chiarotto A, Maxwell LJ, Ostelo RW, Boers M, Tugwell P, Terwee CB. Measurement properties of visual analogue scale, numeric rating scale, and pain severity subscale of the brief pain inventory in patients with low back pain: a systematic review. J Pain. 2019;20(3):245–63.
49. Hall KR, Stanley AY. Literature review: assessment of opioidrelated sedation and the pasero opioid sedation scale. J Perianesth Nurs. 2019;34(1):132–42.
50. Schroeppel TJ, Clement LP, Barnard DL, Guererro W, Ferguson MD, Sharpe JP, et al. Propofol infusion syndrome: efficacy of a prospective screening protocol. Am Surg. 2018;84(8):1333–8.
51. Guervilly C, Bisbal M, Forel JM, Mechati M, Lehingue S, Bourenne J, et al. Effects of neuromuscular blockers on transpulmonary pressures in moderate to severe acute respiratory distress syndrome. Intensive Care Med. 2017;43(3):408–18.
52. Hodgson CL, Berney S, Harrold M, Saxena M, Bellomo R. Clinical review: early patient mobilization in the ICU. Crit Care. 2013;17(1):207.
53. Nydahl P, Sricharoenchai T, Chandra S, Kundt FS, Huang M, Fischill M, et al. Safety of patient mobilization and rehabilitation in the intensive care unit. Systematic review with meta-analysis. Ann Am Thorac Soc. 2017;14(5):766–77.
54. Stiller K. Physiotherapy in intensive care: an updated systematic review. Chest. 2013;144(3):825–47.
55. Zang K, Chen B, Wang M, Chen D, Hui L, Guo S, et al. The effect of early mobilization in critically ill patients: a meta-analysis. Nurs Crit Care. 2020;25(6):360–7.
56. Liu M, Luo J, Zhou J, Zhu X. Intervention effect of neuromuscular electrical stimulation on ICU acquired weakness: a metaanalysis. Int J Nurs Sci. 2020;7(2):228–37.
57. Toledo DO, Giorelli G, Castro MG. The critically ill patient: an athlete who never rest. World J Adv Healthc Res. 2019;3(2):69–72.
58. Marik PE, Bellomo R. Stress hyperglycemia: an essential survival response! Crit Care Med. 2013;41(6):e93–4.
59. Freire AX, Bridges L, Umpierrez GE, Kuhl D, Kitabchi AE. Admission hyperglycemia and other risk factors as predictors of hospital mortality in a medical ICU population. Chest. 2005;128(5):3109–16.
60. Singer P, Doig GS, Pichard C. The truth about nutrition in the ICU. Intensive Care Med. 2014;40(2):252–5.

61. Mesinovic J, Zengin A, De Courten B, Ebeling PR, Scott D. Sarcopenia and type 2 diabetes mellitus: a bidirectional relationship. Diab Metab Syndr Obes. 2019;12:1057–72.
62. Moghissi ES, Korytkowski MT, DiNardo M, Einhorn D, Hellman R, Hirsch IB, et al. American Association of Clinical Endocrinologists; American Diabetes Association. American Association of Clinical Endocrinologists and American Diabetes Association consensus statement on inpatient glycemic control. Diabetes Care. 2009;32(6):1119–31.
63. Rhodes A, Evans LE, Alhazzani W, Levy MM, Antonelli M, Ferrer R, et al. Surviving Sepsis Campaign: international guidelines for management of sepsis and septic shock: 2016. Crit Care Med. 2017;45(3):486–552.
64. Alhazzani W, Møller MH, Arabi YM, Loeb M, Gong MN, Fan E, et al. Surviving Sepsis Campaign: guidelines on the management of critically ill adults with coronavirus disease 2019 (COVID19). Intensive Care Med. 2020;46(5):854–87.
65. Barbas CSV, Ísola AM, Farias AMC, Cavalcanti AB, Gama AMC, Duarte ACM, et al. Brazilian recommendations of mechanical ventilation 2013 (part 1). Rev Bras Ter Intensiva. 2014;26(2):89–121.
66. Barbas CSV, Ísola AM, Farias AMC, Cavalcanti AB, Gama AMC, Duarte ACM, et al. Brazilian recommendations of mechanical ventilation 2013 (part 2). Rev Bras Ter Intensiva. 2014;26(3):215–39.
67. Fan E, Del Sorbo L, Goligher EC, Hodgson CL, Munshi L, Walkey AJ, et al. American Thoracic Society, European Society of Intensive Care Medicine, and Society of Critical Care Medicine. An official American Thoracic Society/European Society of Intensive Care Medicine/Society of Critical Care Medicine Clinical Practice Guideline: mechanical ventilation in adult patients with acute respiratory distress syndrome. Am J Respir Crit Care Med. 2017;195(9):1253–63.
68. Girard TD, Alhazzani W, Kress JP, Ouellette DR, Schmidt GA, Truwit JD, et al. An official American Thoracic Society/American College of Chest Physicians Clinical Practice Guideline: liberation from mechanical ventilation in critically ill adults. Rehabilitation protocols, ventilator liberation protocols, and cuff leak tests. Am J Respir Crit Care Med. 2017;195(1):120–33.
69. Vignaux L, Vargas F, Roeseler J, Tassaux D, Thille AW, Kossowsky MP, et al. Patient-ventilator asynchrony during noninvasive ventilation for acute respiratory failure: a multicenter study. Intensive Care Med. 2009;35(5):840–6.
70. Epstein SK. How often does patient-ventilator asynchrony occur and what are the consequences? Respir Care. 2011;56(1):25–38.
71. Bickenbach J, Fritsch S, Cosler S, Simon Y, Dreher M, Theisen S, et al. Effects of structured protocolized physical therapy on the duration of mechanical ventilation in patients with prolonged weaning. J Crit Care. 2024;80:154491.
72. Lippi L, de Sire A, D'Abrosca F, Polla B, Marotta N, Castello LM, et al. Efficacy of physiotherapy interventions on weaning in mechanically ventilated critically ill patients: a systematic review and meta-analysis. Front Med. 2022;9:889218.
73. Wu RY, Hj Y, Chang KJ, Tsai MW. Effects of different types and frequencies of early rehabilitation on ventilator weaning among patients in intensive care units: a systematic review and meta-analysis. PLoS One. 2023;18(4):e0284923.
74. Dong Z, Liu Y, Gai Y, Meng P, Lin H, Zhao Y, et al. Early rehabilitation relieves diaphragm dysfunction induced by prolonged mechanical ventilation: a randomised control study. BMC Pulm Med. 2021;21:106.
75. Lai CC, Chou W, Chan KS, Cheng KC, Yuan KS, Chao CM, et al. Early mobilization reduces duration of mechanical ventilation and intensive care unit stay in patients with acute respiratory failure. Arch Phys Med Rehabil. 2017;98:931–9.
76. Pinkaew D, Wonglanga K, Ueawattanasirikul C, Wongpalee T, Chanritwattana S, Jaiwongpeng P, et al. The effect of early mobilization with elastic band exercise on the duration of mechanical ventilator weaning of critically ill patients. Indian J Public Health Res Dev. 2020;11:237–43.
77. McCaughey EJ, Jonkman AH, Boswell-Ruys CL, McBain RA, Bye EA, Hudson AL, et al. Abdominal functional electrical stimulation to assist ventilator weaning in critical illness: a double-blinded, randomised, sham-controlled pilot study. Crit Care. 2019;23:261. https://doi.org/10.1186/s13054-019-2544-0.

78. Xu C, Yang F, Wang Q, Gao W, et al. Effect of neuromuscular electrical stimulation in critically ill adults with mechanical ventilation: a systematic review and network meta-analysis. BMC Pulm Med. 2024;24:56.
79. Jung B, Moury PH, Mahul M, de Jong A, Galia F, Prades A, et al. Diaphragmatic dysfunction in patients with ICU-acquired weakness and its impact on extubation failure. Intensive Care Med. 2016;42:853–61.
80. Peñuelas O, Frutos-Vivar F, Fernández C, Anzueto A, Epstein SK, Apezteguía C, et al. Characteristics and outcomes of ventilated patients according to time to liberation from mechanical ventilation. Am J Respir Crit Care Med. 2011;184:430–7.
81. Elkins M, Dentice R. Inspiratory muscle training facilitates weaning from mechanical ventilation among patients in the intensive care unit: a systematic review. J Physiother. 2015;61:125–34.
82. Cader SA, de Vale RGS, Castro JC, Bacelar SC, Biehl C, Gomes MCV, et al. Inspiratory muscle training improves maximal inspiratory pressure and may assist weaning in older intubated patients: a randomised trial. J Physiother. 2010;56:171–7.
83. Martin AD, Smith BK, Davenport PD, Harman E, Gonzalez-Rothi RJ, Baz M, et al. Inspiratory muscle strength training improves weaning outcome in failure to wean patients: a randomized trial. Crit Care. 2011;15:R84.
84. Guimarães BS, Souza LC, Cordeiro HF, Regis TL, Leite CA, Puga FP, et al. Inspiratory muscle training with an electronic resistive loading device improves prolonged weaning outcomes in a randomized controlled trial. Crit Care Med. 2021;49(4):589–97.

Chapter 15
Diaphragm Dysfunction and Weaning

Catherine A. Bellissimo and Ewan C. Goligher

15.1 Introduction to Diaphragm Mechanics

The act of breathing is easy to take for granted, but it represents a complex and coordinated activity involving a combination of neural activation and mechanical action of the respiratory muscles. The diaphragm is a thin, umbrella-shaped muscular structure that separates the abdominal and thoracic cavities and acts as the main respiratory pump during inspiration. It ensures that sufficient negative pressures can be maintained to inflate the lungs during the inspiratory phase of the respiratory cycle. While thought to be one muscle, the diaphragm is comprised of three separate segments: the central tendon, the costal diaphragm, and the crural diaphragm. The central tendon of the diaphragm is a noncontractile structure that allows major blood vessels, including the inferior vena cava, to pass through from the thoracic to the abdominal cavity. The costal and crural diaphragm have distinct innervation and mechanical actions on the rib cage. The costal diaphragm projects from the central tendon, inserting on the xiphoid process of the sternum and the upper margins of the lower six ribs. The crural diaphragm inserts on the ventrolateral aspect of the first three lumbar vertebrae and on the aponeurotic arcuate ligament. During inspiration, the costal diaphragm contracts, lowering the dome of the diaphragm and expanding the lower rib cage to increase intrathoracic volume.

C. A. Bellissimo
Toronto General Hospital Research Institute, University Health Network, Toronto, ON, Canada

E. C. Goligher (✉)
Division of Respirology, Department of Medicine, Toronto General Hospital, University Health Network, Toronto, ON, Canada

Interdepartmental Division of Critical Care Medicine, Department of Physiology, Faculty of Medicine, University of Toronto, Toronto, ON, Canada
e-mail: ewan.goligher@utoronto.ca

A. R. Baptistella et al. (eds.), *Weaning from Mechanical Ventilation*,
https://doi.org/10.1007/978-3-032-01145-9_15

The motion of the diaphragm can be compared to that of a piston within a cylinder. During inspiration, the dome of the diaphragm descends, allowing for the expansion of the pleural cavity and caudal displacement of the chest wall. During this time, intrapleural pressure falls and, if the airway is open, allows for inflation of the lungs. As the primary muscle of inspiration, the diaphragm is essential for the maintenance of adequate ventilation, especially when respiratory loads are elevated. When respiratory mechanics are compromised, diaphragm weakness may predispose patients to ventilator-induced diaphragm injury (myotrauma). This predisposition is not from mechanical ventilation per se, but a mismatch in applied ventilatory support and patient efforts that may result in injury (myotrauma) to the diaphragm and or lungs. This can ultimately contribute to a vicious cycle of diaphragm weakness that leads to dependence on ventilatory support which further perpetuates the weakness. Understanding the mechanisms of diaphragm myotrauma is critical for the development of ventilation and rehabilitation strategies in critical illness. This chapter focuses on the concepts of diaphragm myotrauma in mechanical ventilation and their impact on weaning.

15.2 Diaphragm Myotrauma in Mechanical Ventilation

Respiratory muscle weakness, either intrinsic weakness or weakness linked to fatigue, has widely been thought to contribute to respiratory failure and inabilities to wean from mechanical ventilation [1]. Increasing evidence has shown that the diaphragm is especially susceptible to fatigue during critical illness; thus, initial practice was to "rest" the diaphragm with the use of mechanical ventilation. However, this paradigm was shifted when it was demonstrated that disuse of the muscle during mechanical ventilation contributes to maladaptive changes leading to weakness and atrophy [2]. This dysfunction in the diaphragm is a progressively common phenomenon in critical illness. Studies show that between 63% and 80% [3–5] of critically ill patients experience some level of diaphragm dysfunction at time of weaning, based on a pressure-based definition of diaphragm weakness ($P_{et} < 11$ cmH_2O) [6, 7]. Concerningly, diaphragm dysfunction is twice as prevalent as limb weakness in critically ill patients and has a direct impact on weaning outcomes [3] and long-term outcomes including increased hospital readmission and mortality [8–10].

More recently, the term myotrauma has been used to describe basic muscle injury [11, 12] and has been extended to describe diaphragm injury, given the injury-like phenotype [13, 14]. The mechanisms by which diaphragm myotrauma is caused can be varied, yet they remain important mediators of patient trajectory in critical illness. This chapter focuses on the various models of diaphragm myotrauma and their impact on weaning outcomes (Fig. 15.1).

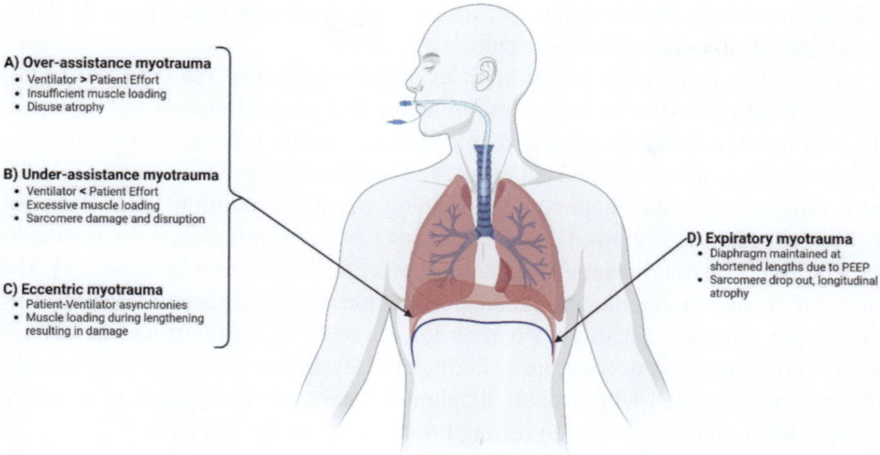

Fig. 15.1 Summary of diaphragmatic myotrauma. (**a**) Over-assistance myotrauma is a result of insufficient loading of the diaphragm. This may be due to impaired patient efforts, over-sedation, or the over-application of ventilator support, leading to the rapid onset of atrophy. (**b**) Contrarily, when the diaphragm is not sufficiently unloaded, load-induced injury may occur leading to sarcomere damage and contractile apparatus disruption, termed under-assistance myotrauma. (**c**) Eccentric myotrauma may occur while the diaphragm is loaded in a lengthened position. Several forms of patient-ventilatory asynchronies may predispose patients to eccentric diaphragm contractions. (**d**) Prolonged application of high positive end-expiratory pressure (PEEP) results in adaptation of the diaphragm to a shortened length and sarcomere drop out termed "longitudinal atrophy." Rapid withdrawal of PEEP may lead to diaphragm weakness due to impaired length-tension

15.2.1 Over-Assistance Myotrauma

The balance of patient efforts and ventilatory support by mechanical ventilation is critical to maintaining respiratory function and oxygenation. However, when an imbalance occurs, for example, when ventilatory support is beyond what is required by the patient and or the patient's efforts are suppressed, over-assistance myotrauma can occur. The first evidence of ventilator-induced diaphragm atrophy in humans was identified in 1988 in young neonates [15]. Levine et al. supported this finding histologically in brain-dead organ donors [2]. Further, these effects were exclusive to the diaphragm, as biopsies obtained from the pectoralis were unaffected despite the same period of inactivity. Subsequently, numerous studies have identified that controlled mechanical ventilation results in rapid onset of diaphragmatic atrophy and weakness in pre-clinical models [16–19] and humans alike [2, 13, 20–25]. Diaphragm muscle biopsies taken from diverse ICU patient populations demonstrate that diaphragm dysfunction is not only due to atrophy [21]. Indeed, reductions in force-generating capacity of the muscle fibers (even when protein loss is accounted for), increased proteolysis (MuRF-1, caspase-3), and the presence of inflammatory cells within the muscle are observed [2, 21]. Mitochondrial dysfunction and oxidative stress have also been thought to be contributors to ventilator-induced diaphragm atrophy, yet these results are conflicting [2, 26]. Understanding the mechanisms by which diaphragm atrophy may occur may reveal possible therapeutic targets to combat over-assistance myotrauma.

As diaphragm biopsies are difficult to obtain in patients, more recent studies have utilized point-of-care ultrasound to assess diaphragm function and structure. This noninvasive determination of diaphragmatic atrophy is feasible and reproducible in mechanically ventilated patients [24, 27] and can be used to quantify inspiratory efforts with tidal diaphragm thickening during inspiration [13]. Work by Goligher et al. (2015) showed that over the first week of ventilation, 44% of patients experienced a loss of diaphragm thickness greater than 10% from baseline [13]. The rate and change in diaphragm thickness over time was significantly influenced by diaphragm contractile activity, whereby lower contractile activity was associated with decreasing thickness over time. Further, the level of contractility activity in the diaphragm associated with a stable diaphragm thickness corresponds to a normal level of inspiratory effort during resting breathing in healthy subjects.

Although over-assistance diaphragm myotrauma has been well documented in animal models [17, 18, 28] and fully controlled ventilation in brain-dead organ donors [2, 20], the clinical significance of this myotrauma is unclear, given the common use of partially assisted modes of ventilation [29, 30]. Sassoon et al. observed that assisted mechanical ventilation blunts the loss of tetanic force that occurs as a result of controlled mechanical ventilation [31]. Further, intermittent spontaneous breathing in ventilated rats showed similar effects in mitigating the deleterious effects of controlled mechanical ventilation [29]. However, some maintenance of patient inspiratory effort does not guarantee that atrophy will be mitigated completely. Use of high-pressure support ventilation for 18 h in rats showed similar atrophy to control mechanical ventilation of the same duration. This atrophy also presented with increases in proteolysis and oxidative damage [30]. In humans, decreases in end-expiratory thickness [13] and fiber cross-sectional area [21, 32] are still observed in patients undergoing partially assisted ventilation.

Avoiding over-assistance myotrauma seems to be a more complex process than expected, as 50% of ventilated patients experience this form of myotrauma. More recently, intermittent phrenic nerve stimulation (PNS) has been explored as a possible therapeutic option to maintain diaphragm activity during mechanical ventilation. Experimental evidence showed that continuous PNS mitigated diaphragmatic atrophy and weakness [33–35]. Use of PNS in patients has had promising results. In a series of patients undergoing open cardiothoracic surgery, maintaining diaphragm activity by means of unilateral PNS applied intraoperatively prevented diaphragm weakness [36]. Intraoperative PNS pacing also mitigates mitochondrial dysfunction in the diaphragm, a potential contributor to ventilator-induced diaphragm dysfunction [37]. In the RESCUE 2 multi-center randomized clinical trial, patients with difficulties weaning from mechanical ventilation underwent PNS delivered through a transvenous technique. PNS increased maximal inspiratory pressure compared to standard of care, suggesting that this technique may be useful to maintain or improve diaphragm function in mechanically ventilated patients [38]. Further trials are underway to examine if PNS can improve patient-centered outcomes. Early data from the STIMULUS I phase I clinical trial indicates that continuous on-demand

PNS is feasible and that temporary PNS can ensure continuous diaphragmatic activity during MV [39]. Avoiding disuse of the diaphragm via PNS may limit over-assistance myotrauma, by preserving diaphragm strength and structure, resulting in earlier liberation from MV and, therefore, reductions associated with adverse events.

It should be noted that suppression of patient inspiratory efforts by sedation and neuromuscular blockade also contributes to over-assistance myotrauma. Excessive sedation may suppress respiratory drive and effort, leading to diaphragm atrophy and weakness [40]. In ICU patients, the dose of propofol was correlated with the severity of diaphragm weakness [41]. Neuromuscular blockades, which are typically used to adapt patients to mechanical ventilation, also have concerning effects on diaphragm activity and may contribute to diaphragm disuse. Rocuronium (an aminosteroidal non-depolarizing neuromuscular blocker) has been shown to exacerbate diaphragm weakness induced by controlled mechanical ventilation in rats [42]. Current sedations practices operate independent from ventilation, when ideally sedation and mechanical ventilation should be managed together to modulate respiratory effort and drive [43].

15.2.2 Under-Assistance Myotrauma

While over-assistance myotrauma affects nearly half of all ventilated patients, under-assistance by the ventilator is also associated with detrimental effects on diaphragm function. An important goal of mechanical ventilation is to provide support to patients to lessen the work of breathing, reduce oxygen consumption by respiratory muscles, and avoid diaphragmatic fatigue. Unfortunately, if ventilatory support is insufficient or the diaphragm is not adequately unloaded, respiratory drive may become elevated. When respiratory drive becomes too high, vigorous inspiratory efforts can result in global or regional excessive lung tension and strain [44], leading to lung injury and systemic inflammation. This mechanism is termed "patient self-inflicted lung injury" (P-SILI) and can result in distribution of ventilation without changes to tidal volume leading to pendelluft and regional hyperinflation [44, 45]. At this same time, systemic inflammation sensitizes the diaphragm to mechanical stress and load-induced injury [46]. Excessive inspiratory loads have resulted in sarcolemmal rupture, sarcomeric disorganization, and inflammatory infiltration [47–49] with similar findings in clinical studies [20, 22].

Interestingly, moderate elevations in respiratory efforts for prolonged periods can result in diaphragmatic injury and weakness [50]. Experimental evidence from hamsters undergoing tracheal banding showed that increased resistive loading resulted in diaphragm injury and ventilatory failure [20, 22, 50, 51]. Finally, the diaphragm may be more susceptible to injury during cases of sepsis and systemic inflammation [52]. Acute endotoxemia and subacute peritonitis models of sepsis lead to significant impairments in sarcolemmal damage and altered resting membrane potential of diaphragm myofibrils, which may be linked to increased nitric oxide synthase activity [52, 53].

However, careful consideration of patient needs should be examined as mechanical ventilation has been shown to mitigate load-induced diaphragm injury. In patients with exacerbations of chronic obstructive pulmonary disease, resulting in an increase in respiratory load, the initiation of mechanical ventilation results in the rapid decrease of inflammatory cytokines such as IL-6 and IL-10 [54], which have been linked to the control of breathing [55]. Furthermore, this increase in respiratory load may result in a load-induced injury to the diaphragm. Early during mechanical ventilation, Goligher et al. observed that 25% of patients had a rapid increase in diaphragm muscle thickness observed through ultrasound. This increase was associated with prolonged mechanical ventilation and may be related to tissue edema and inflammation [56]. Although still a hypothesis in the diaphragm, similar effects have been observed in load-induced injuries inflicted on the biceps brachii during exhaustive exercise [57]. While experimental evidence strongly suggests the existence of under-assistance myotrauma, further clinical evidence is required to support this hypothesis.

15.2.3 Eccentric Myotrauma

While under-assistance myotrauma may occur when a concentric contraction of the diaphragm occurs, eccentric loading may be just as injurious to the diaphragm. Eccentric muscle contractions occur when a load is applied while the muscle is lengthening, typically in response to slow a movement, such as downhill walking. This phenomenon can also occur in respiratory muscles such as the diaphragm after inspiration. While the damaging effects of eccentric contraction in limb muscles have long been examined [58] only recently has this been studied in the diaphragm [59].

Previously, the diaphragm was thought to be inactive during expiration; however, it is now known to maintain activity during this "post-inspiratory" phase [59]. In healthy volunteers [60] and mechanically ventilated patients (both adults and neonates) [60–62], post-inspiration diaphragm activity is present and increases with inspiratory load. The diaphragm in this fashion is thought to act as an "expiratory brake," to preserve lung volume and to protect against lung collapse [63, 64], particularly when lung consolidation and atelectasis are present [64]. During positive pressure ventilation, eccentric contractions may occur when the ventilator initiates its expiratory phase before the inspiratory phase is complete, leading to "post-inspiratory" loading of the diaphragm. This dyssynchrony between the diaphragm and ventilator may contribute to diaphragm weakness, but the specific mechanism has yet to be elucidated.

Despite this uncertainty in the mechanism underlying eccentric myotrauma, studies have shown that the prevalence of eccentric contractions of the diaphragm is high [65], likely occurring during patient-ventilator asynchronies including ineffective triggering, premature cycling, and reverse triggering [66, 67]. Ineffective triggering may be observed in 38% of mechanically ventilated patients and represents the most common of the patient-ventilator asynchronies in mechanically ventilated patients [68, 69]. Similarly, 30%–55% of patients under controlled mechanical ventilation exhibited reverse triggering [70]. Collectively, this suggests that eccentric activity is highly prevalent in mechanical ventilation, especially during episodes of dyssynchrony between the patient and the ventilator. Although highly speculative, the associated myotrauma due to such dyssynchronies may contribute to the link between patient–ventilator dyssynchrony and poor outcomes, especially ineffective efforts during expiration [69, 71]. The abdominal muscles and rib cage may experience an additional form of dyssynchrony that also results in eccentric contractions. In healthy subjects, breathing against severe resistance resulted in asynchrony between the rib cage and abdominal muscles, termed an "abdominal paradox." The visible efforts of abdominal muscles during inspiration have been indicative of diaphragmatic fatigue and would result in upward movement of the even as it attempts to generate inspiratory flow (i.e., shorten) [72].

Preclinical models have revealed some of the implications of eccentric myotrauma in other models of muscle dysfunction. In a murine model of impaired membrane repair (dysferlin-lacking mice), when eccentric contractions are applied ex vivo to the diaphragm, immediate reductions in force are observed followed by sarcolemmal damage [73]. Similar results are obtained in canine models when supramaximal twitches are applied via phrenic nerve stimulation while the abdominal wall is being compressed. These functional impairments lasted for over 12 h and happened in conjunction with sarcomeric and sarcolemmal damage [74]. In a porcine model of lung injury, reverse triggering in combination with high respiratory effort resulted in impaired diaphragm function and an increase in abnormal myofibers. When respiratory effort was low (average pressure-time product <150 cm H_2O/s/min), diaphragmatic force was maintained compared to fully passive modes of mechanical ventilation [75]. Collectively, these results indicate that eccentric myotrauma results in rapid and persistent impairments to diaphragm structure and function.

In mechanically ventilated patients, preliminary evidence demonstrates that eccentric contractions are common and are strongly associated with reverse triggering dyssynchronies [61]. Similar to preclinical models, reverse triggering in combination with low respiratory efforts resulted in better oxygenation and were more likely to progress to assisted ventilatory mode, or be extubated within the next 24 h compared with patients with a low frequency of reverse triggering [76]. Supporting this, Rodriguez et al. observed that the reverse triggering was associated with a decrease in hospital mortality, suggesting that it may be a marker of better outcomes in patients on mechanical ventilation [77]. In a more recent study of mechanically ventilated patients, evaluation of the influence of inspiratory loading of the diaphragm and dyssynchronous post-inspiratory muscle loading revealed that post-inspiratory loading was present in roughly 13% of examined hours with its prevalence progressively increasing with time. Post-inspiratory loading was likely to occur when dyssynchronies were present and were well correlated with inspiratory effort [78]. Additionally, a higher proportion of hours with post-inspiratory loading per day was associated with a progressive impairment in diaphragm neuromuscular coupling, a measure of efficiency of diaphragm muscle performance by normalizing force generation to the level of muscle activation. Diaphragm thickness tended to increase over time with a greater duration of post-inspiratory loading per day, although not statistically significant, and changes to diaphragm thickness (both increases and decreases) were associated with reduced diaphragm neuromuscular coupling [79–81]. This study highlighted the need to maintain patient-ventilator synchrony rather than overt respiratory efforts. However, more evidence is required to fully elucidate the influence of eccentric myotrauma and its long-term effect on mechanically ventilated patients.

15.2.4 Expiratory Myotrauma

An additional potential form of myotrauma is termed expiratory myotrauma. Here, excessive positive end-expiratory pressure (PEEP) alters diaphragm length and impairs function. PEEP is applied to mechanically ventilated patients to improve gas exchange and respiratory mechanics by increasing end-expiratory lung volume, preventing alveolar collapse [82]. Indeed, high levels of PEEP during controlled modes of ventilation have been utilized to reduce ventilator-induced lung injury in patients with ARDS [83]. However, increasing levels of PEEP may flatten the shape of the diaphragm dome while limiting inspiratory efforts [84]. Indeed, short-term increases in PEEP resulted in changes to diaphragm geometry [85–89] and results in caudal movement of the diaphragm in ventilated ICU patients [90].

In pre-clinical models, prolonged use of PEEP has been shown to induce diaphragm remodeling that resulted in significant impairments to force production and reductions at the length in which maximal force was produced [90]. These reductions were related to alterations in both fiber length and sarcomere length that were related to titin compliance (a major protein in muscle that is responsible for passive elasticity) [91]. Additionally, this study revealed that elevated levels of PEEP resulted in a reduction in the numbers of sarcomeres (the smallest contractile unit in muscle) in series, termed longitudinal atrophy. Similar declines have been observed in other studies [92, 93] but are still debated in the literature [94]. Interestingly, the PEEP level used in this experimental model would be equivalent to 5–6 cm H_2O PEEP in humans (estimation based on respiratory system compliance of 64 ml/cm H_2O and TLC of 5167 ml for humans [95] versus 0.51 ml/cm H_2O and TLC of 16.7 ml for rats) [96]. As the cohort of mechanically ventilated patients in this study had a nearly twofold higher average PEEP, there may be significant detrimental effects on sarcomere length in the diaphragm at common PEEP levels used during mechanical ventilation. The authors speculated that longitudinal atrophy is likely to occur early within humans and contribute to the observed diaphragm weakness in critically ill patients. The acute reductions or withdrawal of PEEP may stretch the remodeled diaphragm, resulting in the diaphragm operating at compromised force-length relationship. Finally, the authors suggested that a slow reduction in PEEP may be advisable to allow for the reversal of longitudinal atrophy but requires further testing in humans.

15.3 Effect on Weaning

Mechanical ventilation is a lifesaving intervention that is associated with several complications including prolonged weaning. Approximately 40% of time spent on the ventilator on mechanical ventilation is devoted to weaning [97] with 20%–50% of patients experiencing difficulties in discontinuing ventilatory support [98]. Weaning failure stems from an imbalance in the loads applied to the respiratory system and its capacity. Respiratory muscle function is thought to be a factor in weaning outcome, with diaphragm weakness being strongly associated with difficult weaning from mechanical ventilation, prolonged ICU stay, and long-term mortality risk [3, 24, 56, 99]. However, the impact of diaphragm dysfunction is somewhat debated, given that some patients with diaphragm dysfunction are still successfully extubated [5]. While this somewhat complicates an interpretation of the impact of diaphragm weakness on weaning success, it is still very likely that mechanically ventilated patients still experience some form of diaphragm myotrauma that contributes to their long-term outcomes including weaning success.

Diaphragm dysfunction is an increasingly common phenomenon during mechanical ventilation with 63%–80% patients being affected and is more prevalent than limb muscle weakness (ICU-acquired weakness) [5, 100–102]. Given that delays in weaning success predispose patients to more adverse outcomes, including prolonging mechanical ventilation, patients are further exposed to protracted immobilization and sedation that leads to peripheral muscle weakness and in turn contributes to more progressive diaphragm weakness. Ultimately, this creates a vicious cycle for patients that may contribute to lengthy hospital stays and increase morbidity and mortality. Diaphragm weakness itself is strongly associated with weaning failure and mortality [3]. This next section focuses on the described diaphragm myotrauma and its associated impacts on weaning outcomes.

While few studies explicitly characterize the form of diaphragm myotrauma in relation to its effect on weaning, rapid changes in diaphragm thickness (>10% decreases and increases), which may be indicative of over-assistance and under-assistance myotrauma, respectively, are associated with poor clinical outcomes. Over-assistance myotrauma is well document in the clinical setting with approximately 50% of ventilated patients experiencing this myotrauma and is associated with lower daily probability of liberation from mechanical ventilation [56]. Similarly, under-assistance myotrauma (demonstrated by an increase in diaphragm thickness) is associated with prolonged mechanical ventilation when adjusted for competing risk of death [56]. Collectively, changes to diaphragm thickness (either an increase or decrease) are associated with prolonged ventilator dependence, reintubation, and extended hospitalization. Therefore, all efforts must be taken to prevent and treat over- and under-assistance myotrauma given.

Preserving some diaphragm activity during mechanical ventilation can mitigate atrophy but may have limited effects on supporting successful weaning. Results from the RESCUE-2 randomized clinical trial using transvenous phrenic nerve stimulation in difficult-to-wean patients (failed at least two attempts of liberation) did not increase the proportion of successfully weaned patients from mechanical ventilation, though the trial was not powered for that endpoint [38]. Bilateral phrenic nerve stimulation improved maximal inspiratory pressure compared to standard of care [38]. Preliminary work with on-demand phrenic nerve stimulation has demonstrated feasibility [39] but further work is needed to optimize delivery and stimulation strategies. Further, mediation analysis has shown that over-assistance and under-assistance myotrauma contribute in part to the effect of mechanical ventilation on clinical outcomes [103], and more information is still required to fully understand the implications of all forms of myotrauma on the ability to wean patients from the ventilator.

Synchrony between the ventilator and patient is a key factor in mechanical ventilation, and loss of this balance predisposes patients to injurious contractions of the diaphragm. However, the nature of each dyssynchrony may have differential effects on weaning outcomes. Ineffective triggering and double-triggering asynchronies, two of the main patterns observed, may lead to increased energy expenditure, abnormal diaphragm patters and problems identify if patients are ready-to-wean [104]. Additionally, several forms of patient-ventilator dyssynchrony (ineffective triggering, premature cycling, and reverse triggering) have been associated with eccentric contraction and poorer patient outcomes [71, 105–108].

Reverse triggering, for example, has potentially favorable effects depending on its triggering characteristics, that may influence outcomes. Specifically, when reverse triggering occurs during inspiration in pressure- and volume- control modes of ventilation, diaphragm disuse atrophy (over-assistance myotrauma) may be prevented. Higher frequency of reverse triggering events previously increased the likelihood of patients progressing to assisted modes of ventilation or being extubated within the following 24 h. However, this must be balanced with monitoring the phase of respiration in which this dyssynchrony occurs and the patient's effort level [70], as reverse triggering during high efforts may yield damage to the diaphragm [75]. To date, no prospective study has evaluated the impact of eccentric activation of the diaphragm on weaning outcomes.

Finally, little is known about expiratory myotrauma and its influence on weaning outcomes. High levels of PEEP have been shown to improve lung function [109] and lower mortality when not combined with a lung recruit maneuver [83]. However, it is plausible that the associated remodeling due to sustained high PEEP may predispose the diaphragm to operating at a compromised force-length relationship once PEEP is withdrawn or reduced [90, 103]. However, it is unknown if this negatively impacts weaning outcomes. Further research is required to ascertain the influence of expiratory myotrauma on weaning.

While still a developing field, identification and management of diaphragm myotrauma should be a consideration for clinicians given the impact on weaning and patient-centered outcomes. Clinicians should aim to manage both patient efforts and ventilatory support to maintain some diaphragm activity that is synchronous with the ventilator, while minimizing volumes and pressures applied. The goal of future research should be to determine the underlying mechanisms of diaphragm myotrauma (more specifically in eccentric and expiratory myotrauma) and to further understand the clinical implications for all forms.

References

1. Jubran A, Tobin MJ. Pathophysiologic basis of acute respiratory distress in patients who fail a trial of weaning from mechanical ventilation. Am J Respir Crit Care Med. 1997;155(3):906–15. https://doi.org/10.1164/ajrccm.155.3.9117025.
2. Levine S, Nguyen T, Taylor N, et al. Rapid disuse atrophy of diaphragm fibers in mechanically ventilated humans. N Engl J Med. 2008;358(13):1327–35. https://doi.org/10.1056/NEJMoa070447.
3. Dres M, Dubé BP, Mayaux J, et al. Coexistence and impact of limb muscle and diaphragm weakness at time of liberation from mechanical ventilation in medical intensive care unit patients. Am J Respir Crit Care Med. 2017;195(1):57–66. https://doi.org/10.1164/rccm.201602-0367OC.
4. Laghi F, Cattapan SE, Jubran A, et al. Is weaning failure caused by low-frequency fatigue of the diaphragm? Am J Respir Crit Care Med. 2003;167(2):120–7. https://doi.org/10.1164/rccm.200210-1246OC.
5. Jung B, Moury PH, Mahul M, et al. Diaphragmatic dysfunction in patients with ICU-acquired weakness and its impact on extubation failure. Intensive Care Med. 2016;42(5):853–61. https://doi.org/10.1007/s00134-015-4125-2.
6. ATS/ERS. ATS/ERS statement on respiratory muscle testing. Am J Respir Crit Care Med. 2002;166(4):518–624. https://doi.org/10.1164/rccm.166.4.518.
7. Hamnegåard CH, Wragg S, Kyroussis D, et al. Mouth pressure in response to magnetic stimulation of the phrenic nerves. Thorax. 1995;50(6):620–4. https://doi.org/10.1136/thx.50.6.620.
8. Medrinal C, Prieur G, Frenoy É, et al. Respiratory weakness after mechanical ventilation is associated with one-year mortality – a prospective study. Crit Care. 2016;20(1):231. https://doi.org/10.1186/s13054-016-1418-y.
9. Demoule A, Jung B, Prodanovic H, et al. Diaphragm dysfunction on admission to the intensive care unit. Prevalence, risk factors, and prognostic impact-a prospective study. Am J Respir Crit Care Med. 2013;188(2):213–9. https://doi.org/10.1164/rccm.201209-1668OC.
10. Adler D, Dupuis-Lozeron E, Richard JC, Janssens JP, Brochard L. Does inspiratory muscle dysfunction predict readmission after intensive care unit discharge? Am J Respir Crit Care Med. 2014;190(3):347–50. https://doi.org/10.1164/rccm.201404-0655LE.
11. Hawke TJ, Garry DJ. Myogenic satellite cells: physiology to molecular biology. J Appl Physiol (1985). 2001;91(2):534–51. https://doi.org/10.1152/jappl.2001.91.2.534.
12. McKay BR, Toth KG, Tarnopolsky MA, Parise G. Satellite cell number and cell cycle kinetics in response to acute myotrauma in humans: immunohistochemistry versus flow cytometry. J Physiol. 2010;588(Pt 17):3307–20. https://doi.org/10.1113/jphysiol.2010.190876.
13. Goligher EC, Fan E, Herridge MS, et al. Evolution of diaphragm thickness during mechanical ventilation. Impact of inspiratory effort. Am J Respir Crit Care Med. 2015;192(9):1080–8. https://doi.org/10.1164/rccm.201503-0620OC.
14. Fan E, Brodie D, Slutsky AS. Acute respiratory distress syndrome: advances in diagnosis and treatment. JAMA. 2018;319(7):698–710. https://doi.org/10.1001/jama.2017.21907.
15. Knisely AS, Leal SM, Singer DB. Abnormalities of diaphragmatic muscle in neonates with ventilated lungs. J Pediatr. 1988;113(6):1074–7. https://doi.org/10.1016/s0022-3476(88)80585-7.

16. Le Bourdelles G, Viires N, Boczkowski J, Seta N, Pavlovic D, Aubier M. Effects of mechanical ventilation on diaphragmatic contractile properties in rats. Am J Respir Crit Care Med. 1994;149(6):1539–44. https://doi.org/10.1164/ajrccm.149.6.8004310.
17. Sassoon CS, Caiozzo VJ, Manka A, Sieck GC. Altered diaphragm contractile properties with controlled mechanical ventilation. J Appl Physiol (1985). 2002;92(6):2585–95. https://doi.org/10.1152/japplphysiol.01213.2001.
18. Powers SK, Shanely RA, Coombes JS, et al. Mechanical ventilation results in progressive contractile dysfunction in the diaphragm. J Appl Physiol (1985). 2002;92(5):1851–8. https://doi.org/10.1152/japplphysiol.00881.2001.
19. Anzueto A, Peters JI, Tobin MJ, et al. Effects of prolonged controlled mechanical ventilation on diaphragmatic function in healthy adult baboons. Crit Care Med. 1997;25(7):1187–90. https://doi.org/10.1097/00003246-199707000-00021.
20. Jaber S, Petrof BJ, Jung B, et al. Rapidly progressive diaphragmatic weakness and injury during mechanical ventilation in humans. Am J Respir Crit Care Med. 2011;183(3):364–71. https://doi.org/10.1164/rccm.201004-0670OC.
21. Hooijman PE, Beishuizen A, Witt CC, et al. Diaphragm muscle fiber weakness and ubiquitin-proteasome activation in critically ill patients. Am J Respir Crit Care Med. 2015;191(10):1126–38. https://doi.org/10.1164/rccm.201412-2214OC.
22. van den Berg M, Hooijman PE, Beishuizen A, et al. Diaphragm atrophy and weakness in the absence of mitochondrial dysfunction in the critically ill. Am J Respir Crit Care Med. 2017;196(12):1544–58. https://doi.org/10.1164/rccm.201703-0501OC.
23. Schepens T, Verbrugghe W, Dams K, Corthouts B, Parizel PM, Jorens PG. The course of diaphragm atrophy in ventilated patients assessed with ultrasound: a longitudinal cohort study. Crit Care. 2015;19:1–8.
24. Grosu HB, Lee YI, Lee J, Eden E, Eikermann M, Rose KM. Diaphragm muscle thinning in patients who are mechanically ventilated. Chest. 2012;142(6):1455–60. https://doi.org/10.1378/chest.11-1638.
25. Zambon M, Beccaria P, Matsuno J, et al. Mechanical ventilation and diaphragmatic atrophy in critically ill patients: an ultrasound study. Crit Care Med. 2016;44(7):1347–52. https://doi.org/10.1097/ccm.0000000000001657.
26. Picard M, Jung B, Liang F, et al. Mitochondrial dysfunction and lipid accumulation in the human diaphragm during mechanical ventilation. Am J Respir Crit Care Med. 2012;186(11):1140–9. https://doi.org/10.1164/rccm.201206-0982OC.
27. Goligher EC, Laghi F, Detsky ME, et al. Measuring diaphragm thickness with ultrasound in mechanically ventilated patients: feasibility, reproducibility and validity. Intensive Care Med. 2015;41(4):642–9. https://doi.org/10.1007/s00134-015-3687-3.
28. Gayan-Ramirez G, de Paepe K, Cadot P, Decramer M. Detrimental effects of short-term mechanical ventilation on diaphragm function and IGF-I mRNA in rats. Intensive Care Med. 2003;29(5):825–33. https://doi.org/10.1007/s00134-003-1688-0.
29. Gayan-Ramirez G, Testelmans D, Maes K, et al. Intermittent spontaneous breathing protects the rat diaphragm from mechanical ventilation effects. Crit Care Med. 2005;33(12):2804–9. https://doi.org/10.1097/01.ccm.0000191250.32988.a3.
30. Hudson MB, Smuder AJ, Nelson WB, Bruells CS, Levine S, Powers SK. Both high level pressure support ventilation and controlled mechanical ventilation induce diaphragm dysfunction and atrophy. Crit Care Med. 2012;40(4):1254–60. https://doi.org/10.1097/CCM.0b013e31823c8cc9.
31. Sassoon CS, Zhu E, Caiozzo VJ. Assist-control mechanical ventilation attenuates ventilator-induced diaphragmatic dysfunction. Am J Respir Crit Care Med. 2004;170(6):626–32. https://doi.org/10.1164/rccm.200401-042OC.
32. Hooijman PE, Beishuizen A, de Waard MC, et al. Diaphragm fiber strength is reduced in critically ill patients and restored by a troponin activator. Am J Respir Crit Care Med. 2014;189(7):863–5. https://doi.org/10.1164/rccm.201312-2260LE.

33. Masmoudi H, Coirault C, Demoule A, et al. Can phrenic stimulation protect the diaphragm from mechanical ventilation-induced damage? Eur Respir J. 2013;42(1):280–3. https://doi.org/10.1183/09031936.00045613.
34. Yang M, Wang H, Han G, et al. Phrenic nerve stimulation protects against mechanical ventilation-induced diaphragm dysfunction in rats. Muscle Nerve. 2013;48(6):958–62. https://doi.org/10.1002/mus.23850.
35. Reynolds SC, Meyyappan R, Thakkar V, et al. Mitigation of Ventilator-induced Diaphragm Atrophy by Transvenous Phrenic Nerve Stimulation. Am J Respir Crit Care Med. 2017;195(3):339–48. https://doi.org/10.1164/rccm.201502-0363OC.
36. Ahn B, Beaver T, Martin T, et al. Phrenic nerve stimulation increases human diaphragm fiber force after cardiothoracic surgery. Am J Respir Crit Care Med. 2014;190(7):837–9. https://doi.org/10.1164/rccm.201405-0993LE.
37. Martin AD, Joseph AM, Beaver TM, et al. Effect of intermittent phrenic nerve stimulation during cardiothoracic surgery on mitochondrial respiration in the human diaphragm. Crit Care Med. 2014;42(2):e152–6. https://doi.org/10.1097/CCM.0b013e3182a63fdf.
38. Dres M, de Abreu MG, Merdji H, et al. Randomized clinical study of temporary Transvenous phrenic nerve stimulation in difficult-to-wean patients. Am J Respir Crit Care Med. 2022;205(10):1169–78. https://doi.org/10.1164/rccm.202107-1709OC.
39. Morris IS, Bassi T, Bellissimo CA, et al. Proof of concept for continuous on-demand phrenic nerve stimulation to prevent diaphragm disuse during mechanical ventilation (STIMULUS): a phase 1 clinical trial. Am J Respir Crit Care Med. 2023;208 https://doi.org/10.1164/rccm.202305-0791LE.
40. Kim WY, Suh HJ, Hong SB, Koh Y, Lim CM. Diaphragm dysfunction assessed by ultrasonography: influence on weaning from mechanical ventilation. Crit Care Med. 2011;39(12):2627–30. https://doi.org/10.1097/CCM.0b013e3182266408.
41. Hermans G, Agten A, Testelmans D, Decramer M, Gayan-Ramirez G. Increased duration of mechanical ventilation is associated with decreased diaphragmatic force: a prospective observational study. Crit Care. 2010;14(4):R127. https://doi.org/10.1186/cc9094.
42. Testelmans D, Maes K, Wouters P, et al. Rocuronium exacerbates mechanical ventilation-induced diaphragm dysfunction in rats. Crit Care Med. 2006;34(12):3018–23. https://doi.org/10.1097/01.Ccm.0000245783.28478.Ad.
43. Chanques G, Kress JP, Pohlman A, et al. Impact of ventilator adjustment and sedation-analgesia practices on severe asynchrony in patients ventilated in assist-control mode. Crit Care Med. 2013;41(9):2177–87. https://doi.org/10.1097/CCM.0b013e31828c2d7a.
44. Brochard L, Slutsky A, Pesenti A. Mechanical ventilation to minimize progression of lung injury in acute respiratory failure. Am J Respir Crit Care Med. 2017;195(4):438–42. https://doi.org/10.1164/rccm.201605-1081CP.
45. Yoshida T, Nakahashi S, Nakamura MAM, et al. Volume-controlled ventilation does not prevent injurious inflation during spontaneous effort. Am J Respir Crit Care Med. 2017;196(5):590–601. https://doi.org/10.1164/rccm.201610-1972OC.
46. Ebihara S, Hussain SN, Danialou G, Cho WK, Gottfried SB, Petrof BJ. Mechanical ventilation protects against diaphragm injury in sepsis: interaction of oxidative and mechanical stresses. Am J Respir Crit Care Med. 2002;165(2):221–8. https://doi.org/10.1164/ajrccm.165.2.2108041.
47. Reid WD, Huang J, Bryson S, Walker DC, Belcastro AN. Diaphragm injury and myofibrillar structure induced by resistive loading. J Appl Physiol (1985). 1994;76(1):176–84. https://doi.org/10.1152/jappl.1994.76.1.176.
48. Vassilakopoulos T, Petrof BJ. Ventilator-induced diaphragmatic dysfunction. Am J Respir Crit Care Med. 2004;169(3):336–41. https://doi.org/10.1164/rccm.200304-489CP.
49. Wang X, Jiang TX, Road JD, Redenbach DM, Reid WD. Granulocytosis and increased adhesion molecules after resistive loading of the diaphragm. Eur Respir J. 2005;26(5):786–94. https://doi.org/10.1183/09031936.05.00105204.

50. Reid WD, Belcastro AN. Chronic resistive loading induces diaphragm injury and ventilatory failure in the hamster. Respir Physiol. 1999;118(2–3, 203):–18. https://doi.org/10.1016/s0034-5687(99)00089-4.
51. Reid WD, Noonan J, Chung F, Tesler-Mabe C. Ventilatory failure induced by tracheal banding in the hamster. J Appl Physiol (1985). 1992;73(4):1671–5. https://doi.org/10.1152/jappl.1992.73.4.1671.
52. Lin MC, Ebihara S, El Dwairi Q, et al. Diaphragm sarcolemmal injury is induced by sepsis and alleviated by nitric oxide synthase inhibition. Am J Respir Crit Care Med. 1998;158(5 Pt 1):1656–63. https://doi.org/10.1164/ajrccm.158.5.9803112.
53. Boczkowski J, Lanone S, Ungureanu-Longrois D, Danialou G, Fournier T, Aubier M. Induction of diaphragmatic nitric oxide synthase after endotoxin administration in rats: role on diaphragmatic contractile dysfunction. J Clin Invest. 1996;98(7):1550–9. https://doi.org/10.1172/jci118948.
54. Hillas G, Perlikos F, Toumpanakis D, et al. Controlled mechanical ventilation attenuates the systemic inflammation of severe chronic obstructive pulmonary disease exacerbations. Am J Respir Crit Care Med. 2016;193(6):696–8. https://doi.org/10.1164/rccm.201508-1700LE.
55. Sigala I, Makropoulou M, Karavana V, et al. Glucose transport in the strenuously contracting diaphragm. Eur Respir J. 2015;46(suppl 59):PA3914. https://doi.org/10.1183/13993003.congress-2015.PA3914.
56. Goligher EC, Dres M, Fan E, et al. Mechanical ventilation-induced diaphragm atrophy strongly impacts clinical outcomes. Am J Respir Crit Care Med. 2018;197(2):204–13. https://doi.org/10.1164/rccm.201703-0536OC.
57. Yasuda T, Fukumura K, Iida H, Nakajima T. Effect of low-load resistance exercise with and without blood flow restriction to volitional fatigue on muscle swelling. Eur J Appl Physiol. 2015;115(5):919–26. https://doi.org/10.1007/s00421-014-3073-9.
58. Proske U, Morgan DL. Muscle damage from eccentric exercise: mechanism, mechanical signs, adaptation and clinical applications. J Physiol. 2001;537(Pt 2):333–45. https://doi.org/10.1111/j.1469-7793.2001.00333.x.
59. García-Valdés P, Fernández T, Jalil Y, Peñailillo L, Damiani LF. Eccentric contractions of the diaphragm during mechanical ventilation. Respir Care. 2023;68(12):1757–62. https://doi.org/10.4187/respcare.11040.
60. de Vries HJ, Jonkman AH, Holleboom MC, et al. Diaphragm activity during expiration in ventilated critically ill patients. Am J Respir Crit Care Med. 2024;209(7):881–3. https://doi.org/10.1164/rccm.202310-1845LE.
61. Goligher EC, Urrea C, Vorona SL, et al. Diaphragm inactivity and eccentric contractile activity are common and impair diaphragm function during mechanical ventilation. D105 respiratory failure: role of the diaphragm and skeletal muscles. 2016. p. A7642–A7642.
62. Emeriaud G, Beck J, Tucci M, Lacroix J, Sinderby C. Diaphragm electrical activity during expiration in mechanically ventilated infants. Pediatr Res. 2006;59(5):705–10. https://doi.org/10.1203/01.pdr.0000214986.82862.57.
63. Shee CD, Ploy-Song-Sang Y, Milic-Emili J. Decay of inspiratory muscle pressure during expiration in conscious humans. J Appl Physiol (1985). 1985;58(6):1859–65. https://doi.org/10.1152/jappl.1985.58.6.1859.
64. Pellegrini M, Hedenstierna G, Roneus A, Segelsjö M, Larsson A, Perchiazzi G. The diaphragm acts as a brake during expiration to prevent lung collapse. Am J Respir Crit Care Med. 2017;195(12):1608–16. https://doi.org/10.1164/rccm.201605-0992OC.
65. Rolland-Debord C, Bureau C, Poitou T, et al. Prevalence and prognosis impact of patient-ventilator asynchrony in early phase of weaning according to two detection methods. Anesthesiology. 2017;127(6):989–97. https://doi.org/10.1097/aln.0000000000001886.
66. Chao DC, Scheinhorn DJ, Stearn-Hassenpflug M. Patient-ventilator trigger asynchrony in prolonged mechanical ventilation. Chest. 1997;112(6):1592–9. https://doi.org/10.1378/chest.112.6.1592.

67. Akoumianaki E, Lyazidi A, Rey N, et al. Mechanical ventilation-induced reverse-triggered breaths: a frequently unrecognized form of neuromechanical coupling. Chest. 2013;143(4):927–38. https://doi.org/10.1378/chest.12-1817.
68. Mellott KG, Grap MJ, Munro CL, et al. Patient ventilator asynchrony in critically ill adults: frequency and types. Heart Lung. 2014;43(3):231–43. https://doi.org/10.1016/j.hrtlng.2014.02.002.
69. Vaporidi K, Babalis D, Chytas A, et al. Clusters of ineffective efforts during mechanical ventilation: impact on outcome. Intensive Care Med. 2017;43(2):184–91. https://doi.org/10.1007/s00134-016-4593-z.
70. Rodrigues A, Telias I, Damiani LF, Brochard L. Reverse triggering during controlled ventilation: from physiology to clinical management. Am J Respir Crit Care Med. 2023;207(5):533–43. https://doi.org/10.1164/rccm.202208-1477CI.
71. Blanch L, Villagra A, Sales B, et al. Asynchronies during mechanical ventilation are associated with mortality. Intensive Care Med. 2015;41(4):633–41. https://doi.org/10.1007/s00134-015-3692-6.
72. Cohen CA, Zagelbaum G, Gross D, Roussos C, Macklem PT. Clinical manifestations of inspiratory muscle fatigue. Am J Med. 1982;73(3):308–16.
73. Barton ER, Wang BJ, Brisson BK, Sweeney HL. Diaphragm displays early and progressive functional deficits in dysferlin-deficient mice. Muscle Nerve. 2010;42(1):22–9. https://doi.org/10.1002/mus.21645.
74. Gea J, Zhu E, Gáldiz JB, et al. Functional consequences of eccentric contractions of the diaphragm. Arch Bronconeumol. 2009;45(2):68–74. Consecuencias de las contracciones excéntricas del diafragma sobre su función. https://doi.org/10.1016/j.arbres.2008.04.003.
75. Damiani LF, Engelberts D, Bastia L, et al. Impact of reverse triggering dyssynchrony during lung-protective ventilation on diaphragm function: an experimental model. Am J Respir Crit Care Med. 2022;205(6):663–73. https://doi.org/10.1164/rccm.202105-1089OC.
76. Mellado Artigas R, Damiani LF, Piraino T, et al. Reverse triggering dyssynchrony 24 h after initiation of mechanical ventilation. Anesthesiology. 2021;134(5):760–9. https://doi.org/10.1097/aln.0000000000003726.
77. Rodriguez PO, Tiribelli N, Fredes S, et al. Prevalence of reverse triggering in early ARDS: results from a multicenter observational study. Chest. 2021;159(1):186–95. https://doi.org/10.1016/j.chest.2020.08.018.
78. Coiffard B, Dianti J, Telias I, et al. Dyssynchronous diaphragm contractions impair diaphragm function in mechanically ventilated patients. Crit Care. 2024;28(1):107. https://doi.org/10.1186/s13054-024-04894-3.
79. Singh B, Panizza JA, Finucane KE. Diaphragm electromyogram root mean square response to hypercapnia and its intersubject and day-to-day variation. J Appl Physiol (1985). 2005;98(1):274–81. https://doi.org/10.1152/japplphysiol.01380.2003.
80. Finucane KE, Panizza JA, Singh B. Efficiency of the normal human diaphragm with hyperinflation. J Appl Physiol (1985). 2005;99(4):1402–11. https://doi.org/10.1152/japplphysiol.01165.2004.
81. Doorduin J, van Hees HW, van der Hoeven JG, Heunks LM. Monitoring of the respiratory muscles in the critically ill. Am J Respir Crit Care Med. 2013;187(1):20–7. https://doi.org/10.1164/rccm.201206-1117CP.
82. Acosta P, Santisbon E, Varon J. The use of positive end-expiratory pressure in mechanical ventilation. Crit Care Clin. 2007;23(2):251–61, x. https://doi.org/10.1016/j.ccc.2006.12.012.
83. Dianti J, Tisminetzky M, Ferreyro BL, et al. Association of positive end-expiratory pressure and lung recruitment selection strategies with mortality in acute respiratory distress syndrome: a systematic review and network meta-analysis. Am J Respir Crit Care Med. 2022;205(11):1300–10.
84. Widing H, Pellegrini M, Chiodaroli E, Persson P, Hallén K, Perchiazzi G. Positive end-expiratory pressure limits inspiratory effort through modulation of the effort-to-drive ratio: an experimental crossover study. Intensive Care Med Exp. 2024;12(1):10. https://doi.org/10.1186/s40635-024-00597-9.

85. Loring SH, Mead J, Griscom NT. Dependence of diaphragmatic length on lung volume and thoracoabdominal configuration. J Appl Physiol (1985). 1985;59(6):1961–70. https://doi.org/10.1152/jappl.1985.59.6.1961.
86. Wait JL, Nahormek PA, Yost WT, Rochester DP. Diaphragmatic thickness-lung volume relationship in vivo. J Appl Physiol (1985). 1989;67(4):1560–8. https://doi.org/10.1152/jappl.1989.67.4.1560.
87. Wait JL, Staworn D, Poole DC. Diaphragm thickness heterogeneity at functional residual capacity and total lung capacity. J Appl Physiol (1985). 1995;78(3):1030–6. https://doi.org/10.1152/jappl.1995.78.3.1030.
88. Gauthier AP, Verbanck S, Estenne M, Segebarth C, Macklem PT, Paiva M. Three-dimensional reconstruction of the in vivo human diaphragm shape at different lung volumes. J Appl Physiol (1985). 1994;76(2):495–506. https://doi.org/10.1152/jappl.1994.76.2.495.
89. Jansen D, Jonkman AH, Vries HJ, et al. Positive end-expiratory pressure affects geometry and function of the human diaphragm. J Appl Physiol (1985). 2021;131(4):1328–39. https://doi.org/10.1152/japplphysiol.00184.2021.
90. Lindqvist J, van den Berg M, van der Pijl R, et al. Positive end-expiratory pressure ventilation induces longitudinal atrophy in diaphragm fibers. Am J Respir Crit Care Med. 2018;198(4):472–85. https://doi.org/10.1164/rccm.201709-1917OC.
91. Herzog W. The multiple roles of titin in muscle contraction and force production. Biophys Rev. 2018;10(4):1187–99. https://doi.org/10.1007/s12551-017-0395-y.
92. Yang L, Luo J, Bourdon J, Lin MC, Gottfried SB, Petrof BJ. Controlled mechanical ventilation leads to remodeling of the rat diaphragm. Am J Respir Crit Care Med. 2002;166(8):1135–40. https://doi.org/10.1164/rccm.2202020.
93. Supinski GS, Kelsen SG. Effect of elastase-induced emphysema on the force-generating ability of the diaphragm. J Clin Invest. 1982;70(5):978–88. https://doi.org/10.1172/jci110709.
94. Sassoon CS, Zhu E, Fang L, Sieck GC, Powers SK. Positive end-expiratory airway pressure does not aggravate ventilator-induced diaphragmatic dysfunction in rabbits. Crit Care. 2014;18(5):494. https://doi.org/10.1186/s13054-014-0494-0.
95. Henderson WR, Chen L, Amato MBP, Brochard LJ. Fifty years of research in ARDS. Respiratory mechanics in acute respiratory distress syndrome. Am J Respir Crit Care Med. 2017;196(7):822–33. https://doi.org/10.1164/rccm.201612-2495CI.
96. Rubini A, El-Mazloum D, Morra F, Bosco G. The effect of body cooling on respiratory system mechanics and hysteresis in rats. Respir Physiol Neurobiol. 2013;189(1):52–8.
97. Esteban A, Alía I, Ibañez J, Benito S, Tobin MJ. Modes of mechanical ventilation and weaning. A national survey of Spanish hospitals. The Spanish Lung Failure Collaborative Group. Chest. 1994;106(4):1188–93. https://doi.org/10.1378/chest.106.4.1188.
98. Esteban A, Frutos F, Tobin MJ, et al. A comparison of four methods of weaning patients from mechanical ventilation. Spanish Lung Failure Collaborative Group. N Engl J Med. 1995;332(6):345–50. https://doi.org/10.1056/nejm199502093320601.
99. Peñuelas O, Muriel A, Frutos-Vivar F, et al. Prediction and outcome of intensive care unit-acquired paresis. J Intensive Care Med. 2018;33(1):16–28. https://doi.org/10.1177/0885066616643529.
100. Dot I, Pérez-Teran P, Samper MA, Masclans JR. Diaphragm dysfunction in mechanically ventilated patients. Arch Bronconeumol. 2017;53(3):150–6. Disfunción diafragmática: una realidad en el paciente ventilado mecánicamente https://doi.org/10.1016/j.arbres.2016.07.008.
101. Demoule A, Molinari N, Jung B, et al. Patterns of diaphragm function in critically ill patients receiving prolonged mechanical ventilation: a prospective longitudinal study. Ann Intensive Care. 2016;6(1):75. https://doi.org/10.1186/s13613-016-0179-8.
102. Supinski GS, Callahan LA. Diaphragm weakness in mechanically ventilated critically ill patients. Crit Care. 2013;17(3):R120. https://doi.org/10.1186/cc12792.
103. Goligher EC, Brochard LJ, Reid WD, et al. Diaphragmatic myotrauma: a mediator of prolonged ventilation and poor patient outcomes in acute respiratory failure. Lancet Respir Med. 2019;7(1):90–8. https://doi.org/10.1016/s2213-2600(18)30366-7.

104. Thille AW, Rodriguez P, Cabello B, Lellouche F, Brochard L. Patient-ventilator asynchrony during assisted mechanical ventilation. Intensive Care Med. 2006;32(10):1515–22. https://doi.org/10.1007/s00134-006-0301-8.
105. de Wit M, Miller KB, Green DA, Ostman HE, Gennings C, Epstein SK. Ineffective triggering predicts increased duration of mechanical ventilation. Crit Care Med. 2009;37(10):2740–5. https://doi.org/10.1097/ccm.0b013e3181a98a05.
106. Thille AW, Cabello B, Galia F, Lyazidi A, Brochard L. Reduction of patient-ventilator asynchrony by reducing tidal volume during pressure-support ventilation. Intensive Care Med. 2008;34(8):1477–86. https://doi.org/10.1007/s00134-008-1121-9.
107. Damiani LF, Bruhn A, Retamal J, Bugedo G. Patient-ventilator dyssynchronies: are they all the same? A clinical classification to guide actions. J Crit Care. 2020;60:50–7. https://doi.org/10.1016/j.jcrc.2020.07.016.
108. Pham T, Telias I, Piraino T, Yoshida T, Brochard LJ. Asynchrony consequences and management. Crit Care Clin. 2018;34(3):325–41. https://doi.org/10.1016/j.ccc.2018.03.008.
109. Mercat A, Richard J-CM, Vielle B, et al. Positive end-expiratory pressure setting in adults with acute lung injury and acute respiratory distress syndrome: a randomized controlled trial. JAMA. 2008;299(6):646–55. https://doi.org/10.1001/jama.299.6.646.

Chapter 16
Airway Clearance Techniques and Weaning

Fernando Silva Guimarães and Marcia Souza Volpe

16.1 Introduction

In mechanically ventilated patients, the primary mechanisms of respiratory secretions clearance—mucociliary transport and cough—are impaired. The presence of the artificial airway [1], poor humidification of inspired gases [2], relative immobility [3], and weak cough strength [4] are the major causes of respiratory secretion retention in this population. Moreover, patients with underlying diseases associated with increased mucus production and reduced lung ventilatory capacity, such as chronic obstructive pulmonary disease (COPD) [5] and spinal cord injury [6], are at heightened risk of respiratory secretions retention, making it a critical complication to address throughout their recovery.

Accumulated secretion in the airways, if extensive, starts a self-sustaining cycle of ventilation/perfusion mismatch, gas-exchange impairment, increased work of breathing, and subsequent augmented risk of mechanical ventilation dependence, which, in turn, closes a positive loop predisposing to more retention of secretions [7, 8]. In addition, retained secretions are a sequestered growth medium for bacteria, which increases the risk of pneumonia and keeps feeding this cycle [9, 10].

It is also known that the presence of moderate to copious secretion and the inability to clear secretions can contribute significantly to extubation failure [11, 12]. Copious secretions are typically defined as requiring airway suctioning more than twice per hour [12]. Patients with moderate or abundant secretions are three

F. S. Guimarães (✉)
Cardiopulmonary and Musculoskeletal Physiotherapy Department, Federal University of Rio de Janeiro, Rio de Janeiro, Brazil
e-mail: fguimaraes@hucff.ufrj.br

M. S. Volpe
Department of Sciences of Human Movement, Federal University of São Paulo, São Paulo, Brazil

A. R. Baptistella et al. (eds.), *Weaning from Mechanical Ventilation*, https://doi.org/10.1007/978-3-032-01145-9_16

to eight times more likely to experience extubation failure than those with minimal or no secretions [11, 13]. Additionally, moderate to copious secretions have been identified as a predictor of reintubation even in patients who have demonstrated an adequate cough and completed a successful spontaneous breathing trial [12].

Secretion clearance in patients with artificial airways is mainly performed through endotracheal suctioning [14]. It has been recommended to apply shallow suctioning instead of deep suctioning, which limits the insertion of the suction catheter to the tip of the artificial airway and may restrain its level of action. [15] However, when suctioning stimulates effective coughing, this procedure can remove secretions from the large airways up to the third-generation bronchi.

Cough strength is frequently diminished due to the presence of the endotracheal tube, which increases airway resistance and impairs normal laryngeal and vocal cord functions. [14] This impairment inhibits the ability to close the glottis, essential for generating the pressure required for an effective cough. Furthermore, studies have demonstrated that expiratory muscle weakness is common during ventilator weaning, compromising cough strength, and may be associated with extubation failure [12, 16–18]. Systemic inflammation, sepsis, ICU-acquired muscle weakness, sedation, ventilator settings, nutritional status, and co-morbidities like COPD and myopathies were identified as factors contributing to expiratory muscle weakness [19, 20]. The impact of mechanical ventilation on expiratory muscles has not been systematically investigated; however, ventilator settings, including high PEEP, a high level of inspiratory assistance, and asynchronies as delayed cycling, may increase the activity of the expiratory muscles representing an expiratory overload, which, if prolonged, may impair expiratory muscle function [21, 22].

Given these factors, it is advisable to implement strategies that mobilize pulmonary secretions from peripheral to central airways, preserve expiratory muscle function during mechanical ventilation, and utilize cough augmentation techniques in patients with weak cough strength both before and after extubation, to enhance the likelihood of successful weaning from mechanical ventilation.

Several airway clearance techniques for mechanically ventilated patients have been described, such as manual and ventilator hyperinflation. In recent years, the mechanisms underlying effective airway clearance have become clearer, particularly in relation to the use of flow bias and the maneuvers that optimize it [8].

This chapter provides a concise overview of the role of flow bias and dynamic airway compression in airway clearance therapy, along with insights and recommendations on four techniques that apply these principles to enhance secretion clearance and, consequently, may potentially aid in weaning from mechanical ventilation. The techniques discussed—ventilator hyperinflation, expiratory rib cage compression (ERCC), pressure end-expiratory positive-zero end-expiratory pressure (PEEP-ZEEP), and mechanical insufflation-exsufflation (MI-E) have not only the likelihood to effectively clear secretions but also are relatively simple to perform. To conclude, the importance and relationship between cough strength and extubation outcome are explored.

16.2 Flow Bias and Airways Dynamic Compression During Airway Clearance Therapy

The flow bias is a consequence of the continuous "to and fro" movement of gas in the airways. Averaged over several breaths, the net volume of gas moved in either direction must be equal, but the peak (or mean) flow of the inspiratory and expiratory phases can differ greatly, creating the flow bias [23]. When considering which one is greater, peak inspiratory flow (PIF) or peak expiratory flow (PEF), an inspiratory or expiratory flow bias is established and leads the net movement of mucus in its same direction, that is, toward the lungs or the glottis, respectively. In the normal lung, the narrowing of airways on exhalation increases expiratory air velocity, thus increasing the air–liquid interaction and favoring an expiratory/cephalad mucus flow [24]. However, in mechanically ventilated patients, especially on pressure support ventilation and pressure controlled ventilation, it is usual to find ventilation with PIF that is much higher than the PEF, which creates an inspiratory flow bias and an augmented risk of embedding pulmonary secretion [25, 26].

The flow bias moves mucus by using the two-phase gas-liquid transport mechanism and is usually expressed as the ratio (PEF:PIF) or difference (PEF—PIF) between the peak flows. The critical factors that affect mucus transport by this mechanism include inspiratory-expiratory air velocity, viscosity of mucus, and thickness of the mucus layer, which needs to achieve 5%–10% of the airway diameter [27–29].

In the late 1980s, the influence of the flow bias on secretion management in the patient on mechanical ventilation was raised. The first flow bias threshold described in the literature associated with cephalad mucus displacement was a PEF:PIF ratio > 1.11 [30]. Since then, this flow bias threshold has been used to infer the efficacy of airway clearance techniques in critical care patients [31–33]. In 2008, Volpe et al. [23], after a series of experiments using a bench bicompartmental model and mucus simulant, demonstrated that the transport of airway secretions by the two-phase gas–liquid transport mechanism appears to be best explained by the difference between PEF and PIF and not by the PEF:PIF ratio. The authors identified a critical threshold for mucus displacement toward the glottis a PEF-PIF difference of >17 L/min, and that the larger this difference, the greater the mucus displacement [23]. In 2012, Li Bassi et al. [34] conducted a study on mechanically ventilated pigs in the semirecumbent position and found that the animals' own mucus was displaced centrally when an average PEF-PIF difference of 33.0 ± 7.6 L/min was achieved, while the average PEF:PIF ratio was 4.3 ± 1.2, significantly exceeding the threshold of 1.11.

When comparing the flow bias thresholds reported in the literature, the PEF-PIF difference of >33.0 L/min is likely more clinically relevant for mechanically ventilated patients, as it was observed in a live experiment involving the animal's own mucus over prolonged mechanical ventilation (4–72 h), where mucus had to move against gravity [34].

The airways' dynamic compression is also advocated as a valuable way to improve the gas–liquid flow interaction with the premise that expiratory flow is kept constant or higher in narrower airways, resulting in air flow acceleration. This occurs because, according to Bernoulli's principle, gas velocity for the same flow is higher in the narrower airway [35, 36]. During maneuvers that increase the pleural pressure, such as manual ERCC, this effect is accentuated because it reduces even further the airway diameter during exhalation. In these situations, as the intrabronchial pressure is progressively lower from the alveoli to the mouth, there will be a point where it equals the surrounding pleural pressure (i.e., the equal pressure point) [36]. In the upstream airway segment from the equal pressure point (toward the alveoli), there is no dynamic airway compression, whereas downstream (toward the mouth), pleural pressure exceeds intrabronchial pressure and dynamic compression occurs [37]. The site of the equal pressure point is influenced by the airway stability, the expiratory force, and lung volume. For instance, a higher expiratory force and an exhalation starting from small lung volumes shift the equal pressure point more peripherally [37, 38]. On the other hand, an exhalation starting from high lung volumes shifts the equal pressure point more centrally. Independent of where the equal pressure point is initially located, with an ongoing forced expiration, the equal pressure point gradually moves upstream (toward the alveoli), creating a wave of choke points. In theory, to assist with airway clearance, the equal pressure point needs to be shifted to where the mucus is accumulated to catch mucus in such a choke point and thus expel it toward the glottis by the increased expiratory air flow velocity [36]. These physiological principles are the rational basis for the use of low lung volume to remove secretion from distal airways and high lung volumes from central airways [24].

However, patients with unstable airways or reduced lung volumes may be susceptible to expiratory flow limitation during compressive or forced expiratory maneuvers, which is believed to be related to the collapsibility of airways [39, 40]. If the airways collapse, the downstream flow drops to zero and secretion removal is interrupted [24, 39].

16.3 Airway Clearance Techniques for Mechanically Ventilated Patients

Ventilator hyperinflation, ERCC, PEEP-ZEEP, and MI-E are airway clearance techniques that utilize the mechanisms of flow bias and dynamic airway compression to facilitate effective secretion removal [8]. However, there are ongoing debates regarding the optimal application of these techniques, and further clarification is needed. Moreover, there is a lack of studies addressing their effects on long-term clinically relevant outcomes, such as length of stay and duration of mechanical ventilation, highlighting the need for further research. Given the limited evidence, these techniques should be applied when there is clear evidence of secretion retention.

16.3.1 Ventilator Hyperinflation

Ventilator hyperinflation can be defined as the use of the ventilator to deliver increased tidal volume aimed at assisting with secretion removal. This technique was introduced as an alternative to manual hyperinflation, which is performed by delivering a large tidal volume with a resuscitation bag, followed by an inspiratory plateau, and a fast release of the bag to provide high expiratory flows [41]. Both ventilator hyperinflation and manual hyperinflation may be applied with a second aim, to open collapsed lung units that are not necessarily associated with airway secretion retention. In this chapter, we discuss only the use of ventilator hyperinflation as an airway clearance technique.

The first use of the term "ventilator hyperinflation" took place in 2002 [42] and reported that this technique was equivalent to manual hyperinflation in improving secretion removal and static compliance of the respiratory system. Since then, many studies on ventilator hyperinflation have been carried out with general samples of critical care patients [42–46]. These studies confirmed the similarity between ventilator hyperinflation and manual hyperinflation in clearing secretions, improving respiratory mechanics, and gas exchange [42, 44, 45]. Due to the potential advantages of ventilator hyperinflation, we embrace its use instead of manual hyperinflation. When using the ventilator to apply the maneuver, the patient is not disconnected from the mechanical ventilator, which avoids PEEP loss, hypoxemia, and shear stress caused by cyclic opening and closing of small airways. Moreover, different from manual hyperinflation, ventilator hyperinflation makes it possible to monitor and set the parameters of interest for the technique's application, including the expiratory flow bias [44, 45, 47].

Studies on ventilator hyperinflation have used different criteria to determine the inspiratory volume: 50% above the current tidal volume [46], 130% of the set tidal volume [44], 15 mL/kg [45], and volume corresponding to a peak inspiratory pressure of 40 cmH_2O [42, 43, 47]. Regardless of the criteria chosen, the peak inspiratory pressure was limited to 40 cmH_2O. The main modes used for ventilator hyperinflation were volume controlled ventilation [42, 46] and pressure support ventilation [43]. Regarding the inspiratory time or flow settings during ventilator hyperinflation, the following were used: inspiratory time of 3–5 s [45], inspiratory flow of 20 L/min plus an inspiratory pause of 2 s [42], or no modification at all [44].

In 2015, after 232 trials with a bench lung model circuit, Thomas [48] found that volume controlled ventilation proved more effective than pressure support and pressure control ventilation to achieve expiratory flow bias thresholds. Another in vitro study using a mucus simulant showed that longer rise times reduced PIF, improving expiratory flow bias and mucus movement [49]. Also, Ribeiro et al. studied 6 ventilator hyperinflation modes in 30 mechanically ventilated subjects, finding that volume controlled ventilation with a 20 L/min inspiratory flow and pressure support with 10% or 25% cycling off provided the best results [47].

For patients presenting with respiratory drive, some ventilatory modes may cause patient–ventilator asynchrony during ventilator hyperinflation. In the study by

Table 16.1 Suggested procedures for ventilator hyperinflation (VH)

	Optimal procedure for VH	Procedure for VH for patients who present flow asynchrony under optimal VH
Ventilation mode and strategy to decrease PIF	1. Use VCV with square wave flow of and inspiratory flow of 20–30 L/min	1. Use PSV with cycling off of 10% and set the slowest rise time that does not cause flow asynchrony
Target VT and inspiratory pressures	2. Increase VT to reach PIP of 35 cmH_2O and certify that Pplat is ≤30 cmH_2O[a]	2. Increase PSV to reach PIP of 30 cmH_2O
Expiratory flow bias	3. Ensure that PEF-PIF difference >33 L/min; if it is not, consider reducing the inspiratory flow or the rise time	3. Certify that the PEF-PIF difference is >33 L/min; if it is not, consider slowing the rise time
PEEP	4. Set optimal PEEP to maintain airway patency	
Monitor	5. Monitor hemodynamics, oxygen saturation, and ventilator curves throughout the procedure	

VCV volume controlled ventilation, *PSV* pressure support ventilation, *VT* tidal volume, *PEF* peak expiratory flow, *PIF* peak inspiratory flow, *PIP* peak inspiratory pressure, *Pplat* plateau pressure, *PEEP* positive end-expiratory pressure

[a]In patients without respiratory drive, reduce breathing frequency to keep the baseline minute ventilation

Ribeiro et al. [47], the authors also reported that volume controlled ventilation with an inspiratory flow of 20 or 50 L/min and pressure controlled ventilation with prolonged inspiratory time (i.e., 3 s) were associated with a high incidence of flow and phase asynchronies, respectively.

In 2020, recommendations were provided on how to select the ventilator settings to perform an optimized ventilator hyperinflation maneuver—aiming the PEF-PIF difference > 33 L/min, for patients under controlled ventilation, and to those experiencing respiratory discomfort or patient-ventilator asynchrony during the maneuver applied in volume controlled mode [8]. The procedures to perform the ventilator hyperinflation according to recommendations are shown in Table 16.1. Following the publication of these recommendations, two studies reported that ventilator hyperinflation in volume controlled ventilation, compared to pressure control ventilation, was more effective at removing secretions [50] and achieving the expiratory flow bias threshold [26, 50].

16.3.2 Expiratory Rib Cage Compression

ERCC is one of the most commonly applied airway clearance techniques in mechanically ventilated patients [51–54]. However, there is great controversy on how this technique should be performed, which is reflected by the several forms of ERCC found in the literature [55, 56]. Specific details on how the compression is applied (i.e., intensity of the compression, its initiation and duration in relation to the phase of the ventilator cycle, whether performed in association with chest wall vibration, and how chest release is applied at the end of the maneuver) modify the technique greatly. To make this topic even more controversial, there is no consensus on terminology used to distinguish the different forms of ERCC [57].

Regarding its objectives, ERRC is usually applied either to assist with secretion movement from distal to proximal airways or to remove secretion from large airways [58, 59]. In theory, if ERRC is applied with gradual intensity (from gentle to strong) to prolong exhalation after the onset of the expiratory phase, it removes secretions from distal airways. On the other hand, if ERRC is applied with hard compressions to increase PEF and synchronized with the onset of expiration, it removes secretions from proximal airways. Marti et al. [56] named these two techniques soft manual rib cage compression and hard manual rib cage compression, respectively. To facilitate the understanding, we suggest a similar terminology: soft/long ERCC and hard/brief ERCC.

Marti et al. [56] compared these two ERCC forms in pigs under prolonged mechanical ventilation, assessing mucus clearance through fluoroscopy tracking of radio-opaque markers. They found that the hard/brief ERCC increased the PEF by ~9 L/min and significantly improved mucus clearance in the trachea without causing any deleterious effect. On the other hand, the soft/long ERCC did not influence mucus clearance and slightly worsened the static lung elastance and cardiac output. The prolonged chest squeezing probably caused a decrease in the expiratory lung volume and in the venous return, leading to the worsening of respiratory mechanics and hemodynamics, respectively. However, because mucus movement was measured only at the trachea, it is not possible to infer anything about mucus displacement in the lung periphery. It is also worth noting that these assessments were measured only prior to and after each technique, without details on how long they lasted.

Others have investigated the use of the soft/long ERCC form, and the results are diverse. In a study with mechanically ventilated rabbits with induced atelectasis by instillation of artificial mucus, Unoki et al. [60] reported that the use of this technique followed by suctioning worsened the respiratory compliance and gas exchange compared to the control group submitted only to airway suctioning. However, the rabbits were ventilated with no PEEP, which might have predisposed the animals to airway collapse during ERCC. In another study by the same group, the use of the soft/long ERCC in association with lateral decubitus position in 31 ventilated subjects resulted in no changes in pulmonary mechanics, gas exchange, and secretion clearance [61]. Genc et al. [62] also reported that the addition of ERCC to manual hyperinflation did not improve lung compliance and secretion removal in 22 ventilated subjects. On the contrary, another study indicated that the use of the soft/long ERCC combined with abdominal compression in 16 subjects with ventilator-associated pneumonia removed more secretion and resulted in a transient improvement in static lung compliance when compared to the control group [55].

Regarding the hard/brief ERCC form, several studies that investigated this technique in ventilated lung models, animals, and adult subjects reported significant increases in PEF of 8.8 L/min [63], 8.9–13 L/min [56, 64], and 6.7–43.8 L/min [65–68],, respectively. The capacity of the hard/brief ERCC to increase PEF seems to be mainly determined by the timing of the maneuver application, which should be performed in full synchronization with the onset of expiration [63]. However, other factors, such as properties of the respiratory system, inspired tidal volume, and use of one or two hands, also influence the resulting PEF.

Avena et al. [57] reported that the use of the hard/brief ERCC form followed by airway suctioning in surgical subjects resulted in reduced airway resistance and improved oxygenation, indicating the efficacy of the technique in removing secretion. It is important to note that, in the study by Marti et al. [56], the animals were ventilated with an expiratory flow bias already in the baseline and that the ERCC increased this flow bias, favoring secretion removal. In the study by Avena et al. [57], although the peak flows were not reported, the ERCC probably resulted in an expiratory flow bias because the subjects were ventilated in volume-controlled ventilation with a square wave flow and increased inspiratory time. Therefore, in both studies, the efficacy of the hard/brief ERCC form in removing secretion was associated with the presence of an expiratory flow bias.

Gonçalves et al. [69] also reported that the hard/brief ERCC form resulted in greater removal of secretion and improvement of static compliance in 30 mechanically ventilated subjects. In another study with 35 ventilated subjects, the use of the hard/brief ERCC applied in association with an increment on PEEP from 5 cmH_2O to 15 cmH_2O and on inspiratory time from 1 s to 2 s resulted in higher PEF and decreased airway resistance when compared to ERCC alone [66]. The authors postulated that the higher PEEP minimized airway collapse during ERCC and thus allowed higher PEF. However, because the subjects were ventilated in the pressure controlled mode, the increase in the inspiratory time and PEEP could have resulted in higher tidal volume, thus leading to a higher PEF. Guimaraes et al. [67] investigated the application of the hard/long ERCC in 20 mechanically ventilated subjects with pulmonary infection. The maneuver resulted in an increase in the PEF, in the terminal expiratory flow (which reflects the flow pattern in small airways), and in the amount of removed secretion. However, six subjects exhibited expiratory flow limitation during ERCC. This was detected by the superimposition between the baseline (current ventilation) and ERCC flow-volume loops observed on the ventilator display. Because the flow-volume loop is a practical method to detect expiratory flow limitation in ventilated patients [70, 71], the authors suggested that the PEEP level should be increased to stabilize the small airways during ERCC to the point at which there is no superimposition between the baseline and ERCC flow-volume loops (Fig. 16.1) [67].

Considering the methodological limitations of many of the studies mentioned above and the inconsistency in the studies' results, it is not possible to make recommendations regarding the use of the soft/long ERCC. However, the use of the hard/brief ERCC appears to be capable of increasing the PEF and thus the expiratory flow bias. Recommendations on how to perform the hard/brief ERCC are described in Table 16.2. Regardless of which ERCC form is applied, chest release should be performed slowly to avoid increasing the elastic recoil of the respiratory system and

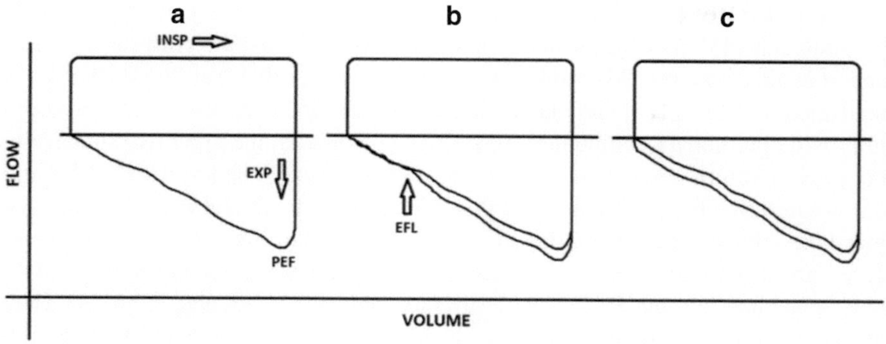

Fig. 16.1 Suggested use of flow-volume curves to set the PEEP level and compressive force during ERCC. (**a**) Baseline flow-volume loop. (**b**) Baseline (internal expiratory curve) and ERCC flow-volume loops (external expiratory curve); the superposition in the terminal part of expiratory flow denotes expiratory flow limitation. (**c**) Baseline (internal expiratory curve) and ERCC flow-volume loops (external expiratory curve) with a PEEP level set to avoid expiratory flow limitation. Note that the flow is increased until the end of expiration. *INSP* inspiration, *EXP* expiration, *PEF* peak expiratory flow, *EFL* expiratory flow limitation, *ERCC* expiratory rib cage compression

Table 16.2 Suggested procedure for hard/brief ERCC indicated to remove secretions from large/central airways

1. Position hands bilaterally on the lower third of the thorax
2. Start compression in full synchronization with the onset of expiration; observe the ventilator curves for better performance
3. Compression should be hard and fast
4. Avoid releasing hands from the chest too quickly to avoid auto-triggering the ventilator and to avoid increasing the transmural pressure, which could increase the PIF of the next cycle
5. Monitor the ventilator screen to observe the increment in the PEF caused by ERCC. If there is no increment, the maneuver is not effective Ensure the PEF-PIF difference > 33 L/min
6. Monitor hemodynamics, oxygen saturation, and ventilator curves throughout the procedure

ERCC expiratory rib cage compression, *PEF* peak expiratory flow, *PIF* peak inspiratory flow

thus prevent the increase in the transpulmonary pressure that could increase the PIF and reduce the expiratory flow bias of the next ventilation cycle.

16.3.3 PEEP-ZEEP

This technique consists of increasing PEEP to 15 cmH_2O during five cycles with peak inspiratory pressure limited to 40 cmH_2O, followed by abrupt reduction of PEEP to 0 cmH_2O [72, 73]. By increasing the delta pressure at the onset of the expiratory phase, this technique increases the PEF and, consequently, the expiratory flow bias. The hard/brief ERRC can be applied in association with PEEP-ZEEP to augment the expiratory flow bias.

The PEEP-ZEEP technique has been proven to be safe in a general sample of ICU subjects [65], in subjects undergoing coronary artery bypass graft surgery [73], and in cardiac patients [74]. Additional studies have reported that PEEP-ZEEP was equivalent to ERCC [72] and manual hyperinflation [75] in removing secretion and improving pulmonary compliance, respectively. However, the latter two studies did not provide information about the ventilation mode used to apply PEEP-ZEEP and did not describe the peak flows and flow bias achieved. Amaral et al. [65] investigated the influence of the ventilation mode (volume controlled ventilation vs. pressure control ventilation) and the effects of applying the hard/brief ERCC on the flow bias generated during PEEP-ZEEP in mechanically ventilated subjects. They reported that the expiratory flow bias was higher in the volume controlled ventilation than in the pressure control ventilation, with a PEF-PIF difference of 39.5 ± 11.5 L/min versus 6.7 ± 5.7 L/min, respectively. This result was caused by a lower PIF in the volume control mode. In addition, in the majority of cycles of PEEP-ZEEP applied in the pressure controlled mode, an inspiratory flow bias was generated, which might embed mucus (Fig. 16.2). Another study from the same group also confirmed that combining the hard/brief ERCC with PEEP-ZEEP increased the expiratory flow bias [59]. PEF was 6.7 ± 3.4 L/min higher with ERCC compared to without ERCC, which increased the PEF-PIF difference by the same amount. Figure 16.3 illustrates the effect of combining ERCC with PEEP-ZEEP.

One limitation of this technique is that using PEEP-ZEEP may induce alveolar collapse in patients with high lung elastance and unstable alveoli. Therefore, it is imperative that PEEP-ZEEP is only applied to carefully selected patients who are not prone to alveolar collapse or acute lung injury [8].

16.3.4 Mechanical Insufflation-Exsufflation

MI-E is used to simulate cough mechanically by applying positive and negative pressure changes to the airways, either noninvasively via a mask or mouthpiece or invasively via a tracheostomy or endotracheal tube. This therapy was developed in the early 1950s and has been used primarily to assist, noninvasively, airway clearance in patients with neuromuscular weakness [76–78].

However, its use in mechanically ventilated patients has been increasing in the past few years [79, 80].

In a study conducted by Coutinho et al., MI-E was compared to traditional tracheal suctioning in mechanically ventilated patients [81]. The results demonstrated no statistically significant difference between the two techniques in lung compliance, pulmonary resistance, hemodynamics, or secretion volume. The study of Kubota et al. compared the effects of MI-E with conventional care on the duration of mechanical ventilation in patients with high sputum retention [82]. The results showed no significant difference in the number of ventilator-free days, ICU length of stay, mortality rate, or tracheostomy rate between the two groups. Therefore, MI-E did not significantly shorten the duration of mechanical ventilation in this

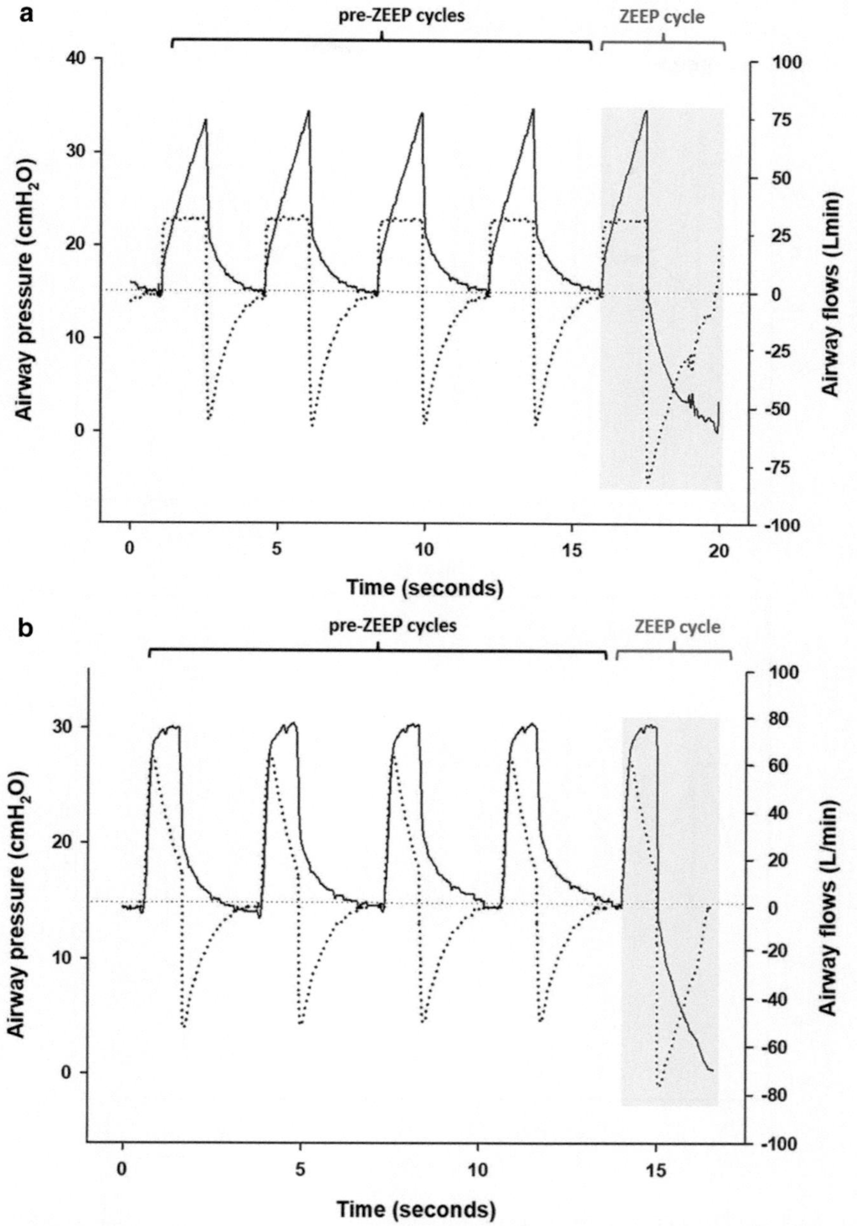

Fig. 16.2 Airway pressure and air flow curves of the PEEP-ZEEP technique applied in (**a**): the volume-controlled mode and in (**b**): the pressure controlled mode, without expiratory rib cage compression, for a representative patient. Pressure curve tracings are continuous, and air flow tracings are interrupted. Note the increment in expiratory flow bias (PEF-PIF difference) during the ZEEP cycle during both ventilation modes caused by PEF augmentation. However, in the pressure controlled mode, the expiratory flow bias (PEF-PIF difference) is 16 L/min, which is enhanced to 50 L/min in the volume controlled mode. Note also that, during the cycles before ZEEP, there is an inspiratory flow bias (PEF-PIF difference) of—11 L/min in the pressure controlled mode, whereas there is an expiratory flow bias of 26 L/min in the volume controlled mode. (From Ref. [65], with permission)

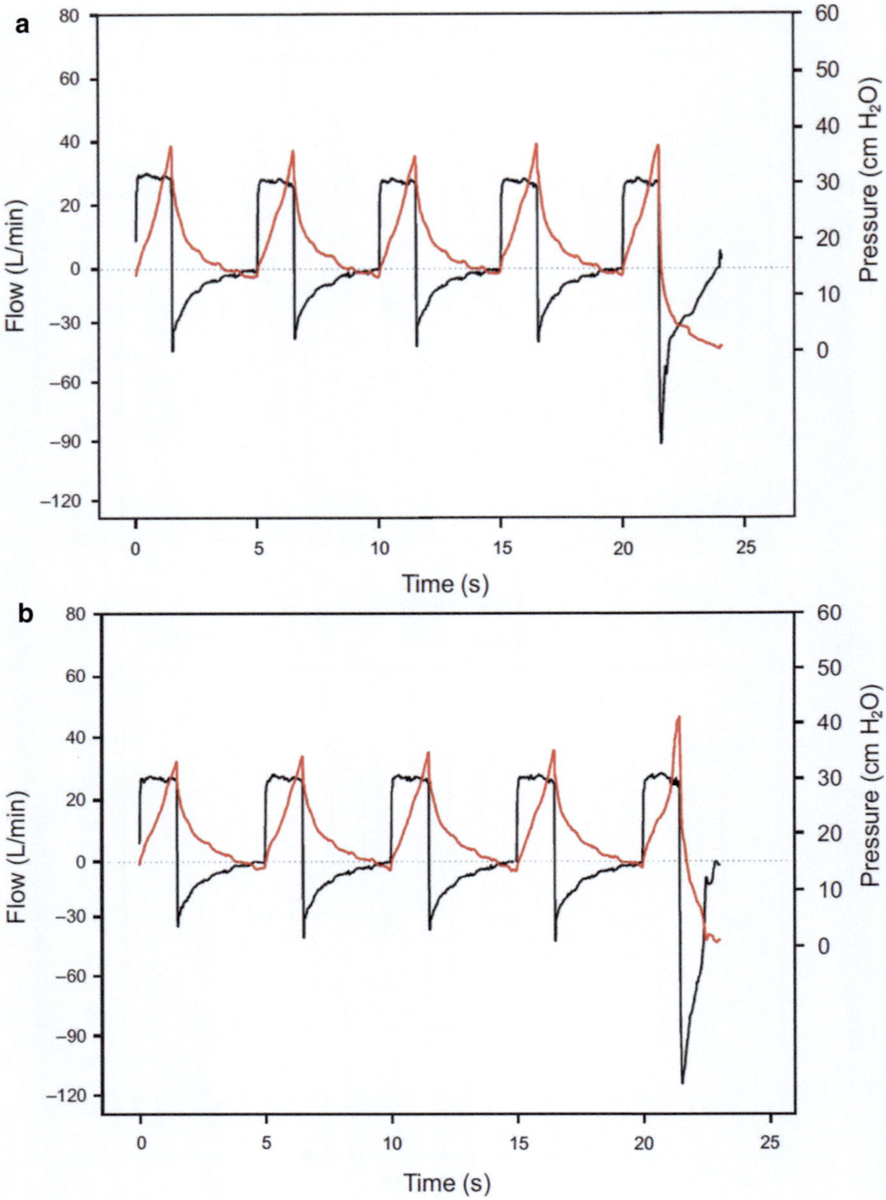

Fig. 16.3 (**a**) The PEEP-ZEEP maneuver without expiratory rib cage compression and (**b**) the PEEP-ZEEP maneuver with expiratory rib cage compression in a representative subject of the study sample. The expiratory flow bias generated during the ZEEP cycle without expiratory rib cage compression (**a**) was ~60 L/min, whereas, with the addition of expiratory rib cage compression (**b**), the expiratory flow bias was ~83 L/min. (From Ref. [59], with permission)

population. However, other studies have reported more favorable outcomes for MI-E. Camillis et al. evaluated MI-E in mechanically ventilated ICU patients and found that it was significantly more efficacious than conventional suctioning in reducing mucus retention and improving lung function [83]. Furthermore, MI-E was associated with a lower incidence of complications, suggesting its potential as a valuable intervention for airway clearance in this population. Alejos et al. investigated the combination of MI-E with ERCC and found that it resulted in significantly higher sputum volume cleared than ERCC alone [84]. This finding suggests that combining these techniques may be particularly effective in improving airway clearance. Sancho et al. compared the effects of MI-E and tracheal suctioning on respiratory variables in patients with amyotrophic lateral sclerosis who required continuous mechanical ventilation via tracheostomy tubes [78]. The results showed that MI-E was more effective than tracheal suctioning in improving respiratory variables, including pulse oxyhemoglobin saturation, peak inspiratory pressure, mean airway pressure, and work of breathing performed by the ventilator [78]. Finally, in the retrospective study of Kurowia et al., the authors compared the incidence of ventilator-associated pneumonia in critically ill patients who received MI-E with those who received chest physical therapy [85]. The results showed that the incidence of VAP was significantly lower in the MI-E group compared to the control group. Therefore, MI-E may be an effective intervention for preventing ventilator-associated pneumonia in critically ill patients.

Overall, most studies indicated that MI-E was more effective than suctioning alone in improving respiratory variables, including secretion removal, pulse oxyhemoglobin saturation, peak inspiratory pressure, mean airway pressure, and work of breathing. This suggests that MI-E is a promising intervention for improving airway clearance in mechanically ventilated patients. Nevertheless, multiple factors may have influenced the study's results, including the inclusion criteria and the methodology of MI-E implementation (parameters, frequency of maneuvers, and daily session count). Consequently, studies that included patients with preserved cough, even hypersecretive, tend to demonstrate minimal or reduced effect size, as the cough peak flow associated with spontaneous cough is sufficient for secretion mobilization.

Regarding MI-E settings (i.e., insufflation-exsufflation pressures, rise time or inspiratory flow, and inspiratory expiratory times), there is no consensus about what settings are optimal for airway clearance. However, adjusting high inspiratory flow might not be indicated in mechanically ventilated patients because it might reduce the expiratory flow bias and, consequently, the efficacy of clearing secretion. Volpe et al. demonstrated this likelihood in a bench study using a lung model simulating a mechanically ventilated patient [86]. The study found that optimizing the MI-E maneuver involved applying slow lung insufflation, which reduced peak inspiratory flow (PIF) and consequently increased the expiratory flow bias. This optimized approach proved far more effective at clearing artificial mucus. Furthermore, the authors observed a significant correlation between the expiratory flow bias (PEF-PIF difference) and the MI-E pressure gradient with mucus displacement, while PEF alone was not significantly correlated. These findings suggest that to optimize airway clearance with MI-E in mechanically ventilated patients, the goal should be to achieve a high PEF-PIF difference. This can be achieved by using slow insufflation (i.e., prolonging inspiratory time) and shorter expiratory times, combined with larger exsufflation pressures (to compensate for the imposed endotracheal tube resistance), within safe pressure limits, such as +30/−40 cmH_2O or + 40/−50 cmH_2O.

Regarding the safety concerns about applying MI-E in mechanically ventilated patients that have been raised, the aforementioned studies have not reported severe complications associated with the use of MI-E in ICU subjects. Nevertheless, MI-E may be detrimental for patients at risk of lung collapse (i.e., using high PEEP levels) or severe hypoxemia due to the utilization of negative pressure and the necessity to disconnect the patient from the mechanical ventilator [87]. Further studies are needed to explore the full potential of MI-E and determine the optimal settings for its use across various intubated critical care patient populations.

16.4 Cough Strength and Cough Augmentation Techniques to Improve the Extubation Outcome

Several studies have demonstrated the value of cough strength measurement in predicting the extubation outcome. In these studies, patients who passed the spontaneous breathing trial and had a cough peak flow (CPF) higher than 55–65 L/min before extubation were successful [88]. With moderate to good predictive power, CPF may be measured using an external spirometer or the ventilator monitor. Although less accurate, the last one offers the advantage of using existing equipment without additional costs or patient disconnection [88]. Moreover, factors such as ventilator parameters, endotracheal tube diameter, circuit resistance, frequency response, sampling frequency, and ventilatory parameters must be carefully considered to ensure reliable CPF measurements [89]. Although there is no defined standardization in the literature, when CPF measurements are taken with a mechanical ventilator, i.e., without an external spirometer, we suggest it be in pressure support ventilation mode (adjusted to avoid under- or over-assistance) and with PEEP equal to zero. It is also essential to adjust the flow versus time curve scale to make the entire expiratory flow curve visible.

Involuntary or reflex cough is generally more reliable since it does not depend on patient motivation. Stimulation can be performed by inserting a catheter through the nasopharynx or by instilling 2–3 mL of saline into the endotracheal tube [90]. CPF can also be measured during spontaneous coughing or suctioning, reducing the discomfort associated with catheter or saline stimulation. However, it is important to note that the suctioning catheter increases airway resistance, potentially leading to underestimating CPF values. In such instances, if the measured values are below 60 L/min, additional stimulation utilizing saline or through the nasopharynx may be necessary to obtain more accurate measurements.

Despite the moderate to high accuracy of cough strength in predicting extubation outcomes, there is no formal recommendation not to extubate a patient with a

CPF of less than 60 L/min. A low CPF means the patient may not protect the airways after extubation, and it is at risk of accumulating pulmonary secretions, resulting in extubation failure. Therefore, CPF measures help to identify patients at a higher risk of extubation failure and those needing special attention post-extubation [89].

When the goal is to increase CPF, the resources that come to mind are physiotherapy techniques or mechanically assisted cough. Also, the impact of expiratory muscles' electrical stimulation on CPF and extubation outcomes is promising but has yet to be consistently evaluated in randomized clinical trials [91–93].

Techniques such as manually assisted coughing or hard/brief ERCC are used to prevent and manage respiratory complications associated with chronic conditions, mainly neuromuscular disease, and may improve short- and long-term outcomes for people with acute respiratory failure [94]. In these techniques, chest and/or abdominal manual compression is performed during the expulsive phase of the cough, preceded or not by positive inspiratory pressure to increase the inspired volume in patients with reduced inspiratory capacity [95].

In a systematic review by Rose et al. [96], the authors found only three clinical trials (one not randomized) on the effect of cough-assisting techniques on the extubation outcome [96]. The largest randomized trial (75 participants) found an 83% extubation success rate with the combination of mechanically and manually assisted cough, compared to 53% in the control group, making successful extubation over 1.5 times more likely. Despite the very low-quality evidence from single-trial findings, the authors concluded that cough-promoting techniques might increase the successful removal of the breathing tube and decrease the time spent on mechanical ventilation while not causing harm.

Regarding MI-E, in 2009, Gonçalves et al. [97] published a randomized study evaluating the effectiveness of MI-E as part of a weaning protocol for patients at risk of respiratory failure after extubation. Patients mechanically ventilated for over 48 h were divided into two groups: one receiving standard weaning therapy and the other receiving MI-E sessions alongside standard therapy. The study found significantly lower re-intubation rates in the group treated with MI-E (14%) compared to the control group (50%), particularly among patients using noninvasive ventilation, where re-intubation rates were 6% for the MI-E group versus 80% for the control group. Patients from the MI-E group also experienced shorter post-extubation ICU stays. The findings suggest that MI-E improves airway clearance, reduces noninvasive ventilation failure, and decreases ICU length of stay, making it a valuable addition to weaning protocols for high-risk patients.

Although there remains a paucity of research supporting the implementation of interventions to enhance cough effectiveness and mitigate the risk of reintubation failure, many services have adopted MI-E as a way to prevent extubation based on the little evidence available and on the theoretical rationale [98, 99].

In conclusion, when implementing cough augmentation techniques for patients with reduced CPF after extubation, the following recommendations presented in Table 16.3 are suggested.

Table 16.3 Suggested procedure for hard/brief ERCC indicated to remove secretions from large/central airways

1—Limit cough augmentation techniques to patients with CPF <60 L/min, assessed before extubation
2—In patients with reduced vital capacity, administer inspiratory positive pressure (via noninvasive ventilation or techniques like air stacking with a bag-valve-mask) to increase the inspired volume before the expulsive phase of the cough
3—Enhance the expulsive phase by applying hard/brief ERCC synchronized with the patient's cough
4—If a MI-E device is available, a general/initial configuration may be inspiratory/expiratory pressures of +30/−40 cmH_2O, an insufflation-exsufflation time ratio of 3:2 s, slow insufflation (to reduce PIF), with 8–10 cycles per session, interspersed with rest periods. Perform 2–3 sessions daily or as needed. Hard/brief ERCC may also be applied during the expiratory phase when using MI-E to augment CPF further

CPF cough peak flow, *ERCC* expiratory rib cage compression, *MI-E* mechanical insufflation-exsufflation

References

1. Pneumatikos IA, Dragoumanis CK, Bouros DE, Warner DS, Warner MA. Ventilator-associated pneumonia or endotracheal tube-associated pneumonia? Anesthesiology. 2009;110(3):673–80. https://doi.org/10.1097/ALN.0b013e31819868e0.
2. Restrepo RD, Walsh BK. Humidification during invasive and noninvasive mechanical ventilation: 2012. Respir Care. 2012;57(5):782–8. https://doi.org/10.4187/respcare.01766.
3. Paratz J, Ntoumenopoulos G. Detection of secretion retention in the ventilated patient. Curr Respir Med Rev. 2015;10(3):151–7. https://doi.org/10.2174/1573398X11666141229230526.
4. Gal TJ. Effects of endotracheal intubation on normal cough performance. Anesthesiology. 1980;52(4) https://doi.org/10.1097/00000542-198004000-00008.
5. Rouzéa A, Cottereaua A, Nseir S. Chronic obstructive pulmonary disease and the risk for ventilator-associated pneumonia. Curr Opin Crit Care. 2014;20(5):525–31. https://doi.org/10.1097/MCC.0000000000000123.
6. Hendershot KA, O'Phelan KH. Respiratory complications and weaning considerations for patients with spinal cord injuries: a narrative review. J Pers Med. 2023;13(1) https://doi.org/10.3390/jpm13010097.
7. Hess DR. Airway clearance: physiology, pharmacology, techniques, and practice. Respir Care. 2007;52(10):1392–6.
8. Volpe MS, Guimarães FS, Morais CCA. Airway clearance techniques for mechanically ventilated patients: insights for optimization. Respir Care. 2020;65(8) https://doi.org/10.4187/respcare.07904.
9. Zamanian M, Marini JJ. Pressure-flow signatures of central-airway mucus plugging. Crit Care Med. 2006;34(1):223–6. https://doi.org/10.1097/01.CCM.0000196216.49407.EE.
10. Konrad F, Schreiber T, Brecht-Kraus D, Georgieff M. Mucociliary transport in ICU patients. Chest. 1994;105(1):237–41. https://doi.org/10.1378/chest.105.1.237.
11. Salam A, Tilluckdharry L, Amoateng-Adjepong Y, Manthous CA. Neurologic status, cough, secretions and extubation outcomes. Intensive Care Med. 2004;30(7):1334–9. https://doi.org/10.1007/s00134-004-2231-7.
12. Mokhlesi B, Tulaimat A, Gluckman TJ, Wang Y, Evans AT, Corbridge TC. Predicting Extubation failure after successful completion of a spontaneous breathing trial. Respir Care. 2007;52(12):1710.

13. Khamiees M, Raju P, DeGirolamo A, Amoateng-Adjepong Y, Manthous CA. Predictors of Extubation outcome in patients who have successfully completed a spontaneous breathing trial. Chest. 2001;120(4):1262–70. https://doi.org/10.1378/chest.120.4.1262.
14. Branson RD, Faarc R. Airway clearance: physiology, pharmacology, techniques, and practice. Respir Care. 2007;52(10):1392–6.
15. American Association for Respiratory Care. AARC clinical practice guidelines. Endotracheal suctioning of mechanically ventilated patients with artificial airways 2010. Respir Care. 2010;55(6):758–64.
16. Thille AW, Harrois A, Schortgen F, Brun-Buisson C, Brochard L. Outcomes of extubation failure in medical intensive care unit patients. Crit Care Med. 2011;39(12) https://doi.org/10.1097/CCM.0b013e3182282a5a.
17. Rothaar RC, Epstein SK. Extubation failure: magnitude of the problem, impact on outcomes, and prevention. Curr Opin Crit Care. 2003;9(1) https://doi.org/10.1097/00075198-200302000-00011.
18. Thille AW, Boissier F, Muller M, et al. Role of ICU-acquired weakness on extubation outcome among patients at high risk of reintubation. Crit Care. 2020;24(1) https://doi.org/10.1186/s13054-020-2807-9.
19. Vishwas P, Amara V, Maddani SS, Chaudhuri S, Podder S. Risk factors of decreased abdominal expiratory muscle thickness in mechanically ventilated critically ill patients—the mNUTRIC score is an independent predictor. Indian J Crit Care Med. 2023;27(1) https://doi.org/10.5005/jp-journals-10071-24375.
20. Dres M, Goligher EC, Heunks LMA, Brochard LJ. Critical illness-associated diaphragm weakness. Intensive Care Med. 2017;43(10) https://doi.org/10.1007/s00134-017-4928-4.
21. Zakynthinos SG, Vassilakopoulos T, Zakynthinos E, Mavrommatis A, Roussos C. Contribution of expiratory muscle pressure to dynamic intrinsic positive end-expiratory pressure: validation using the Campbell diagram. Am J Respir Crit Care Med. 2000;162(5) https://doi.org/10.1164/ajrccm.162.5.9903084.
22. Shi ZH, Jonkman A, de Vries H, et al. Expiratory muscle dysfunction in critically ill patients: towards improved understanding. Intensive Care Med. 2019;45(8) https://doi.org/10.1007/s00134-019-05664-4.
23. Volpe MS, Adams AB, Amato MBP, Marini JJ. Ventilation patterns influence airway secretion movement. Respir Care. 2008;53(10):1287.
24. Fink JB. Forced expiratory technique, directed cough, and autogenic drainage. Respir Care. 2007;52
25. Ntoumenopoulos G, Shannon H, Main E. Do commonly used ventilator settings for mechanically ventilated adults have the potential to embed secretions or promote clearance? Respir Care. 2011;56(12) https://doi.org/10.4187/respcare.01229.
26. Thomas P, Paratz J. Ventilator hyperinflation – what settings generate an expiratory flow rate bias? Physiother (UK). 2023;119:44–53. https://doi.org/10.1016/j.physio.2022.11.006.
27. Freitag L, Long WM, Kim CS, Wanner A. Removal of excessive bronchial secretions by asymmetric high-frequency oscillations. J Appl Physiol. 1989;67(2) https://doi.org/10.1152/jappl.1989.67.2.614.
28. Kim CS, Greene MA, Sankaran S, Sackner MA. Mucus transport in the airways by two-phase gas-liquid flow mechanism: continuous flow model. J Appl Physiol. 1986;60(3) https://doi.org/10.1152/jappl.1986.60.3.908.
29. Kim CS, Rodriguez CR, Eldridge MA, Sackner MA. Criteria for mucus transport in the airways by two-phase gas-liquid flow mechanism. J Appl Physiol. 1986;60(3) https://doi.org/10.1152/jappl.1986.60.3.901.
30. Kim CS, Iglesias AJ, Sackner MA. Mucus clearance by two-phase gas-liquid flow mechanism: asymmetric periodic flow model. J Appl Physiol. 1987;62(3) https://doi.org/10.1152/jappl.1987.62.3.959.
31. Maxwell L, Ellis ER. The effects of three manual hyperinflation techniques on pattern of ventilation in a test lung model. Anaesth Intensive Care. 2002;30(3) https://doi.org/10.1177/0310057x0203000304.

32. Maxwell LJ, Ellis ER. Pattern of ventilation during manual hyperinflation performed by physiotherapists. Anaesthesia. 2007;62(1) https://doi.org/10.1111/j.1365-2044.2006.04898.x.
33. Jones AM, Thomas PJ, Paratz JD. Comparison of flow rates produced by two frequently used manual hyperinflation circuits: a benchtop study. Heart Lung J Acute Crit Care. 2009;38(6) https://doi.org/10.1016/j.hrtlng.2009.06.002.
34. Li Bassi G, Saucedo L, Marti JD, et al. Effects of duty cycle and positive end-expiratory pressure on mucus clearance during mechanical ventilation*. Crit Care Med. 2012;40(3):895–902. https://doi.org/10.1097/CCM.0b013e318236efb5.
35. Kallet RH. Adjunct therapies during mechanical ventilation: airway clearance techniques, therapeutic aerosols, and gases. Respir Care. 2013;58(6) https://doi.org/10.4187/respcare.02217.
36. Oberwaldner B. Physiotherapy for airway clearance in paediatrics. Eur Respir J. 2000;15(1) https://doi.org/10.1034/j.1399-3003.2000.15a36.x.
37. Holland AE, Button BM. Is there a role for airway clearance techniques in chronic obstructive pulmonary disease? Chron Respir Dis. 2006;3(2) https://doi.org/10.1191/1479972306cd097rs.
38. Osadnik CR, McDonald CF, Holland AE. Advances in airway clearance technologies for chronic obstructive pulmonary disease. Expert Rev Respir Med. 2013;7(6) https://doi.org/10.1586/17476348.2013.847368.
39. Van Der Schans CP, Postma DS, Koëter GH, Rubin BK. Physiotherapy and bronchial mucus transport. Eur Respir J. 1999;13(6) https://doi.org/10.1034/j.1399-3003.1999.13f37.x.
40. Junhasavasdikul D, Telias I, Grieco DL, et al. Expiratory flow limitation during mechanical ventilation. Chest. 2018;154(4) https://doi.org/10.1016/j.chest.2018.01.046.
41. Paulus F, Binnekade JM, Vroom MB, Schultz MJ. Benefits and risks of manual hyperinflation in intubated and mechanically ventilated intensive care unit patients: a systematic review. Crit Care. 2012;16(4) https://doi.org/10.1186/cc11457.
42. Berney S, Denehy L. A comparison of the effects of manual and ventilator hyperinflation on static lung compliance and sputum production in intubated and ventilated intensive care patients. Physiother Res Int. 2002;7(2) https://doi.org/10.1002/pri.246.
43. Lemes DA, Zin WA, Guimarães FS. Hyperinflation using pressure support ventilation improves secretion clearance and respiratory mechanics in ventilated patients with pulmonary infection: a randomised crossover trial. Aust J Physiother. 2009;55(4) https://doi.org/10.1016/S0004-9514(09)70004-2.
44. Savian C, Paratz J, Davies A. Comparison of the effectiveness of manual and ventilator hyperinflation at different levels of positive end-expiratory pressure in artificially ventilated and intubated intensive care patients. Heart Lung J Acute Crit Care. 2006;35(5) https://doi.org/10.1016/j.hrtlng.2006.02.003.
45. Dennis D, Jacob W, Budgeon C. Ventilator versus manual hyperinflation in clearing sputum in ventilated intensive care unit patients. Anaesth Intensive Care. 2012;40(1) https://doi.org/10.1177/0310057x1204000117.
46. Assmann CB, Vieira PJC, Kutchak F, De Mello RM, Forgiarini SGI, Forgiarini LA. Lung hyperinflation by mechanical ventilation versus isolated tracheal aspiration in the bronchial hygiene of patients undergoing mechanical ventilation. Rev Bras Ter Intensiva. 2016;28(1) https://doi.org/10.5935/0103-507X.20160010.
47. Ribeiro BS, Lopes AJ, Menezes SLS, Guimarães FS. Selecting the best ventilator hyperinflation technique based on physiologic markers: a randomized controlled crossover study. Heart Lung. 2019;48(1) https://doi.org/10.1016/j.hrtlng.2018.09.006.
48. Thomas PJ. The effect of mechanical ventilator settings during ventilator hyperinflation techniques: a bench-top analysis. Anaesth Intensive Care. 2015;43(1) https://doi.org/10.1177/0310057x1504300112.
49. Chapman RL, Shannon H, Koutoumanou E, Main E. Effect of inspiratory rise time on sputum movement during ventilator hyperinflation in a test lung model. Physiotherapy. 2019;105(2):283–9. https://doi.org/10.1016/j.physio.2018.06.003.
50. Bonczynski GS, Novo JS, Dias AS, et al. Ventilator hyperinflation associated with flow bias optimization in the bronchial hygiene of mechanically ventilated patients. Heart Lung. 2024;64:64. https://doi.org/10.1016/j.hrtlng.2023.10.011.

51. van der Lee L, Patman S, Hill AM. Development of a clinical practice guideline for physiotherapy management of adults invasively ventilated with community-acquired pneumonia. Physiotherapy (UK). 2024;122:57–67. https://doi.org/10.1016/j.physio.2023.12.003.
52. Rich J, Coman M, Sharkey A, Church D, Pawson J, Thomas A. A single center observational study of the incidence, frequency and timing of critical care physiotherapy intervention during the COVID-19 pandemic. J Intensive Care Soc. 2022;23(3):273–80. https://doi.org/10.1177/1751143721991060.
53. Trojman A, Hough J, Hides J, Gustafsson L, Flores O, Paratz J. Physiotherapy practices when treating patients with COVID-19 during a pandemic: a survey study. Heart Lung. 2023;57:152–60. https://doi.org/10.1016/j.hrtlng.2022.09.012.
54. Jalil Y, Damiani LF, Basoalto R, Bachmman MC, Bruhn A. A deep look into the rib cage compression technique in mechanically ventilated patients: a narrative review. Rev Bras Ter Intensiva. 2022;34(1) https://doi.org/10.5935/0103-507x.20220012-en.
55. Freynet A, Gobaille G, Joannes-Boyau O, et al. Effects of chest physiotherapy by expiratory flow increase on secretion removal and lung mechanics in ventilated patients: a randomized crossover study. Intensive Care Med. 2016;42(6) https://doi.org/10.1007/s00134-016-4315-6.
56. Martí JD, Li Bassi G, Rigol M, et al. Effects of manual rib cage compressions on expiratory flow and mucus clearance during mechanical ventilation. Crit Care Med. 2013;41(3):850–6. https://doi.org/10.1097/CCM.0b013e3182711b52.
57. Avena KDM, Duarte ACM, Cravo SLD, Sologuren MJJ, Gastaldi AC. Effects of manually assisted coughing on respiratory mechanics in patients requiring full ventilatory support. J Bras Pneumol. 2008;34(6) https://doi.org/10.1590/S1806-37132008000600008.
58. Guimarães FS, Silveira de Menezes SL, ucia, Lopes AJ. Expiratory rib cage compressions to improve secretion clearance during mechanical ventilation: not only a matter of squeezing the chest-reply. Respir Care. 2014;59(8) https://doi.org/10.4187/respcare.03522.
59. Oliveira ACO, Lorena DM, Gomes LC, Amaral BLR, Volpe MS. Effects of manual chest compression on expiratory flow bias during the positive end-expiratory pressure–zero end-expiratory pressure maneuver in patients on mechanical ventilation. J Bras Pneumol. 2019;45(3) https://doi.org/10.1590/1806-3713/e20180058.
60. Unoki T, Mizutani T, Toyooka H. Effects of expiratory rib cage compression combined with endotracheal suctioning on gas exchange in mechanically ventilated rabbits with induced atelectasis. Respir Care. 2004;49(8):896.
61. Unoki T, Kawasaki Y, Mizutani T, et al. Effects of expiratory rib-cage compression on oxygenation, ventilation, and airway-secretion removal in patients receiving mechanical ventilation. Respir Care. 2005;50(11):1430.
62. Genc A, Akan M, Gunerli A. The effects of manual hyperinflation with or without rib-cage compression in mechanically ventilated patients. Ital J Physiother. 2011;1(2)
63. Shannon H, Stiger R, Gregson RK, Stocks J, Main E. Effect of chest wall vibration timing on peak expiratory fl{ligature}ow and inspiratory pressure in a mechanically ventilated lung model. Physiotherapy. 2010;96(4) https://doi.org/10.1016/j.physio.2010.02.007.
64. Ouchi A, Sakuramoto H, Unoki T, et al. Effects of manual rib cage compressions on mucus clearance in mechanically ventilated pigs. Respir Care. 2020;65(8) https://doi.org/10.4187/respcare.07249.
65. Amaral BLR, de Figueiredo AB, Lorena DM, Oliveira ACO, Carvalho NC, Volpe MS. Effects of ventilation mode and manual chest compression on flow bias during the positive end- and zero end-expiratory pressure manoeuvre in mechanically ventilated patients: a randomised crossover trial. Physiotherapy (UK). 2020;106 https://doi.org/10.1016/j.physio.2018.12.007.
66. Silva ARB, Fluhr SA, De Lemos BA, De Valois Correia Júnior MA, De França ET, De Andrade FMID. Expiratory peak flow and respiratory system resistance in mechanically ventilated patients undergoing two different forms of manually assisted cough. Rev Bras Ter Intensiva. 2012;24(1) https://doi.org/10.1590/S0103-507X2012000100009.
67. Guimarães FS, Lopes AJ, Constantino SS, Lima JC, Canuto P, de Menezes SLS. Expiratory rib cage in mechanically ventilated subjects: a randomized crossover trial. Respir Care. 2014;59(5) https://doi.org/10.4187/respcare.02587.

68. MacLean D, Drummond G, Macpherson C, McLaren G, Prescott R. Maximum expiratory airflow during chest physiotherapy on ventilated patients before and after the application of an abdominal binder. Intensive Care Med. 1989;15(6) https://doi.org/10.1007/BF00261500.
69. Gonçalves EC, Souza HCD, Tambascio J, Almeida MB, Filho AB, Gastaldi AC. Effects of chest compression on secretion removal, lung mechanics, and gas exchange in mechanically ventilated patients: a crossover, randomized study. Intensive Care Med. 2016;42(2) https://doi.org/10.1007/s00134-015-4117-2.
70. Calverley PMA, Koulouris NG. Flow limitation and dynamic hyperinflation: key concepts in modern respiratory physiology. Eur Respir J. 2005;25(1) https://doi.org/10.1183/09031936.04.00113204.
71. Koutsoukou A, Armaganidis A, Stavrakaki-Kallergi C, et al. Expiratory flow limitation and intrinsic positive end-expiratory pressure at zero positive end-expiratory pressure in patients with adult respiratory distress syndrome. Am J Respir Crit Care Med. 2000;161(5) https://doi.org/10.1164/ajrccm.161.5.9904109.
72. Dos Santos FRA, Schneider Júnior LC, Forgiarini Junior LA, Veronezi J. Effects of manual rib-cage compression versus PEEP-ZEEP maneuver on respiratory system compliance and oxygenation in patients receiving mechanical ventilation. Rev Bras Ter Intensiva. 2009;21(2):155.
73. Herbst-Rodrigues MV, Carvalho VO, Auler JOC, Feltrim MIZ. PEEP-ZEEP technique: cardiorespiratory repercussions in mechanically ventilated patients submitted to a coronary artery bypass graft surgery. J Cardiothorac Surg. 2011;6(1) https://doi.org/10.1186/1749-8090-6-108.
74. de Oliveira TF, Peringer VS, Forgiarini Junior LA, Eibel B. PEEP-ZEEP compared with bag squeezing and chest compression in mechanically ventilated cardiac patients: randomized crossover clinical trial. Int J Environ Res Public Health. 2023;20(4) https://doi.org/10.3390/ijerph20042824.
75. Lobo DML, Cavalcante LA, Mont'Alverne DGB. Applicability of bag squeezing and zeep maneuvers in mechanically ventilated patients. Rev Bras Ter Intensiva. 2010;22(2):186.
76. Barach AL, Beck GJ, Bickerman HA, Seanor HE. Physical methods simulating cough mechanisms: use in poliomyelitis, bronchial asthma, pulmonary emphysema, and bronchiectasis. JAMA J Am Med Assoc. 1952;150(14) https://doi.org/10.1001/jama.1952.03680140018004.
77. Chatwin M, Ross E, Hart N, Nickol AH, Polkey MI, Simonds AK. Cough augmentation with mechanical insufflation/exsufflation in patients with neuromuscular weakness. Eur Respir J. 2003;21(3) https://doi.org/10.1183/09031936.03.00048102.
78. Sancho J, Servera E, Vergara P, Marín J. Mechanical insufflation-exsufflation vs. tracheal suctioning via tracheostomy tubes for patients with amyotrophic lateral sclerosis: a pilot study. Am J Phys Med Rehabil. 2003;82(10) https://doi.org/10.1097/01.PHM.0000087456.28979.2E.
79. Branson RD, Benditt JO. Optimizing mechanical insufflation-exsufflation—much more than cough peak flow. Respir Care. 2020;65(2) https://doi.org/10.4187/respcare.07682.
80. Sánchez-García M, Santos P, Rodríguez-Trigo G, et al. Preliminary experience on the safety and tolerability of mechanical "insufflation-exsufflation" in subjects with artificial airway. Intensive Care Med Experim. 2018;6(1) https://doi.org/10.1186/s40635-018-0173-6.
81. Coutinho W, Vieira P, Kutchak F, Dias A, Rieder M, Forgiarini L. Comparison of mechanical insufflation-exsufflation and endotracheal suctioning in mechanically ventilated patients: effects on respiratory mechanics, hemodynamics, and volume of secretions. Indian J Crit Care Med. 2018;22(7) https://doi.org/10.4103/ijccm.IJCCM_164_18.
82. Kubota S, Hashimoto H, Yoshikawa Y, et al. Effects of mechanical insufflation-exsufflation on ventilator-free days in intensive care unit subjects with sputum retention; a randomized clinical trial. PLoS One. 2024;19(5) https://doi.org/10.1371/journal.pone.0302239.
83. de Camillis MLF, Savi A, Rosa RG, et al. Effects of mechanical insufflation-exsufflation on airway mucus clearance among mechanically ventilated icu subjects. Respir Care. 2018;63(12) https://doi.org/10.4187/respcare.06253.
84. Martínez-Alejos R, Martí JD, Li Bassi G, et al. Effects of mechanical insufflation-exsufflation on sputum volume in mechanically ventilated critically ill subjects. Respir Care. 2021;66(9) https://doi.org/10.4187/respcare.08641.

85. Kuroiwa R, Tateishi Y, Oshima T, et al. Mechanical insufflation-exsufflation for the prevention of ventilator-associated pneumonia in intensive care units: a retrospective cohort study. Indian J Crit Care Med. 2021;25(1) https://doi.org/10.5005/jp-journals-10071-23508.
86. Volpe MS, Naves JM, Ribeiro GG, Ruas G, Amato MBP. Airway clearance with an optimized mechanical insufflation-exsufflation maneuver. Respir Care. 2018;63(10) https://doi.org/10.4187/respcare.05965.
87. Guimarães FS, Rocha ÂRM. Weak cough strength and secretion retention in mechanically ventilated patients: is there a role for cough-assist devices? Respir Care. 2018;63(12) https://doi.org/10.4187/respcare.06527.
88. Duan J, Zhang X, Song J. Predictive power of extubation failure diagnosed by cough strength: a systematic review and meta-analysis. Crit Care. 2021;25(1) https://doi.org/10.1186/s13054-021-03781-5.
89. de Araújo FN, de Sá FA, Guimarães FS. Cough peak flow to predict extubation outcome: a systematic review and meta-analysis. Rev Bras Ter Intensiva. 2021;33(3) https://doi.org/10.5935/0103-507X.20210060.
90. Almeida CM, Lopes AJ, Guimarães FS. Cough peak flow to predict the extubation outcome: comparison between three cough stimulation methods. Can J Resp Ther. 2020;56 https://doi.org/10.29390/CJRT-2020-037.
91. Jonkman AH, Frenzel T, McCaughey EJ, et al. Breath-synchronized electrical stimulation of the expiratory muscles in mechanically ventilated patients: a randomized controlled feasibility study and pooled analysis. Crit Care. 2020;24(1) https://doi.org/10.1186/s13054-020-03352-0.
92. McCaughey EJ, Jonkman AH, Boswell-Ruys CL, et al. Abdominal functional electrical stimulation to assist ventilator weaning in critical illness: a double-blinded, randomised, sham-controlled pilot study. Crit Care. 2019;23(1) https://doi.org/10.1186/s13054-019-2544-0.
93. Dall'Acqua AM, Sachetti A, Santos LJ, et al. Use of neuromuscular electrical stimulation to preserve the thickness of abdominal and chest muscles of critically ill patients: a randomized clinical trial. J Rehabil Med. 2017;49(1) https://doi.org/10.2340/16501977-2168.
94. Morrow B, Argent A, Zampoli M, Human A, Corten L, Toussaint M. Cough augmentation techniques for people with chronic neuromuscular disorders. Cochrane Database Syst Rev. 2021;2021(4) https://doi.org/10.1002/14651858.CD013170.pub2.
95. Spinou A. A review on cough augmentation techniques: assisted inspiration, assisted expiration and their combination. Physiol Res. 2020;69 https://doi.org/10.33549/physiolres.934407.
96. Rose L, Adhikari NKJ, Leasa D, Fergusson DA, Mckim D. Cough augmentation techniques for extubation or weaning critically ill patients from mechanical ventilation. Cochrane Database Syst Rev. 2017;2017(1) https://doi.org/10.1002/14651858.CD011833.pub2.
97. Gonçalves MR, Honrado T, Winck JC, Paiva JA. Effects of mechanical insufflation-exsufflation in preventing respiratory failure after extubation: a randomized controlled trial. Crit Care. 2012;16(2) https://doi.org/10.1186/cc11249.
98. Swingwood E, Tume L, Cramp F. A survey examining the use of mechanical insufflation-exsufflation on adult intensive care units across the UK. J Intensive Care Soc. 2020;21(4) https://doi.org/10.1177/1751143719870121.
99. Rose L, Adhikari NK, Poon J, Leasa D, McKim DA. Cough augmentation techniques in the critically ill: a Canadian national survey. Respir Care. 2016;61(10) https://doi.org/10.4187/respcare.04775.

Chapter 17
Inspiratory Muscle Training for Weaning

Bruno Leonardo da Silva Guimarães, Leonardo Cordeiro de Souza, and Mellina Tamy Fagundes Fujihara

Abbreviations

MV	Mechanical ventilation
VIDD	Ventilator-induced diaphragmatic dysfunction
IMT	Inspiratory muscle training
TIE index	Timed inspiratory effort
PImax	Maximal inspiratory pressure
P0.1	Inspiratory muscle effort and occlusion pressure at 100 ms
ICU	Intensive care unit
PSV	Pressure-supported ventilation
RASS	Richmond Agitation-Sedation Scale; Apache II: Acute Physiology and Chronic Health Evaluation II
RMD	Respiratory muscle dysfunction
COPD	Chronic obstructive pulmonary disease

17.1 Introduction

Ventilation-induced diaphragm dysfunction (VIDD) has been identified as a major cause of ventilator weaning failure and prolongation [1–4]. It is estimated that approximately 15% of patients undergoing weaning progress to prolonged weaning

B. L. da Silva Guimarães (✉) · M. T. F. Fujihara
Physical Therapy Hospital Niterói D'or, Niterói, RJ, Brazil

L. C. de Souza
Physical Therapy School, Universidade Estácio de Sá, Rio de Janeiro, RJ, Brazil

A. R. Baptistella et al. (eds.), *Weaning from Mechanical Ventilation*,
https://doi.org/10.1007/978-3-032-01145-9_17

[2, 5, 6], resulting in increased ICU length of stay, hospitalization costs, and hospital mortality. [7].

Despite being a widely discussed topic in the scientific community, the diagnosis and treatment of respiratory muscle dysfunction (RMD) in critically ill patients remain controversial. Furthermore, interventions to restore inspiratory muscle function could significantly contribute to this scenario by increasing the success rate of ventilator weaning and intensive care unit (ICU) survival [8–12].

The search for an appropriate diagnosis of RMD in the ICU has been a long one. Since 1973, when the first study on the measurement of maximum inspiratory pressure (PImax) was published, numerous researchers have investigated the correlation between inspiratory weakness and ventilatory dependence, but few studies have demonstrated good technical accuracy and clinical relevance that could guide treatment prescriptions. Among the existing bedside diagnostic methods, two are particularly noteworthy: diaphragmatic ultrasound, which measures excursion and muscle thickening, and the timed inspiratory effort method index (TIE index), which evaluates inspiratory muscle effort and closing pressure at 100 ms (P0.1) intervals over time.

The most common treatment is inspiratory muscle training (IMT), but its protocol is not fully established. Therefore, finding a reliable source for the diagnosis of RMD and improving the management of the IMT program will help critical care physiotherapists achieve increasingly successful results in the near future.

17.2 History and Background

Inspiratory muscle weakness has been associated with difficulty weaning from the ventilator [13], and the degree of weakness correlates with the duration of MV [14]. MV is known to increase proteolysis and promote diaphragmatic atrophy [5]. Thus, diaphragm weakness is considered one of the major causes of difficulty and prolongation of mechanical ventilation [15].

The contractile activity of skeletal muscles, such as the diaphragm, can be modified by neuromuscular activity, hormones, age, electrical stimulation, and the presence or absence of stress and exercise. Changes in contractile activity are accompanied by structural and molecular changes that affect the number of mitochondria, enzymatic activity, types of myofibrils present, number of capillaries, type and number of neuromuscular junctions, and number of cell nuclei [16].

The idea of training inspiratory muscles is not new, and the use of devices connected to ventilator prostheses has been limited to basic devices with different characteristics, mainly related to the type of load applied [17]. The first devices used for training were characterized as linear airflow devices, with holes of different sizes that generated different training loads. However, this approach relied on the patient's cooperation and, as a result, training could be ineffective if there was not a strong inspiratory effort during inspiration [17].

17.3 Current Trends

Over the past 7 years, literature reviews have been published specifically addressing the topic of respiratory muscle training in intubated and tracheostomized critical care patients undergoing various forms of intervention. In 2019, Bissett and colleagues described a multidisciplinary approach for these patients and concluded that IMT is safe and feasible, especially for patients with a ventilator duration of more than 7 days [18]. However, there is inconsistency regarding when and how to initiate it, how often it should be performed, the duration and load to be implemented, and the best type of equipment for each situation [9].

In a systematic review published in 2018, the authors demonstrated that it is possible to use IMT in critically ill patients with good tolerance and highlighted the technique as one of the possible strategies to reverse and rehabilitate respiratory muscle weakness in patients undergoing invasive mechanical ventilation. The authors also showed that IMT can be performed with two strategies, endurance or strength training, with strength training being the most commonly used among the studies included in the review. The timing of starting IMT also varies; it can be early when weaning is classified as difficult, or a little later in prolonged weaning or after extubation [8, 19].

Cader et al. [20, 21] suggested that respiratory muscle training with Threshold IMT® (Health Scan Products Inc.; Cedar Grove, USA) should be indicated early in intubated patients and in elderly populations. On the other hand, other authors have shown that starting IMT after the transition to spontaneous mode of mechanical ventilation can increase PImax, improve rapid and shallow breathing index (RSBI) values, reduce weaning time, and determine a lower need for noninvasive mechanical ventilation in the post-extubation period [20, 21].

Among the studies that have performed IMT with the Threshold IMT® device in tracheostomized patients, four publications stand out:

1. Martin M et al. in [12] observed an increase in PImax and favorable outcomes in patients with weaning failure.
2. Pascotini et al. in [11] concluded that IMT could be an important ally in weaning as well as in maintaining respiratory parameters such as respiratory rate.
3. Bissett BM et al. in [4] suggest that IMT may be an effective strategy to reverse residual muscle weakness after prolonged mechanical ventilation and improve quality of life in patients who received 2 weeks of training.
4. Bissett BM et al. in 2022 concluded that even without achieving ventilator independence or improvements in muscle strength, IMT with mechanical threshold exercise improves quality of life and reduces dyspnea in ventilator-dependent patients.

Given these principles of muscle training, several studies described in the systematic review and meta-analysis by Vorona et al. [8] analyzed different IMT methods in critical patients, with different devices, loads, intensities, and frequencies. The Threshold® device was the most commonly used, and PImax was the parameter used as a guide to determine the load used. In most studies, IMT was initiated with a shorter MV time, in patients still intubated, preserving diaphragmatic functional capacity and attenuating the impairments associated with VIDD [4, 8, 11, 12, 22].

One promising therapy is the use of IMT with linear pressure-loaded devices. This modality has been successfully used for the outpatient treatment of respiratory muscle weakness, primarily in patients with chronic lung disease, with the goal of reducing dyspnea, increasing respiratory muscle strength and fatigue resistance, improving exercise tolerance, and improving quality of life [23, 24].

Since 2002, several studies have demonstrated that the use of IMT may have a positive effect on ventilator weaning [24–26]. Increased inspiratory force, decreased time on mechanical ventilation, and increased successful weaning have been reported in patients with prolonged ventilation [12, 25, 27]. As mentioned above, it is still unclear what type of protocol (load, duration, intensity, and frequency) should be used, especially in patients with little or no cooperation.

In a systematic review of 1513 articles on IMT in weaning from mechanical ventilation, only ten studies were selected for meta-analysis. It was clear that only patients who had difficulty with ventilator weaning benefited from inspiratory muscle training [28]. Thus, inspiratory muscle training is emerging as a therapeutic option to address weaning failure in patients with prolonged mechanical ventilation.

Technological advances have reached IMT devices, and today electronic devices with isokinetic load control can be used. The first case report using this type of device (Powerbreathe® K-5) in critically ill ICU patients to facilitate prolonged weaning was published by Leonardo Cordeiro de Souza in 2014 [29]. In this case, a patient with inclusion body myositis achieved complete ventilatory independence after 3 weeks of daily training with progressive incremental loads and was subsequently discharged from the hospital. In 2017, Tonella and colleagues published a randomized trial evaluating the safety and efficacy of the electronic device by analyzing respiratory and hemodynamic variables. They reported that IMT was safe and useful for critically ill, tracheostomized patients with prolonged ventilation and difficult weaning [30]. Furthermore, in 2021, the first randomized controlled trial using the TIE index and electronic resistors was published in Critical Care Medicine by Guimarães and colleagues, highlighting a high weaning success rate and a reduction in ICU mortality [31].

Not only does diaphragm weakness affect weaning, but scalene and sternocleidomastoid weakness can also affect spontaneous breathing [32, 33]. Hollebeke et al. (2022) found improvements in sternocleidomastoid muscle oxygen saturation index, peak inspiratory flow, and forced vital capacity after high-intensity IMT compared to low-intensity IMT. Further research is needed to assess whether these results also represent a better weaning outcome and to elucidate the physiological mechanism behind them [34].

17.4 Protocols for Weaning

The two most important parameters of any exercise program are intensity and frequency of sessions, as these elements determine the effectiveness of muscle stimulation [35]. To produce significant changes in inspiratory muscle function in healthy individuals, these two factors can be adjusted in a program consisting of 30 breaths twice a day. However, there is still a lack of standardization for hospitalized and critically ill patients [35].

To avoid detrimental effects of training, it is important to emphasize the importance of finding the ideal load, frequency, and intensity for these patients, so as not to negatively affect the quality of muscle stimulation and adaptations, thereby limiting its effectiveness [35].

Researchers recommend training twice a day with 6 h of rest to allow for minimal recovery time, which is a fundamental part of the adaptation process [36]. During IMT, the goal is 60 repetitions per day. Beyond this limit, the inspiratory muscles become susceptible to fatigue, resulting in progressively lower volumetric loads compared to previous efforts. This is a direct result of the inspiratory muscles being stronger at the beginning of inspiration than at the end [36].

With the aim of introducing IMT with electronic loads in the ICU, guided by the TIE index, Souza et al. published two clinical case reports [29, 37] with promising results that motivated their group to develop a new protocol consisting of incremental and interval IMT with 60 repetitions once a day. This protocol allowed the use of electronic devices in critically ill patients with severe muscle dysfunction and reduced cognitive function.

The first case report was of a 43-year-old patient with inclusion body myositis [29]. Two daily sessions were performed with three sets of 10 repetitions for a total of 30 breaths. Training load was 30% of PImax, and PImax and TIE index were assessed weekly to adjust load and intensity. IMT was performed for 4 weeks in conjunction with upper and lower body rehabilitation. The protocol increased inspiratory muscle strength and resistance and, most importantly, resulted in successful ventilator weaning.

The second case report involved a patient with Guillain-Barre after Zika virus [37]. In this case, IMT was initiated 25 days after the start of MV due to the patient's clinical condition. Training was performed with an electronic device (POWERbreathe® K-5), 6 sets of 10 repetitions once a day. Each set consisted of five increasing efforts and 5 breaths at target load, creating an interval and incremental program. After 2 weeks, the patient achieved ventilatory independence.

Guimarães et al. [31] developed a different protocol and evaluated the effects of IMT with an electronic device on muscle strength, weaning outcomes, and survival. IMT resulted in a significantly greater increase in muscle strength as measured by PImax and TIE index. After 60 days in the ICU, the IMT group showed significantly better outcomes in both survival and weaning success. The protocol consisted of 60 breaths divided into 2 sets of 30 repetitions. Each set was divided into 3 subsets of 10 breaths each. The target load was set at 40% of PImax and was applied gradually from 50% to 100% of the target load as shown (Fig. 17.1):

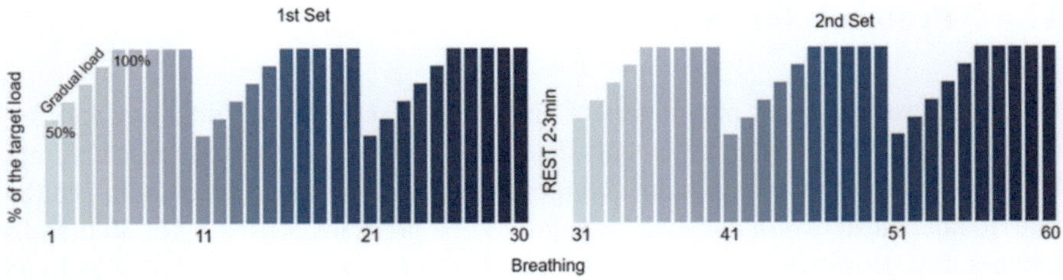

Fig. 17.1 IMT protocol. (Guimarães et al. [31]. Adapted from Fig. 1)

17.5 Conclusion

The effectiveness of IMT depends on precisely calibrated parameters such as intensity and frequency of sessions. While healthy subjects may benefit from standard protocols of 30 breaths twice daily, critically ill patients require careful individualization. As mentioned above, there are some conflicts regarding the parameters and equipment for weaning protocols. However, these studies collectively suggest that IMT for weaning is safe and feasible in critically ill patients, may improve inspiratory muscle strength and quality of life, and may lead to better clinical outcomes such as successful weaning and increased survival rates.

References

1. Levine S, Nguyen T, Taylor N, Frscia ME, et al. Rapid disuse atrophy of diaphragm fibers in mechanically ventilated humans. N Engl J Med. 2008;358:1327–35.
2. Jubran A, Grant BJB, Duffner LA, et al. Effect of pressure support vs unassisted breathing through a tracheostomy collar on weaning duration in patients requiring prolonged mechanical ventilation: a randomized trial. JAMA. 2013;309:671–7.
3. Souza LC, Guimaraes FS, Lugon JR. The timed inspiratory effort: a promising index of mechanical ventilation weaning for patients with neurologic or neuromuscular diseases. Respir Care. 2015a;60:231–8.
4. Bissett BM, Leditschke IA, Neeman T, et al. Inspiratory muscle training to enhance recovery from mechanical ventilation: a randomised trial. Thorax. 2016;71:812–9.
5. Boles JM, Bionc J, Connors A, et al. Weaning from mechanical ventilation. Statement of the sixth international consensus conference on intensive care medicine. Eur Respir J. 2007;29:1033–56.
6. Souza LC, Guimarães FS, Lugon JR. Evaluation of a new index of mechanical ventilation weaning: the timed inspiratory effort. J Intensive Care Med. 2015b;30:37–43.
7. Zilberberg MD, Luippold RS, Sulsky S, et al. Prolonged acute mechanical ventilation, hospital resource utilization, and mortality in the United States. Crit Care Med. 2008;36:724–30.
8. Vorona S, Sabatini U, Al-Maqbali S, et al. Inspiratory muscle rehabilitation in critically ill adults. A systematic review and meta-analysis. Ann Am Thorac Soc. 2018;15:735–44.
9. Elkins M, Dentice R. Inspiratory muscle training facilitates weaning from mechanical ventilation among patients in the intensive care unit: a systematic review. J Physiother. 2015;61:125–34.

10. Schellekens WJM, van Hees HWH, Doorduin J, et al. Strategies to optimize respiratory muscle function in ICU patients. Crit Care. 2016;20:1–9.
11. Pascotini FDS, Denardi C, Nunes GO, et al. Respiratory muscle training in patients weaning from mechanical ventilation. ABCS Heal Sci. 2014;39:12–6.
12. Martin AD, Smith BK, Davenport PD, et al. Inspiratory muscle strength training improves weaning outcome in failure to wean patients: a randomized trial. Crit Care. 2011;15:R 84.
13. Blackman DK, Kamimoto LA, Smith SM. Overview: surveillance for selected public health indicators affecting older adults--United States. MMWR CDC Surveill Summ. 1999;48(8):1-6. PMID: 10634268.
14. Maureen MG, Guyatt D, Cook L, Griffith T, Sinuff C, Kergl J, Mancebo A, Esteban Scott, Epstein. Predicting Success in Weaning From Mechanical Ventilation Chest 2001;120(6):400S-424S 10.1378/chest.120.6_suppl.400S
15. Pedro, Caruso Celena, Friedrich Silvia DC, Denari Soraia AL, Ruiz Daniel, Deheinzelin. The Unidirectional Valve Is the Best Method To Determine Maximal Inspiratory Pressure During Weaning Chest 1999;115(4):1096-1101. https://doi.org/10.1378/chest.115.4.1096.
16. B, Polla. Respiratory muscle fibres: specialisation and plasticity Thorax. 2004;59(9):808-817. https://doi.org/10.1136/thx.2003.009894.
17. Volpe MS. Treinamento muscular inspiratório em Unidade de Terapia Intensiva. In: Associação Brasileira de Fisioterapia Cardiorrespiratória e Fisioterapia em Terapia Intensiva; Martins JA, Andrade FMD, Dias CM, Organizadores. PROFISIO Programa de Atualização em Fisioterapia Intensiva Adulto: ciclo 5. Porto Alegre: Artmed Panamericana; 2015. p. 9/30. (Sistema de Educação Continuada à distância, v. 4)
18. Bernie BIA, Leditschke M, Green V, Marzano S, Collins F, Van H. Inspiratory muscle training for intensive care patients: A multidisciplinary practical guide for clinicians Australian Critical Care 2019;32(3):249-255 https://doi.org/10.1016/j.aucc.2018.06.001.
19. Martin, Dres Ewan C., Goligher Leo M. A., Heunks Laurent J., Brochard (2017) Critical illness-associated diaphragm weakness Intensive Care Medicine. 2017;43(10):1441-1452. https://doi.org/10.1007/s00134-017-4928-4.
20. Samária Ali, Cader Rodrigo Gomes Souza, de Vale Juracy Correa, Castro Silvia Corrêa, Bacelar Cintia, Biehl Maria Celeste Vega, Gomes Walter Eduardo, Cabrera Estélio Henrique Martin, Dantas.Inspiratory muscle training improves maximal inspiratory pressure and may assist weaning in older intubated patients: a randomised trial Journal of Physiotherapy. 2010;56(3):171-177. https://doi.org/10.1016/S1836-9553(10)70022-9.
21. Samária, Samária Ali Cader Vale Zamora Costa Dantas Extubation process in bed-ridden elderly intensive care patients receiving inspiratory muscle training: a randomized clinical trial Clinical Interventions in Aging 437.https://doi.org/10.2147/CIA.S36937.
22. Daniel Martin A, Smith BK, Gabrielli A. Mechanical ventilation, diaphragm weakness and weaning: a rehabilitation perspective. Respir Physiol Neurobiol. 2013;189(2):377-83.https://doi.org/10.1016/j.resp.2013.05.012. Epub 2013 May 18. PMID: 23692928; PMCID: PMC3808482.
23. Green M, Road J, Sieck GC, Similowski T. Tests of respiratory muscle strength. American journal of respiratory and critical care medicine. 2002;166(4):528-547.
24. Thomas L, Clanton Philip T, Diaz (1995) Clinical Assessment of the Respiratory Muscles Physical Therapy. 1995;75(11):983-995. https://doi.org/10.1093/ptj/75.11.983.
25. S., Epstein. Decision to extubate Intensive Care Medicine 2002;28(5):535-546.https://doi.org/10.1007/s00134-002-1268-8.
26. Decramer M, Gayan-Ramirez G. Editorial: Ventilator-induced diafragmatic dysfunction. Toward a better treatment? AM J Respir Crit Care Med. 2004;170:1141-1142.
27. J. Ferdinand, Fiastro Michael P., Habib Brian Y., Shon Sammy C., Campbell. Comparison of Standard Weaning Parameters and the Mechanical Work of Breathing in Mechanically Ventilated Patients Chest. 1988;94(2):232-238. https://doi.org/10.1378/chest.94.2.232.

28. Mark, Elkins Ruth, Dentice. Inspiratory muscle training facilitates weaning from mechanical ventilation among patients in the intensive care unit: a systematic review Journal of Physiotherapy. 2015;61(3):125-134. https://doi.org/10.1016/j.jphys.2015.05.016.
29. Souza LC, Campos JF, Daher LP, et al. Feasibility of isokinetic inspiratory muscle training as an adjunct therapy. Case Reports Crit Care. 2014;14:1–4.
30. Rodrigo Marques, Tonella Ligia, Dos Santos Roceto Ratti Lilian Elisabete Bernardes, Delazari Carlos Fontes, Junior Paula Lima, Da Silva Aline Ribeiro Da Silva, Herran Daniela Cristina, Dos Santos Faez Ivete Alonso Bredda, Saad Luciana Castilho, De Figueiredo Rui, Moreno Desanka, Dragosvac Antonio Luis Eiras, Falcao. Inspiratory Muscle Training in the Intensive Care Unit: A New Perspective Journal of Clinical Medicine Research. 2017;9(11):929-934. https://doi.org/10.14740/jocmr3169w.
31. Guimarães BL, de Souza LC, Cordeiro HF, Regis TL, Leite CA, Puga FP. Inspiratory muscle training with an electronic resistive loading device improves prolonged weaning outcomes in a randomized controlled trial. Crit Care Med. 2021;49:589–97.
32. Parthasarathy S, Jubran A, Tobin MJ. Applied physiology and respiratory mechanics of weaning from mechanical ventilation. In: Tobin MJ, editor. Principles and practice of mechanical ventilation. 2nd ed. New York: McGraw-Hill; 2007. p. 1195–1220.
33. André, De Troyer Aladin M., Boriek Y. S., Prakash Comprehensive Physiology Mechanics of the Respiratory Muscles Wiley 1273-1300.
34. Mariana, Hoffman Marine, Van Hollebeke Beatrix, Clerckx Johannes, Muller Zafeiris, Louvaris Rik, Gosselink Greet, Hermans Daniel, Langer. Can inspiratory muscle training improve weaning outcomes in difficult to wean patients? A protocol for a randomised controlled trial (IMweanT study) BMJ Open. 2018;8(6):e021091. https://doi.org/10.1136/bmjopen-2017-021091.
35. Rasmi, Magadle Alison K., McConnell Marinella, Beckerman Paltiel, Weiner. Inspiratory muscle training in pulmonary rehabilitation program in COPD patients Respiratory Medicine. 2007;101(7):1500-1505.https://doi.org/10.1016/j.rmed.2007.01.010.
36. Peter I, Brown Alison K, McConnell. Respiratory-Related Limitations in Physically Demanding Occupations Aviation Space and Environmental Medicine. 2012;83(4):424-430. https://doi.org/10.3357/ASEM.3163.2012.
37. Souza LC, Souza AA, Almeida EEP, et al. Inspiratory muscle training with isokinetic device to help ventilatory weaning in a patient with Guillain-Barré Syndrome by Zika Virus. Case Reports Crit Care. 2018;18:1–5.

Chapter 18
Weaning from Mechanical Ventilation in Patients with COVID-19

Luis Felipe da Fonseca Reis and Flávio Maciel de Andrade

18.1 Introduction

The Coronavirus disease 2019 (COVID-19) pandemic, caused by Severe Acute Respiratory Syndrome Coronavirus 2 (SARS-CoV-2), has had a profound impact on global health, creating unprecedented challenges for healthcare systems worldwide. By the end of 2023, more than 600 million cases of COVID-19 had been reported worldwide, with more than 6 million deaths, according to the World Health Organization (WHO) [1]. A significant proportion of hospitalized COVID-19 patients develop severe respiratory failure requiring intensive care unit (ICU) admission and mechanical ventilation.

Early reports suggested that approximately 14% of those infected experienced severe illness requiring oxygen therapy, with approximately 5% requiring intensive care and mechanical ventilation [2]. During the peak waves of the pandemic, thousands of patients worldwide required mechanical ventilation simultaneously, raising significant concerns about ICU capacity and resource allocation. For example, a global analysis found that 18.5% of hospitalized COVID-19 patients required ICU admission, and of these, 75.4% received mechanical ventilation [3]. Prolonged

L. F. da Fonseca Reis (✉)
University Center Augusto Motta, Rio de Janeiro, RJ, Brazil

Intensive Care Unit of the Central Hospital of the Military Police of the State of Rio de Janeiro, Rio de Janeiro, RJ, Brazil

Intensive Care Unit of the Gafrée Guinle University Hospital – Federal University of the State of Rio de Janeiro, Rio de Janeiro, RJ, Brazil

F. M. de Andrade
Pernambuco State Health Department, Recife, Brazil

Regional Council of Physiotherapy and Occupational Therapy of the 1st Region, Recife, Brazil

A. R. Baptistella et al. (eds.), *Weaning from Mechanical Ventilation*,
https://doi.org/10.1007/978-3-032-01145-9_18

mechanical ventilation (MV) is associated with several complications, including ventilator-associated pneumonia, muscle weakness, and increased mortality. Weaning from mechanical ventilation is a critical step in the management of ventilated patients and requires careful assessment to ensure readiness and minimize complications.

18.2 Pathophysiology of Severe Acute Respiratory Syndrome Caused by COVID-19

The pathophysiology of severe COVID-19 is characterized by a series of respiratory complications, often culminating in acute respiratory distress syndrome (ARDS). SARS-CoV-2 primarily infects the respiratory tract and enters host cells via the angiotensin-converting enzyme 2 (ACE2) receptor [4]. This viral entry triggers a cascade of inflammatory responses leading to a hyperinflammatory state often referred to as a "cytokine storm." This is characterized by elevated levels of pro-inflammatory cytokines such as interleukin-6 (IL-6), IL-1β, TNF-α, and various chemokines that contribute to widespread tissue damage and multi-organ dysfunction [5].

In the lung, viral infection leads to diffuse alveolar damage, increased vascular permeability, and pulmonary edema, which manifests clinically as ARDS [6]. Histopathologic studies of COVID-19 patients have shown severe endothelial injury and widespread thrombosis, with microangiopathy and angiogenesis being hallmarks of the severe disease [7]. This unique vascular pathology distinguishes COVID-19-induced ARDS from ARDS of other etiologies and complicates management and weaning from mechanical ventilation.

18.3 Factors Interfering with Weaning from Mechanical Ventilation

Weaning from mechanical ventilation in patients with COVID-19 is influenced by several factors, including patient-related factors, disease-related factors, and ventilator-related factors.

Patient-Related Factors Patients recovering from severe COVID-19 often have prolonged ICU stays and experience progressive muscle weakness, known as ICU-acquired weakness (ICUAW) [8, 9]. This muscle weakness can significantly impede spontaneous breathing efforts, making the weaning process more challenging. In addition, neuromuscular complications, including critical illness myopathy and neuropathy, are common and further complicate ventilator weaning [10]. Another important patient-related factor is the presence of comorbidities such as chronic obstructive pulmonary disease (COPD), obesity, diabetes, and cardiovascular disease, which are prevalent in critically ill COVID-19 patients. These conditions may exacerbate respiratory insufficiency and delay the weaning process [10].

Disease-Related Factors The hyperinflammatory state associated with severe COVID-19 contributes significantly to weaning difficulties. Persistent inflammation can lead to refractory hypoxemia and decreased lung compliance, requiring prolonged ventilatory support [11]. In addition, secondary bacterial infections, including ventilator-associated pneumonia (VAP), are common in this patient population, complicating the clinical course and prolonging the duration of mechanical ventilation [12].

Ventilator-Related Factors Ventilator settings and strategies also play a critical role in the weaning process. Strategies that minimize ventilator-induced lung injury (VILI) and optimize gas exchange are essential. However, achieving this balance is challenging in the context of COVID-19-associated ARDS. High levels of positive end-expiratory pressure (PEEP) may be necessary to maintain alveolar recruitment, but may also impede venous return and cause hemodynamic instability, complicating weaning efforts [13]. In addition, practices such as prolonged prone positioning, which have been shown to improve oxygenation in severe COVID-19, may have delayed effects on the weaning process due to the complexity of returning patients to a supine position while maintaining stability [14]. Therefore, weaning COVID-19 patients from mechanical ventilation was a multifactorial challenge influenced by the unique pathophysiologic characteristics of the disease, the presence of comorbid conditions, and mechanical ventilation strategies. Successful weaning required a comprehensive and individualized approach that addressed these multiple factors to optimize patient outcomes.

18.4 Weaning Readiness Assessment

Assessment of weaning readiness involves evaluation of both the underlying pathophysiology of COVID-19 and the general principles of weaning from mechanical ventilation. Key considerations include pulmonary, cardiovascular, and neurological stability, as well as the functional status of the diaphragm and other respiratory muscles. Assessment of readiness is multifaceted and includes both subjective and objective criteria [15–20]:

18.4.1 Respiratory Criteria

Patients must demonstrate adequate respiratory function to be considered for weaning:

- PaO_2/FiO_2 ratio: A ratio greater than 150–200 mmHg is generally accepted as an indication of adequate oxygenation.
- Spontaneous breathing trial (SBT): This remains the gold standard for assessing weaning ability. It involves placing the patient on minimal ventilator support, typically CPAP, pressure support of 5–7 cmH_2O with or without PEEP, for a period of 30–120 min. Success in maintaining stable respiratory parameters during this trial is predictive of successful extubation.
- Rapid Shallow Breathing Index (RSBI): The RSBI, calculated as respiratory rate (RR) divided by tidal volume (VT), is a reliable predictor of weaning success. An RSBI <105 breaths/min indicates readiness for extubation.
- Mechanical stress and compliance: In COVID-19 patients, assessment of lung compliance and airway resistance is essential as many patients have reduced compliance due to the fibrotic and stiff nature of their lungs. A static compliance greater than 30 mL/cm H_2O may indicate readiness for weaning. *Cardiovascular Stability.*
- Cardiovascular stability is essential to ensure that the patient can tolerate weaning from MV without hemodynamic compromise. The following parameters are important to evaluate:
- Absence of myocardial ischemia or arrhythmia: Episodes of new or unstable arrhythmias should be addressed before attempting weaning.
- Adequate blood pressure and heart rate control: Systolic blood pressure (SBP) between 90 and 160 mmHg and heart rate between 60 and 120 beats/min during SBT is indicative of cardiovascular stability.

18.4.2 Neurological and Cognitive Function

Adequate neurological function is required for successful weaning, as patients must have sufficient cognitive and motor control to protect their airway and maintain adequate respiratory effort:

- Glasgow Coma Scale (GCS): A GCS score of ≥13 is generally considered favorable for weaning.
- Delirium and sedation: Any sedation should be minimized or discontinued, and delirium must be managed to prevent impairment of respiratory drive.

18.4.3 Diaphragm and Respiratory Muscle Strength

Weakness of the respiratory muscles, especially the diaphragm, is a common consequence of prolonged MV. The following indicators should be considered:

- Maximal inspiratory pressure (MIP): A value lower than −30 cmH_2O indicates adequate respiratory muscle strength.

- Ultrasound of the diaphragm: Diaphragm thickness and contractility measured by ultrasound can predict weaning success, with thinner and poorly contractile diaphragms indicating a higher risk of weaning failure [21].

18.5 Specific Considerations for Weaning in COVID-19 Patients

COVID-19 presents unique challenges that influence weaning readiness [18, 19]:

- Persistent lung damage and fibrosis: Many patients develop significant pulmonary fibrosis, which reduces lung compliance and increases the work of breathing.
- Inflammatory and immune responses: The hyperinflammatory state seen in severe COVID-19 can impair diaphragmatic function and contribute to muscle atrophy. Monitoring inflammatory markers such as C-reactive protein (CRP) or interleukin-6 (IL-6) levels may provide insight into readiness for weaning.
- Prone positioning and oxygenation: Many COVID-19 patients are placed in the prone position to improve oxygenation. Reverting these patients to a supine position and assessing their ability to maintain stable oxygenation is crucial for weaning readiness.

18.6 Weaning Strategies for COVID-19 Patients

Given the heterogeneity of COVID-19 pathology, the weaning process must be tailored to the individual patient.

Protocol-Driven Weaning Protocol-driven weaning involves standardized procedures and assessments designed to ensure consistency and effectiveness in the weaning process. A study by Shang et al. [22] compared protocol-driven weaning with traditional clinician-driven methods in COVID-19 patients. The results showed that protocol-driven weaning resulted in higher success rates, shorter ventilation durations, and shorter ICU stays. Protocols typically include elements such as daily spontaneous breathing tests (SBTs), objective readiness criteria, and gradual reduction of ventilatory support [17–20, 22].

The following strategies were used in COVID-19 patients:

Gradual Weaning vs. Spontaneous Breathing Trials (SBT)
Spontaneous Breathing Trials (SBTs)

Spontaneous breathing tests are considered the gold standard for assessing a patient's readiness for extubation. During an SBT, ventilatory support is reduced or withdrawn to test whether the patient can sustain spontaneous breathing. Recent studies have focused on the outcomes of SBTs in COVID-19 patients, who often have compromised respiratory mechanics due to pulmonary fibrosis or persistent inflammation. SBTs assess a patient's ability to breathe independently through periodic trials in which ventilatory support is reduced or removed for a period of time. SBTs involve transitioning the patient to minimal ventilatory support settings such as T-piece, CPAP, or pressure support ventilation (PSV) modes. A positive SBT, characterized by stable vital signs and adequate gas exchange, is a critical predictor of successful extubation [17, 20, 23].

In patients who show signs of recovery, daily SBTs may facilitate earlier weaning from MV. This is particularly useful in patients with preserved respiratory drive but reduced lung compliance. Studies have shown that daily SBTs correlate with a higher likelihood of successful weaning [23–25]. Evidence from observational studies suggests that patients with COVID-19 may have a lower success rate with SBTs compared to patients without COVID-19 ARDS. Some guidelines recommend extending the duration of SBT beyond the typical 30–120 min to 4 h or longer in COVID-19 patients due to their increased risk of respiratory muscle fatigue. In addition, the use of pressure support ventilation (PSV) during SBTs may reduce the risk of aerosol production and reduce the risk of respiratory fatigue by providing minimal assistance to overcome airway resistance, which may be particularly beneficial in COVID-19 patients with residual lung injury.

Gradual Weaning Gradual reduction of ventilatory support involves progressively decreasing the amount of assistance provided by the ventilator, allowing the patient's respiratory muscles to adapt and strengthen gradually. A common strategy is pressure support weaning (PSV), in which inspiratory pressure support is gradually reduced. In patients with severe lung injury, a gradual reduction in ventilator support (i.e., a daily reduction in pressure support or time spent on SBT) may be more appropriate than abrupt SBT because it allows the respiratory muscles to adapt gradually to the increased workload. Evidence suggests that PSV is effective in reducing ventilator dependence and promoting patient breathing autonomy [17, 20, 23, 26].

Ventilator Modes in Weaning The choice of ventilator mode during weaning has a significant impact on patient outcomes. Several modes have been studied in the context of weaning COVID-19 patients from mechanical ventilation, with pressure support ventilation (PSV) and proportional assist ventilation (PAV) being the most commonly discussed. In PSV, patients receive a predetermined level of positive pressure during inspiration, which reduces the work of breathing. PAV, on the other hand, adjusts the level of ventilatory support in proportion to the effort. A recent randomized controlled trial (RCT) compared the efficacy of PSV and PAV in COVID-19 patients and found that PAV resulted in shorter weaning times and a lower incidence of reintubation. The adaptability of PAV to the patient's inspiratory effort appears to be particularly beneficial in patients with varying degrees of respiratory muscle weakness and lung compliance, which are common in post-COVID ARDS. However, PAV requires more advanced ventilators and clinician expertise, which may limit its widespread use, particularly in resource-limited settings [17, 20].

18.7 Extubation

It is important to emphasize that the method of extubation should be discussed with the service team according to a strict protocol that ensures the safety of the professionals and the patient. Before extubation, it is necessary to prepare the place (unit, bed, etc.) and have all the materials that will be used ready. Make a checklist of the materials needed to ensure that there is no need to leave the room during the procedure. Ideally, extubation should be performed in pairs to reduce the risk of failure and the duration of the procedure. Finally, monitor for signs of extubation failure and adjust the flow of oxygen from the ventilator interface to maintain adequate oxygenation if indicated ($SpO_2 < 90\%$) [17, 20, 25].

- The use of masks or high-flow systems after extubation and/or any procedure that produces mist or aerosol should be used with caution.
- Minimize the risk of coughing or exposure to secretions. Avoid procedures that irritate the airway and stimulate coughing.
- The use of supraglottic airway devices should be avoided as they stimulate coughing.

The following flowchart is a suggested sequence of extubation steps for patients with COVID-19 [25].

Before
Enter the room only in full protective clothing. Check equipment on site: 10 mL syringe to deflate the cuff. Nasal cannula (up to 6 L/min) or non-rebreathing mask (up to 10 L/min). Equipment for suctioning the airway and oral cavity. Material to remove the tube fixation, if necessary.
During
Perform preoxygenation at 100% FiO_2 for 3 min. Elevate the head of the bed to at least 30°. Perform adequate endotracheal suctioning (using a closed suction system) and oral suctioning. Remove the endotracheal tube fixation. Deflate the cuff. Turn off the ventilator and disconnect the patient. Maintain HMEF to minimize aerosolization. Remove the endotracheal tube. DO NOT REQUEST A COUGH OR PERFORM ADDITIONAL ENDOTRACHEAL SUCTIONING. Apply a mask or nasal cannula immediately after extubation.
After
Monitor for possible signs of failure. Adjust ventilation interface flow to maintain $SpO_2 > 90\%$.

Many patients with COVID-19 require prolonged mechanical ventilation and a tracheostomy to maintain an artificial airway. There is still much debate about the best way to manage spontaneous breathing in these patients. Ideally, a HMEF (or a filter with a minimum efficiency of 99.5% for particles smaller than 0.3 μm) should be attached to the closed suction system (Fig. 18.1).

Noninvasive Ventilation (NIV) Post-Extubation Noninvasive ventilation (NIV) has been used as a bridge during the weaning process, particularly in patients at high risk for extubation failure. Patients with COVID-19 who are at risk for extubation failure (e.g., those with residual lung injury or weakened respiratory muscles) may benefit from noninvasive ventilation (NIV) after extubation [27]. NIV may reduce the risk of reintubation by providing ventilatory support during periods of increased work of breathing.

Several studies have evaluated the role of NIV in weaning COVID-19 patients, particularly those with mild to moderate lung injury. NIV, often delivered via continuous positive airway pressure (CPAP) or bilevel positive airway pressure (BiPAP), can provide respiratory support while avoiding the complications associated with prolonged intubation [28]. Recent evidence suggests that early use of NIV after extubation in COVID-19 patients may reduce the risk of reintubation in selected populations, such as those with obesity, cardiac comorbidities, or hypercapnia [28]. However, the decision to use NIV must be balanced against the potential for aerosol generation and nosocomial transmission of SARS-CoV-2, particularly in poorly ventilated settings.

Use of High-Flow Nasal Cannula (HFNC). High-flow nasal cannula (HFNC) has been shown to be particularly effective in maintaining oxygenation in COVID-19 patients during and after weaning. HFNC provides a continuous flow of oxygen and

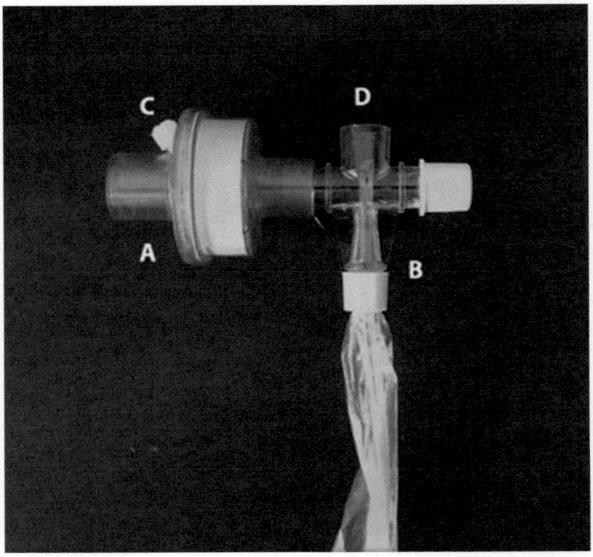

Fig. 18.1 Spontaneous breathing testing device for tracheostomized patients: (**a**) heat humidity exchanger filter (HMEF), (**b**) closed endotracheal suction (Trach-care), (**c**) connection port for oxygen therapy in HMEF, (**d**) tracheostomy port. (The Kelley Circuit in https://tracheostomy.org.uk/storage/files/The%20Kelley%20Circuit%20For%20Tracheostomy.pdf.pdf; [26])

can reduce the work of breathing by providing a small amount of positive end-expiratory pressure (PEEP) and improve patient comfort compared to conventional oxygen therapy [29, 30]. Evidence suggests that HFNC can reduce reintubation rates and support smoother transitions from mechanical ventilation, including alternating with the use of noninvasive ventilation [30, 31].

Successful Weaning Rates Studies suggest that weaning success rates in COVID-19 patients vary and are influenced by factors such as age, comorbidities, and severity of initial illness [12]. Ongoing evaluation and tailored weaning protocols based on individual patient characteristics are critical to improving outcomes [17].

18.8 Other Strategies to Facilitate Ventilatory Weaning in COVID-19

Early Mobilization Early mobilization plays an essential role in improving weaning outcomes, as immobilization can exacerbate ICU-acquired weakness and make the weaning process more challenging. Early physical and occupational therapy interventions, including passive and active mobilization, have been associated with improved functional outcomes and shorter ventilator durations [32]. A narrative review by Wittmer et al. [33] highlighted the role of early rehabilitation in improving weaning success in COVID-19 patients and emphasized the importance of integrating these modalities into weaning protocols.

Inspiratory Muscle Training Inspiratory muscle training as a therapeutic intervention IMT is a noninvasive intervention designed to improve the strength and endurance of the inspiratory muscles through targeted, repetitive exercises. Patients undergoing IMT use devices that provide resistance to inhalation, thereby strengthening the muscles involved in breathing. Studies have shown that IMT can increase diaphragm strength, improve respiratory endurance, and reduce the perceived effort of breathing in patients with respiratory weakness [34–36].

Evidence for IMT in facilitating weaning from MV [34, 35, 37];

In COVID-19 patients who have experienced prolonged MV, IMT may be particularly beneficial. Research in non-COVID populations has shown that IMT may accelerate weaning by:

1. Improving inspiratory muscle strength: IMT increases the contractile ability of the diaphragm, counteracting the effects of VIDD and allowing patients to achieve higher inspiratory pressures. This improvement in muscle strength can help patients achieve spontaneous breathing.
2. Reduce dyspnea: With strengthened respiratory muscles, patients experience less dyspnea, or shortness of breath, which is critical to maintaining patient cooperation and comfort during the weaning process.

3. Reduced weaning time: IMT has been associated with shorter weaning times and reduced ICU stays, which are critical in the context of limited resources during the COVID-19 pandemic.
4. Improved functional outcomes: Improved inspiratory muscle function may contribute to better long-term respiratory outcomes and overall functional status, aiding in post-discharge recovery.

Implementation of IMT in Weaning Protocols While the implementation of IMT during the weaning process in COVID-19 patients has shown potential, individualized protocols are necessary due to the variability in patients' baseline respiratory function and the severity of COVID-19-related lung injury. IMT should be started with low resistance to avoid overexertion and gradually increased as patients' strength improves. Periodic assessments of respiratory muscle strength, such as maximal inspiratory pressure (MIP) measurements, can guide the progression of training intensity [35, 38].

The use of other adjunctive therapies has been explored to support weaning efforts in COVID-19 patients. Neuromuscular electrical stimulation (NMES) of the diaphragm and respiratory muscles has been studied as a means of improving respiratory muscle strength and endurance. Preliminary studies suggest that NMES, in combination with conventional physical therapy, may reduce weaning times in patients with severe respiratory muscle weakness after COVID-19. However, larger studies are needed to confirm these findings.

Pharmacologic therapies, such as dexamethasone and remdesivir, have also played a role in reducing the inflammatory burden during weaning. Dexamethasone in particular has been shown to reduce mortality and shorten the duration of mechanical ventilation in patients with severe COVID-19. Its use during weaning may help modulate the hyperinflammatory response, thereby reducing respiratory muscle fatigue and improving weaning outcomes [39].

18.9 Challenges and Future Directions in Weaning COVID-19 Patients

Prolonged ventilation and ICU-acquired weakness COVID-19 patients often require prolonged mechanical ventilation, resulting in significant muscle wasting and ICU-acquired weakness. This weakness is attributed to critical illness polyneuropathy, myopathy, or a combination of both, and significantly hinders the weaning process [8, 9]. Intervention strategies, including early mobilization and neuromuscular electrical stimulation, have shown promise in mitigating these effects [33].

Ventilator-associated pneumonia (VAP) is a common and serious complication in mechanically ventilated COVID-19 patients, further complicating the weaning process. Infection control measures, including strict oral hygiene protocols, subglottic suctioning, and adherence to ventilator bundles, are critical to preventing VAP and associated morbidity [40].

Novel approaches such as personalized weaning protocols based on real-time monitoring of diaphragm function, lung compliance, and inflammatory markers are under investigation. Telemonitoring and artificial intelligence-based decision support systems are increasingly being integrated into weaning protocols, providing real-time data and predictive analytics to optimize weaning decisions. These systems can help identify patients who are ready for weaning trials and predict potential complications, improving the efficacy and safety of the process [41]. There is also growing interest in the role of rehabilitation during and after mechanical ventilation to prevent muscle wasting and improve recovery. Early mobilization and physiotherapy, even during MV, may improve weaning outcomes.

18.10 Tracheostomy Timing

The timing of tracheostomy in COVID-19 patients is a subject of ongoing debate. While early tracheostomy (within 7–10 days of intubation) may facilitate weaning and reduce the need for sedation (with no effect on mortality), concerns about viral transmission to healthcare workers necessitate a more cautious approach [42]. Studies suggest that performing tracheostomies in a controlled environment with enhanced safeguards may reduce transmission risks and facilitate weaning efforts [43, 44].

18.11 Post-Extubation Complications

COVID-19 patients undergoing prolonged mechanical ventilation are at high risk for post-extubation complications, including upper airway obstruction, laryngeal edema, and dysphagia. Studies have reported that up to 30% of COVID-19 patients may experience significant dysphagia after extubation. Early involvement of speech therapy teams has been shown to improve outcomes by addressing dysphagia and preventing aspiration. Re-intubation rates in COVID-19 patients remain high compared to non-COVID patients. A multicenter cohort study found that approximately 20%–25% of extubated COVID-19 patients required reintubation within 48–72 h, often due to a combination of respiratory muscle fatigue, unresolved inflammation, or ventilator-associated pneumonia. Strategies to mitigate this risk include prophylactic use of corticosteroids to reduce airway edema and close monitoring with repeat SBTs before considering reintubation [43, 45].

18.12 Long-Term Follow-Up After Extubation

Monitoring and rehabilitation are critical to managing potential respiratory and physical sequelae. Long-term follow-up facilitates early detection of complications such as persistent pulmonary function impairment and physical deconditioning [45].

18.13 Conclusion

Weaning strategies for COVID-19 patients include a combination of protocol-driven approaches, individualized patient assessments, and supportive therapies aimed at minimizing complications and optimizing outcomes. Spontaneous breathing trials, gradual reduction of ventilatory support, early mobilization, and vigilant infection control are fundamental components. Special considerations, such as the impact of prone positioning and timing of tracheostomy, require careful attention to balance benefits and risks. Emerging technologies and novel therapies hold promise for further improving the weaning process. Ongoing research and clinical trials will continue to refine these strategies and contribute to improved recovery and survival rates for other viral infections that can cause severe acute respiratory syndrome, as occurred in the COVID-19 pandemic.

References

1. World Health Organization. Clinical management of COVID-19: interim guidance. 2023. Retrieved from [WHO website] (https://www.who.int/publications).
2. Wu Z, McGoogan JM. Characteristics of and important lessons from the coronavirus disease 2019 (COVID-19) outbreak in China: summary of a report of 72 314 cases from the Chinese Center for Disease Control and Prevention. JAMA. 2020;323(13):1239–42. https://doi.org/10.1001/jama.2020.2648.
3. Auld SC, Caridi-Scheible M, Blum JM, Robichaux C, Kraft C, Jacob JT, Jabaley CS, Carpenter D, Kaplow R, Hernandez-Romieu AC, Adelman MW, Martin GS, Coopersmith CM, Murphy DJ, the Emory COVID-19 Quality and Clinical Research Collaborative. ICU and ventilator mortality among critically ill adults with coronavirus disease 2019. Crit Care Med. 2020;48(9):e799–804. https://doi.org/10.1097/CCM.0000000000004457.
4. Hoffmann M, Kleine-Weber H, Schroeder S, Krüger N, Herrler T, Erichsen S, Schiergens TS, Herrler G, Wu NH, Nitsche A, Müller MA, Drosten C, Pöhlmann S. SARS-CoV-2 cell entry depends on ACE2 and TMPRSS2 and is blocked by a clinically proven protease inhibitor. Cell. 2020;181(2):271–280.e8. https://doi.org/10.1016/j.cell.2020.02.052.
5. Tay MZ, Poh CM, Rénia L, MacAry PA, Ng LFP. The trinity of COVID-19: immunity, inflammation and intervention. Nat Rev Immunol. 2020;20(6):363–74. https://doi.org/10.1038/s41577-020-0311-8. Epub 2020 Apr 28
6. Berlin DA, Gulick RM, Martinez FJ. Severe Covid-19. N Engl J Med. 2020;383(25):2451–60. https://doi.org/10.1056/NEJMcp2009575.

7. Ackermann M, Verleden SE, Kuehnel M, Haverich A, Welte T, Laenger F, Vanstapel A, Werlein C, Stark H, Tzankov A, Li WW, Li VW, Mentzer SJ, Jonigk D. Pulmonary vascular endothelialitis, thrombosis, and angiogenesis in Covid-19. N Engl J Med. 2020;383(2):120–8. https://doi.org/10.1056/NEJMoa2015432.
8. Hermans G, Van den Berghe G. Clinical review: intensive care unit acquired weakness. Crit Care. 2015a;19(1):274. https://doi.org/10.1186/s13054-015-0993-7.
9. Hermans G, Van den Berghe G. Clinical review: intensive care unit acquired weakness. Crit Care. 2015b;19:274. https://doi.org/10.1186/s13054-015-0993-7.
10. Grasselli G, et al. Baseline characteristics and outcomes of 1591 patients infected with SARS-CoV-2 admitted to ICUs of the Lombardy region, Italy. JAMA. 2020;323(16):1574–81.
11. Zhou F, Yu T, Du R, Fan G, Liu Y, Liu Z, Xiang J, Wang Y, Song B, Gu X, Guan L, Wei Y, Li H, Wu X, Xu J, Tu S, Zhang Y, Chen H, Cao B. Clinical course and risk factors for mortality of adult inpatients with COVID-19 in Wuhan, China: a retrospective cohort study. Lancet. 2020;395(10229):1054–62. https://doi.org/10.1016/S0140-6736(20)30566-3.
12. Yang X, et al. Clinical course and outcomes of critically ill patients with SARS-CoV-2 pneumonia in Wuhan, China: a single-centered, retrospective, observational study. Lancet Respir Med. 2020;8(5):475–81.
13. Gattinoni L, Chiumello D, Caironi P, Busana M, Romitti F, Brazzi L, Camporota L. COVID-19 pneumonia: different respiratory treatments for different phenotypes? Intensive Care Med. 2020;46(6):1099–102. https://doi.org/10.1007/s00134-020-06033-2.
14. Scaramuzzo G, Gamberini L, Tonetti T, et al. Sustained oxygenation improvement after first prone positioning is associated with liberation from mechanical ventilation and mortality in critically ill COVID-19 patients: a cohort study. Ann Intensive Care. 2021;11:63. https://doi.org/10.1186/s13613-021-00853-1.
15. Bordon J, Akca O, Furmanek S, Cavallazzi RS, Suliman S, Aboelnasr A, Sinanova B, Ramirez JA. Acute respiratory distress syndrome and time to weaning off the invasive mechanical ventilator among patients with COVID-19 pneumonia. J Clin Med. 2021;10:2935. https://doi.org/10.3390/jcm10132935.
16. Chiumello D, Chommeloux J, Langer T, Teniente JRS, Mongero LB, Gattinoni L. *COVID-19: PEEP, pronation, and weaning*. J Thorac Dis. 2020;12(3):105–7. https://doi.org/10.21037/jtd.2020.02.96.
17. Dorado JH, Navarro E, Plotnikow GA, Gogniat E, Accoce M, EpVAr Study Group. Epidemiology of weaning from invasive mechanical ventilation in subjects with COVID-19. Respir Care. 2023;68(1):101–9. https://doi.org/10.4187/respcare.09925.
18. Luo M, Mei Z, Wei L, Cao S, Su S, Wang Y. Precautions for weaning from invasive mechanical ventilation with critically ill COVID-19. Heart Lung. 2020a;49(6):869–71. https://doi.org/10.1016/j.hrtlng.2020.07.005.
19. Luo M, Mei Z, Wei L, Cao S, Su S, Wang Y. Precautions for weaning from invasive mechanical ventilation with critically ill COVID-19. Heart Lung. 2020b;49(6):869–71. https://doi.org/10.1016/j.hrtlng.2020.07.005.
20. de la Fuente IS, de la Fuente JS, Marcos Morales A, Muñoz Calahorro R, Álvaro Valiente E, Sánchez Izquierdo Riera JÁ. Weaning from mechanical ventilation in COVID-19 patients. Med Intensiva (Engl Ed). 2024;48(5):296–8. https://doi.org/10.1016/j.medine.2024.02.001.
21. Vetrugno L, Orso D, Corradi F, et al. Diaphragm ultrasound evaluation during weaning from mechanical ventilation in COVID-19 patients: a pragmatic, cross-section, multicenter study. Respir Res. 2022;23:210. https://doi.org/10.1186/s12931-022-02138-y.
22. Shang Y, Pan C, Yang X, et al. Management of critically ill patients with COVID-19 in ICU: statement from front-line intensive care experts in Wuhan. China Ann Intensive Care. 2020;10:73. https://doi.org/10.1186/s13613-020-00689-1.
23. Fleuren LM, Dam TA, Tonutti M, et al. Predictors for extubation failure in COVID-19 patients using a machine learning approach. Crit Care. 2021;25:448. https://doi.org/10.1186/s13054-021-03864-3.

24. Esteban A, et al. Patients with acute respiratory distress syndrome: what is the mortality today? Intensive Care Med. 2002;28(5):623–33.
25. de Castro LA, Rocha ÂRM, Camillo CA. Weaning from mechanical ventilation in patients with COVID-19. ASSOBRAFIR Ciênc. 2020;11 https://doi.org/10.47066/2177-9333.AC20.covid19.017.
26. Righetti RF, Onoue MA, Politi FVA, Teixeira DT, Souza PN, Kondo CS, Moderno EV, Moraes IG, Maida ALV, Pastore Junior L, Silva FD, Brito CMM, Baia WRM, Yamaguti WP. Physiotherapy care of patients with coronavirus disease 2019 (COVID-19) – a Brazilian experience. Clinics (Sao Paulo). 2020;75:e2017. https://doi.org/10.6061/clinics/2020/e2017. PMID: 32578825
27. Hernández G, Paredes I, Moran F, Buj M, Colinas L, Rodríguez ML, Velasco A, Rodríguez P, Pérez-Pedrero MJ, Suarez-Sipmann F, Canabal A, Cuena R, Blanch L, Roca O. Effect of postextubation noninvasive ventilation with active humidification vs high-flow nasal cannula on reintubation in patients at very high risk for extubation failure: a randomized trial. Intensive Care Med. 2022;48(12):1751–9. https://doi.org/10.1007/s00134-022-06919-3.
28. Boniatti VMC, Pereira CR, Costa GM, Teixeira MC, Werlang AP, Martins FTM, Marques LDS, Nedel WL, Boniatti MM. Extubation failure and the use of noninvasive ventilation during the weaning process in critically ill COVID-19 patients. Crit Care Sci. 2023;35(2):163–7. https://doi.org/10.5935/2965-2774.20230009-en.
29. Li J, Fink JB, Ehrmann S. High-flow nasal cannula for COVID-19 patients: low risk of bioaerosol dispersion. Eur Respir J. 2020;55(5):2000892. https://doi.org/10.1183/13993003.00892-2020.
30. Khanna AK, De Jong A, Myatra SN. High-flow nasal cannula and outcomes in COVID-19: Reading between the lines. Anesth Analg. 2023;136(4):689–91. https://doi.org/10.1213/ANE.0000000000006409.
31. Frat JP, et al. High-flow oxygen through nasal cannula in acute hypoxemic respiratory failure. N Engl J Med. 2015;372:2185–96.
32. Schweickert WD, Pohlman MC, Pohlman AS, Nigos C, Pawlik AJ, Esbrook CL, Spears L, Miller M, Franczyk M, Deprizio D, Schmidt GA, Bowman A, Barr R, McCallister KE, Hall JB, Kress JP. Early physical and occupational therapy in mechanically ventilated, critically ill patients: a randomised controlled trial. Lancet. 2009;373(9678):1874–82. https://doi.org/10.1016/S0140-6736(09)60658-9.
33. Wittmer VL, Paro FM, Duarte H, Capellini VK, Barbalho-Moulim MC. Early mobilization and physical exercise in patients with COVID-19: a narrative literature review. Complement Ther Clin Pract. 2021;43:101364. https://doi.org/10.1016/j.ctcp.2021.101364.
34. Bissett B, Leditschke IA, Green M, Marzano V, Collins S, Van Haren F. Inspiratory muscle training for intensive care patients: a multidisciplinary practical guide for clinicians. Aust Crit Care. 2019;32(3):249–55. https://doi.org/10.1016/j.aucc.2018.06.001. Epub 2018 Jul 11
35. Bissett BM, Wang J, Neeman T, Leditschke IA, Boots R, Paratz J. Which ICU patients benefit most from inspiratory muscle training? Retrospective analysis of a randomized trial. Physiother. Theory Pract. 2020;36(12):1316–21. https://doi.org/10.1080/09593985.2019.1571144. Epub 2019 Feb 9
36. Major ME, Sommers J, Horrevorts E, Buist CM, Dettling-Ihnenfeldt DS, van der Schaaf M. Inspiratory muscle training for mechanically ventilated patients in the intensive care unit: obstacles and facilitators for implementation. A mixed method quality improvement study. Aust Crit Care. 2024 Nov;37(6):851–8. https://doi.org/10.1016/j.aucc.2024.01.005.
37. Abodonya AM, Abdelbasset WK, Awad EA, Elalfy IE, Salem HA, Elsayed SH. Inspiratory muscle training for recovered COVID-19 patients after weaning from mechanical ventilation: a pilot control clinical study. Medicine (Baltimore). 2021;100(13):e25339. https://doi.org/10.1097/MD.0000000000025339.
38. Patsaki I, Kouvarakos A, Vasileiadis I, Koumantakis GA, Ischaki E, Grammatopoulou E, Kotanidou A, Magira EE. Low-medium and high-intensity inspiratory muscle training in critically ill patients: a systematic review and meta-analysis. Medicina (Kaunas). 2024;60(6):869. https://doi.org/10.3390/medicina60060869. PMID: 38929486; PMCID: PMC11205434

39. Recovery Collaborative Group, Horby P, Lim WS, Emberson JR, Mafham M, Bell JL, Linsell L, Staplin N, Brightling C, Ustianowski A, Elmahi E, Prudon B, Green C, Felton T, Chadwick D, Rege K, Fegan C, Chappell LC, Faust SN, Jaki T, Jeffery K, Montgomery A, Rowan K, Juszczak E, Baillie JK, Haynes R, Landray MJ. Dexamethasone in hospitalized patients with Covid-19. N Engl J Med. 2021;384(8):693–704. https://doi.org/10.1056/NEJMoa2021436.
40. Boyd S, Nseir S, Rodriguez A, Martin-Loeches I. Ventilator-associated pneumonia in critically ill patients with COVID-19 infection: a narrative review. ERJ Open Res. 2022;8(3):00046–2022. https://doi.org/10.1183/23120541.00046-2022.
41. Nasa P, Azoulay E, Khanna AK, et al. Expert consensus statements for the management of COVID-19-related acute respiratory failure using a Delphi method. Crit Care. 2021;25:106. https://doi.org/10.1186/s13054-021-03491-y.
42. Angel L, Kon ZN, Chang SH et al. Novel percutaneous tracheostomy for critically ill patients with COVID-19. Ann Thorac Surg. 2020;110:1006–11. https://doi.org/10.1016/j.athoracsur.2020.04.010.
43. Benito DA, Bestourous DE, Tong JY, Pasick LJ, Sataloff RT. Tracheotomy in COVID-19 patients: a systematic review and meta-analysis of weaning, decannulation, and survival. Otolaryngol Head Neck Surg. 2021;165(3):398–405. https://doi.org/10.1177/0194599820984780.
44. McGrath BA, Brenner MJ, Warrillow SJ, Pandian V, Arora A, Cameron TS, Añon JM, Hernández Martínez G, Truog RD, Block SD, Lui GCY, McDonald C, Rassekh CH, Atkins J, Qiang L, Vergez S, Dulguerov P, Zenk J, Antonelli M, Pelosi P, Walsh BK, Ward E, Shang Y, Gasparini S, Donati A, Singer M, Openshaw PJM, Tolley N, Markel H, Feller-Kopman DJ. Tracheostomy in the COVID-19 era: global and multidisciplinary guidance. Lancet Respir Med. 2020 Jul;8(7):717–25. https://doi.org/10.1016/S2213-2600(20)30230-7.
45. Herridge MS, Azoulay É. Outcomes after critical illness. N Engl J Med. 2023;388(10):913–24. https://doi.org/10.1056/NEJMra2104669.

Chapter 19
Tracheostomy and Weaning

Gabriel Manfro and Douglas Pellizzaro

19.1 History of Tracheostomy for Weaning

There are reports of the use of tracheostomy in Egyptian and ancient Greek times, with the first descriptions attributed to the Egyptian Edwin Smith Papyrus (1600 BC) and the Greek Claudius Galen (129–199 AD), the latter responsible for the first anatomical descriptions of the larynx [1, 2]. Tracheostomy was first used in the treatment of airway obstruction at the beginning of the twentieth century. At that time, this technique was not used in the management of patients on mechanical ventilation (MV).

The term tracheostomy refers to the creation of a stoma on the surface of the skin leading to the trachea, while a tracheotomy refers to the corresponding surgical opening into the trachea. A surgical tracheostomy may be performed under local or general anesthesia, may be elective or emergency, and may be temporary or permanent [1].

In the 1950s and 1960s, especially during the polio epidemic, there was a significant increase in the number of patients on MV and the benefits of tracheostomy in patients on MV for prolonged periods began to be recognized [3].

This practice evolved further in the 1970s and 1980s with the advent of intensive care units, which increased the use of prolonged MV and led to the first studies linking tracheostomy to earlier weaning from MV [4] (Figs. 19.1, 19.2 and 19.3).

G. Manfro (✉)
University of Western Santa Catarina – Unoesc, Joaçaba, Santa Catarina, Brazil

D. Pellizzaro
University of Western Santa Catarina – Unoesc, Joaçaba, Santa Catarina, Brazil

Anesthesiology Department, Hospital Universitário Santa Terezinha, Joaçaba, Santa Catarina, Brazil

Unimed Meio Oeste, Joaçaba, Santa Catarina, Brazil

A. R. Baptistella et al. (eds.), *Weaning from Mechanical Ventilation*, https://doi.org/10.1007/978-3-032-01145-9_19

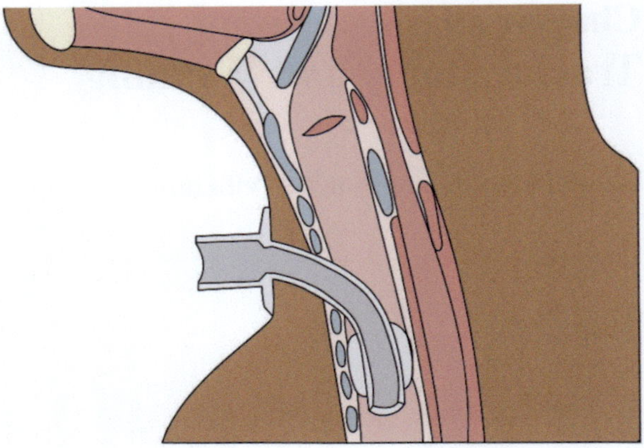

Fig. 19.1 Sagittal plane view of tracheostomy

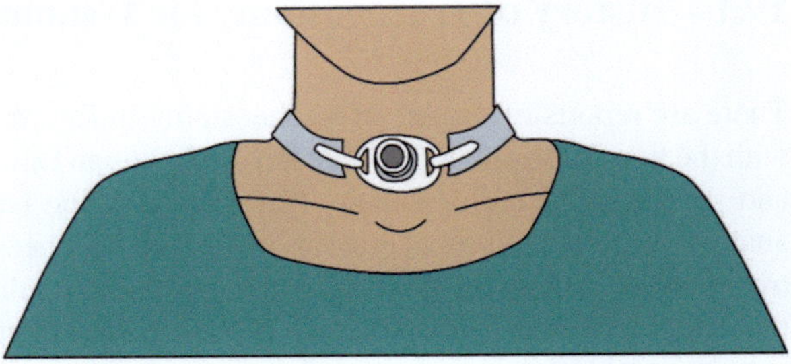

Fig. 19.2 Coronal plane diagram of tracheostomy positioning and fixation

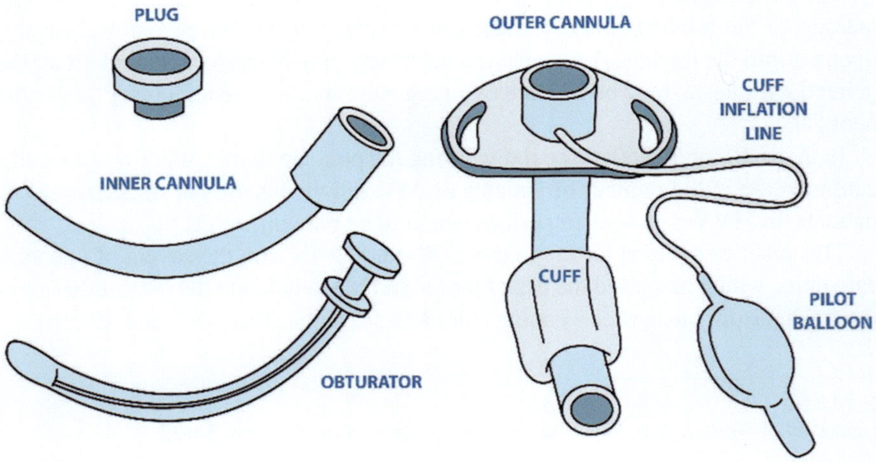

Fig. 19.3 Tracheostomy tube components

19.2 Indications for Tracheostomy

The main indication for tracheostomy is prolonged intubation, a procedure that provides numerous benefits to the patient, such as reducing the risk of subglottic stenosis, improving pulmonary hygiene in the management of secretions, and, most importantly, facilitating weaning of these mechanically ventilated patients [5].

Controlled cuff inflation is essential to allow adequate vascularization of the tracheal and subglottic laryngeal mucosa. In cases where ischemia of the cartilaginous walls occurs, the chances of healing with stenosis increase. The subglottic region, being the smallest region of the airway, has a greater chance of becoming symptomatic if stenosis occurs. In addition, subglottic stenosis is technically more difficult to treat than tracheal stenosis due to the proximity of the vocal cords in the glottic region. Therefore, to protect the subglottic region, in situations where orotracheal intubation is prolonged, performing a tracheostomy aims to remove the aggression from the smaller caliber region of the airway, which is the subglottic region, by positioning the cuff at the level of the trachea, farthest from the vocal cords [6, 7].

Other indications for tracheostomy include airway obstruction due to tumors of the larynx, pharynx, thyroid, or trachea. In cases of bilateral vocal cord paralysis, tracheostomy is also necessary to maintain adequate oxygenation of the patient; inability to intubate, such as in extensive facial trauma, usually after emergency cricothyroidotomy; failure of extubation attempts; and finally, airway protection in neurological diseases and in the treatment of head and neck tumors until swallowing ability is restored without bronchoaspiration (Table 19.1) [8–12].

Table 19.1 Summary of tracheostomy indications

Prolonged intubation (reduced risk of subglottic stenosis)
Airway obstruction from head and neck tumors
Bilateral vocal cord paralysis
Impossibility of tracheal intubation (anticipated difficult airway, facial trauma)
Glottic edema due to burns or anaphylaxis
Failed extubation attempts

Table 19.2 Complications of tracheostomy

Immediate	Early	Late
Bleeding	Bleeding	Granuloma formation
Aspiration	Accidental decannulation	Tracheomalacia
Loss of airway	Pneumothorax	Infection
Hypoxemia	Pneumomediastinum	Tracheoesophageal fistula
Death	Subcutaneous emphysema infection	Tracheoinnominate fistula
	Dysphagia	Tracheal stenosis

Manfro et al. [13]

19.3 Risk of Tracheostomy

Tracheostomy is a surgical procedure whose use has increased significantly in all age groups in recent decades. It has many advantages, but it increases the dependence on professionals who are able to deal with this situation. As with any surgery, there is a risk of complications, which vary depending on the time of occurrence (Table 19.2).

As this is a procedure with a significant number of complications, it should be performed by an experienced team with local anatomical knowledge whenever possible, and should be indicated based on the advantages and disadvantages of this technique.

The length of time the orotracheal tube remains in place varies widely, with the indication for tracheostomy being considered early or late. This lack of definition of the timing of the indication for surgery occurs because of the variables to be considered, such as the evolution of the patient's clinical condition, the reason for the need for mechanical ventilation, the patient's nutritional status, comorbidities, anatomical parameters (obesity, history of difficult airway, cervicofacial deformities), and the patient's clinical prognosis, that is, how long the patient should remain on mechanical ventilation [14–16].

19.4 Does Tracheostomy Improve Outcomes?

The analysis of the benefit of tracheostomy, based on the many situations mentioned above, must be carried out according to several parameters, since the benefit of this technique is significantly increased when it is well indicated, correctly performed, and skillfully managed.

Many advantages can be cited for tracheostomized patients compared to patients with an orotracheal tube during mechanical ventilation:

1. Comfort and tolerance: The tracheostomy, not being in contact with the oropharynx, is much more comfortable for the patient, allowing easier communication and even tolerating oral feeding in some cases [17].
2. Airway resistance: The tracheostomy tube can be larger in caliber and shorter in length, significantly reducing airway resistance and work of breathing [18].
3. Oral hygiene: The absence of an orotracheal tube allows for easier oral and dental hygiene, reducing the risk of oral infections [19].
4. Airway safety: Tracheostomy has a lower risk of airway dislodgement and loss compared to the orotracheal tube [20].
5. Need for sedation: As there is nothing in contact with the oropharynx, which does not trigger a gag reflex, tracheostomized patients require less sedation, which facilitates awakening and anticipates weaning from mechanical ventilation [21].
6. Length of stay in the ICU: Tracheostomized patients typically have a shorter stay on mechanical ventilation and in the ICU [22].
7. Speech and swallowing: Depending on the patient's level of consciousness, tracheostomy allows speech (with the use of an appropriate cannula), in addition to swallowing and analysis of the level of bronchoaspiration, accelerating the patient's complete rehabilitation [23].
8. Airway aspiration: The position of the tracheostomy allows aspiration of more distal regions of the airway, facilitating the removal of secretions and reducing the incidence of pneumonia associated with mechanical ventilation [24].
9. Weaning: The tracheostomy can accelerate independence from mechanical ventilation, through the intermittent use of ventilatory support during the process of initiating the patient's spontaneous ventilation [25].

The advantages of the tracheostomy over the orotracheal tube in the assessment of patients on prolonged ventilation can be explained by several physical principles:

- *Poiseuille's law:* The flow of a fluid in a cylindrical tube is proportional to the radius of this cylinder raised to the fourth power and inversely proportional to the length of the tube and the viscosity of the fluid. The tracheostomy tube is shorter and may have a larger caliber than the orotracheal tube. Even a minimal difference in caliber results in a significant increase in flow for the same pressure gradient [26].
- *Bernoulli's principle:* This principle states that in long, narrow tubes such as the orotracheal tube, an increase in air velocity occurs simultaneously with a decrease in pressure, increasing the resistance to air flow. The Venturi effect is a derivative of Bernoulli's principle and describes how constriction in a tube causes an increase in air velocity and a decrease in pressure, resulting in greater turbulence and resistance to flow. A tracheostomy reduces airflow resistance and turbulence, providing a more stable and efficient airway and facilitating weaning from mechanical ventilation [27].

- *Laplace's law:* It states that the greater the radius of a cylinder, the greater the stress in the cylinder wall. In the context of the airway, this law can help explain how different pressures are needed to keep the airway open or to initiate airflow. The tracheostomy allows an airway of more stable caliber with less risk of collapse under negative pressure compared to the orotracheal tube. This advantage is particularly evident during the weaning period when the patient requires less positive pressure to maintain airway patency [28].
- *Fluid dynamics and turbulence:* Flow in a cylinder can be laminar or turbulent. The former is more efficient, requires less energy, and occurs at lower velocities and in wider tubes. Swirling flow, which occurs at high velocity or in smaller tubes, is less efficient. The tracheostomy tube provides a greater opportunity for laminar flow, which reduces work of breathing and improves gas exchange [29].
- *Pressure-volume relationship:* This relationship is important in understanding lung compliance and resistance. Tracheostomy reduces airway resistance, resulting in a better pressure-volume relationship, facilitating weaning or spontaneous breathing [30].

19.5 Early vs. Standard or Late Tracheostomy and Weaning

Tracheostomy is one of the most common procedures performed on critically ill patients in the ICU, occurring in up to a quarter of patients, mainly in cases of prolonged mechanical ventilation and weaning. However, the ideal time period for its indication remains uncertain. One of the main questions is related to the heterogeneity of definitions of early tracheostomy, which vary widely in the literature from 7 to 21 days [31].

Based on some recent publications, in adult patients with prolonged intubation, early tracheostomy is significantly associated with a reduction in the incidence of hospital-acquired pneumonia, the incidence of mortality, the duration of mechanical ventilation, and the length of stay in the intensive care unit, especially when early tracheostomy is performed in the first 7 days after intubation [31–34]. However, in patients with severe neurological pathology, an early tracheostomy strategy did not significantly improve survival without severe disability at 6 months [35].

Tracheostomy has evolved significantly since its inception to become a critical procedure in the management of patients requiring prolonged ventilation. While it offers benefits such as reduced airway resistance, improved oral hygiene, and reduced sedation, it is important to carefully consider the risks and benefits for each patient. The ideal timing for tracheostomy remains controversial, with recent studies suggesting potential benefits of early tracheostomy in certain cases. As research continues, it is imperative that healthcare professionals stay abreast of best practices to optimize patient outcomes and minimize complications.

References

1. Cooper JD. Surgery of the airway: history notes. J Thorac Dis. 2016;8(Suppl 2):S113–20.
2. CG Kuhn. Galen. Introductio Seu Medicus (trans). Leipzig; 1856. p. 406. Adam F. Areataeus: the therapeutics of acute diseases (trans). London: Syndenham Society; 1856. p. 406.
3. Gale JW, Waters RM. The use of the tracheotomy tube in the treatment of respiratory paralysis in poliomyelitis. JAMA. 1950;144(15):1345–8.
4. Esteban A, Anzueto A, Frutos F, Alía I, Brochard L, Stewart TE, et al. International mechanical ventilation study group. Characteristics and outcomes in adult patients receiving mechanical ventilation: a 28-day international study. JAMA. 2002;287(3):345–55.
5. Trouillet JL, Collange O, Belafia F, Blot F, Capellier G, Cesareo E, et al. Tracheotomy in the intensive care unit: guidelines from a French expert panel. Ann Intensive Care. 2022;12:37.
6. Johnson L, Martinez R. Impact of cuff pressure on tracheal mucosa: a clinical study. Respir Care. 2021;66:789–95. https://doi.org/10.4187/respcare.09234.
7. Lee H, Kim J. Tracheostomy in prolonged intubation: a comparative study. Int J Crit Care. 2021;37:98–105. https://doi.org/10.1097/CCM.0000000000005123.
8. Williams D, Chen L. Tracheostomy in head and neck cancer patients: indications and outcomes. J Otolaryngol Head Neck Surg. 2022;51:145–52. https://doi.org/10.1007/s00405-022-07345-7.
9. Patel R, Singh K. Management of Bilateral Vocal Cord Paralysis: a review. Laryngoscope. 2021;131:987–93. https://doi.org/10.1002/lary.29345.
10. Johnson M, Lee S. Emergency cricothyroidotomy and subsequent tracheostomy in facial trauma. Trauma Surg Acute Care Open. 2022;7:e000823. https://doi.org/10.1136/tsaco-2022-000823.
11. Martinez A, Brown J. Challenges in extubation failure: role of tracheostomy. Respir Care. 2021;66:1023–30. https://doi.org/10.4187/respcare.09345.
12. Garcia P, Thompson M. Airway protection in neurological disorders: indications for tracheostomy. Neurocrit Care. 2022;36:456–63. https://doi.org/10.1007/s12028-022-01456-3.
13. Manfro G, Dias FD, Farias TP. Tracheostomy complications. In: Férias TP, editor. Tracheostomy a surgical guide. 1st ed. Springer; 2018. p. 307–19.
14. Smith J, Brown A. Timing of tracheostomy in mechanically ventilated patients: a systematic review and meta-analysis. Crit Care Med. 2022;50:123–30. https://doi.org/10.1097/CCM.0000000000005123.
15. Johnson L, Martinez R. Factors influencing the timing of tracheostomy in ICU patients. J Intensive Care Med. 2021;36:789–95. https://doi.org/10.1177/08850666211023456.
16. Nguyen T, Patel S. Early vs. late tracheostomy in critically ill patients: outcomes and considerations. Ann Intensive Care. 2022;12:456–62. https://doi.org/10.1186/s13613-022-00945-6.
17. Smith J, Brown L, Johnson M, et al. Patient comfort and tolerance with tracheostomy vs. orotracheal intubation in mechanical ventilation. J Crit Care Med. 2022;37(5):123–30. https://doi.org/10.1016/j.jccm.2022.05.001.
18. Lee H, Kim S, Park J, et al. Airway resistance in tracheostomized patients compared to Orotracheal intubation. Respir Care. 2021;66(4):456–62. https://doi.org/10.4187/respcare.2021.04.002.
19. Martinez A, Lopez R, Gonzalez M, et al. Oral hygiene in Tracheostomized patients: a comparative study. Am J Infect Control. 2022;50(3):145–50. https://doi.org/10.1016/j.ajic.2022.03.005.
20. Patel R, Singh A, Kumar N, et al. Airway security in tracheostomy vs orotracheal intubation. Ann Intensive Care. 2021;11(1):87. https://doi.org/10.1186/s13613-021-00847-3.
21. Johnson M, Davis K, Brown L, et al. Sedation requirements in tracheostomized patients compared to orotracheal intubation. Crit Care. 2022;26(1):98. https://doi.org/10.1186/s13054-022-03987-6.
22. Kim S, Lee H, Park J, et al. ICU stay duration in Tracheostomized vs orotracheal intubated. Patients Intensive Care Med. 2021;47(8):1234–40. https://doi.org/10.1007/s00134-021-06432-9.
23. Brown L, Martinez A, Johnson M, et al. Speech and swallowing outcomes in tracheostomized patients. Dysphagia. 2022;37(2):234–40. https://doi.org/10.1007/s00455-022-10456-7.

24. Davis K, Wilson G, Johnson M, et al. Airway aspiration in tracheostomized patients: a comparative analysis. Respir Med. 2021;176:106543. https://doi.org/10.1016/j.rmed.2021.106543.
25. Wilson G, Brown L, Davis K, et al. Weaning from mechanical ventilation: tracheostomy vs orotracheal intubation. J Intensive Care. 2022;10(1):67. https://doi.org/10.1186/s40560-022-00567-8.
26. Nguyen T, Brown L, Johnson M, et al. Application of Poiseuille's law in tracheostomy vs orotracheal intubation. J Appl Physiol. 2022;132(3):123–30. https://doi.org/10.1152/japplphysiol.2022.00123.
27. Chen Y, Lee H, Park J, et al. Bernoulli's principle and Venturi effect in airway management: tracheostomy vs orotracheal intubation. Respir Physiol Neurobiol. 2021;287:103857. https://doi.org/10.1016/j.resp.2021.103857.
28. Patel R, Singh A, Kumar N, et al. Laplace's law and airway stability in tracheostomy vs orotracheal intubation. Crit Care Med. 2022;50(4):527–34. https://doi.org/10.1097/CCM.0000000000005278.
29. Wilson G, Davis K, Johnson M, et al. Fluid dynamics and turbulence in airway management: benefits of tracheostomy. J Fluid Mech. 2021;912:456–67. https://doi.org/10.1017/jfm.2021.456.
30. Martinez A, Lopez R, Gonzalez M, et al. Pressure-volume relationship in tracheostomized patients: implications for weaning. Am J Respir Crit Care Med. 2022;205(2):100–10. https://doi.org/10.1164/rccm.202201-0100OC.
31. Adly A, Youssef TA, El-Begermy MM, et al. Timing of tracheostomy in patients with prolonged endotracheal intubation: a systematic review. Eur Arch Otorrinolaringol. 2018;275:679–90. https://doi.org/10.1007/s00405-017-4838-7.
32. Chorath K, Hoang A, Rajasekaran K, Moreira A, et al. Association of early vs late tracheostomy placement with pneumonia and ventilator days in critically ill patients: a meta-analysis. JAMA Otolaryngol Head Neck Surg. 2021;147(5):450–9. https://doi.org/10.1001/jamaoto.2021.0025.
33. Andriolo BN, Andriolo RB, Saconato H, et al. Early versus late tracheostomy for critically ill patients. Cochrane Database Syst Rev. 2015 Jan;12;1(1):CD007271 https://doi.org/10.1002/14651858.
34. Young D, Harrison DA, Cuthbertson BH, et al. Effect of early vs late tracheostomy placement on survival in patients receiving mechanical ventilation: the TracMan randomized trial. JAMA. 2013;309(20):2121–9. https://doi.org/10.1001/jama.2013.5154.
35. Bosel J, Niesen WD, Salih F, et al. Effect of early vs standard approach to tracheostomy on functional outcome at 6 months among patients with severe stroke receiving mechanical ventilation: the SETPOINT2 randomized clinical trial. JAMA. 2022;327(19):1899–909. https://doi.org/10.1001/jama.2022.4798.

Chapter 20
Automated Weaning

Aurio Fajardo-Campoverdi and Carmen Chica-Meza

20.1 Introduction

Weaning is a key process in the evolution of the critically ill patient, where the transition from ventilator dependence to recovery of spontaneous ventilation must be carefully managed to minimize the risk of serious complications such as reintubation, prolonged ventilation, and increased mortality rate. Traditionally, weaning has been a process based on clinical judgment, often resulting in considerable variability in outcomes [1].

In recent years, the development of automated systems and the use of artificial intelligence (AI) have transformed the approach to mechanical ventilator weaning, providing tools that allow for a more standardized and even more accurate process. These innovations have promised not only to improve the efficiency of the weaning process, but also to customize it to suit the specific needs of individual patients and even their eventual baseline chronic pathologies. This chapter explores in depth the impact of AI and automated systems on weaning from mechanical ventilation, reviewing the available automated modes and discussing the future perspectives of these technologies applied in intensive ventilatory medicine.

A. Fajardo-Campoverdi (✉)
Universidad de la Frontera, Critical Care Unit, Hospital Biprovincial Quillota-Petorca, Quillota, Chile

International Mechanical Ventilation Group (WeVent), Quillota, Chile

C. Chica-Meza
International Mechanical Ventilation Group (WeVent), Quillota, Chile

URosario, AMCI, Cartagena, Colombia

A. R. Baptistella et al. (eds.), *Weaning from Mechanical Ventilation*,
https://doi.org/10.1007/978-3-032-01145-9_20

20.2 AI and Weaning

20.2.1 Application of AI in Mechanical Ventilation Weaning

AI has emerged as an essential tool in the intensive care environment, enabling the generation of continuous and real-time analysis of patient physiological data, which is crucial for the precise adjustment of ventilator parameters during the weaning process [2]. Modern ventilation systems, such as the IntelliVent-ASV® ventilation mode, use advanced algorithms to automate these settings, optimizing and adjusting specific parameters such as pressure support, inspiratory oxygen fraction (FiO_2), and positive end-expiratory pressure (PEEP) in response to changes in objective physiological variables such as oxygen saturation and partial pressure of CO_2 ($EtCO_2$) [3].

These AI systems not only improve the accuracy of clinical decisions but also significantly reduce the workload of clinical staff. Rather than relying solely on the judgment of medical staff, which can vary widely even within a single critical care unit, AI provides a standardized approach based on averaged epidemiological data and uses it to advance and refine weaning, which could ultimately reduce variability in outcomes and consequently improve patient safety [4].

20.2.2 Advantages and Challenges of AI in Weaning

The primary benefit of integrating AI into weaning is the ability to reduce clinical variability. This is achieved by automating decisions based on real-time physiological data, allowing for accurate and consistent adjustments that can improve patient safety and the efficiency of the ventilator weaning process [5]. In addition, automated systems can adapt and respond to changes in patient status in fractions of a second, even on a cycle-by-cycle basis, which is critical in a critical care setting where patient conditions can deteriorate unexpectedly [6].

However, the implementation of AI in weaning is not without its challenges. One of the main issues is the lack of transparency in the design of AI algorithms, which could lead to a degree of mistrust among healthcare professionals. In addition, there is a risk that over-reliance on technology could undermine essential clinical skills, particularly in situations where automated systems are unavailable or fail [7]. Further clinical trials are therefore needed to validate the efficacy and safety of these systems in a variety of clinical settings at different levels [8].

20.2.3 *Clinical Evidence and Outcomes*

The clinical evidence for the efficacy of AI in the release process is promising. A study by Morato et al. [9] compared three automated release modes: ASV, MRV, and SmartCare, and found that all were able to correctly identify both successes and failures in the process. However, they also observed cross-sectional differences in the stability of pressure support and response to irregular breathing patterns, highlighting the importance of selecting the right mode for each patient while maintaining close clinical supervision of the staff in charge.

An interesting case series by Shimizu et al. [3] documented the successful use of the IntelliVent-ASV® mode in patients with spinal cord injury, raising an interesting hypothesis about how AI could facilitate weaning in complex situations. This approach not only improved patient safety but also minimized the risk of adverse events during the transition to spontaneous ventilation.

In a subsequent study, Neuschwander and Bouneb [7] found that the use of AI significantly reduced the time required for ventilator support and ICU length of stay in postoperative patients compared to nonautomated weaning methods. These findings suggest that integrating AI into weaning not only improves clinical outcomes but also optimizes operational efficiency in the ICU.

20.3 Automated Modes for Weaning

20.3.1 *Description of Automated Modes*

The development of automated modes for weaning from mechanical ventilation represents a significant advance in respiratory critical care. These modes are designed to automatically adjust ventilatory parameters based on continuous monitoring of physiological data collected and interpreted on a cycle-by-cycle basis, such as oxygen saturation and end-expiratory CO_2 partial pressure ($EtCO_2$) [6].

IntelliVent-ASV® is one of the most advanced systems available, using a closed-loop control system to maintain key parameters within predefined ranges set by the operator. The system automatically adjusts not only ventilatory support but also other relevant ventilatory parameters such as positive end-expiratory pressure (PEEP) and inspiratory oxygen fraction (FiO_2), allowing for precise real-time customization of ventilatory management [6].

Another notable example is the SmartCare/PS mode, developed by Dräger. This mode, which is based on pressure support ventilation, is designed for patients with preserved respiratory drive and focuses specifically on the release phase. The SmartCare/PS algorithm continuously assesses the patient's respiratory capacity and adjusts the pressure support to facilitate a gradual and safe release [10] (Fig. 20.1).

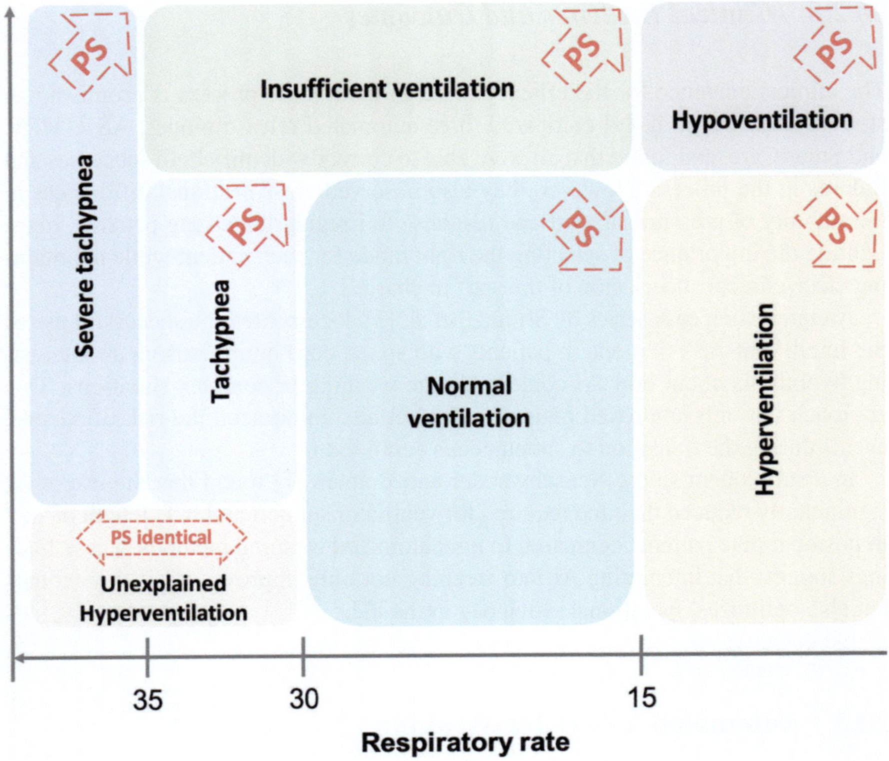

Fig. 20.1 Simplified algorithm of the SmartCare® system. Once ventilatory stability is achieved, with a pressure support level set according to the predetermined threshold settings, and if the patient has a PEEP below 5 cmH_20, a spontaneous ventilation test will be initiated. After 1–2 h and depending on the initially set level of support, if the patient remains stable, the system will suggest to proceed with the release of the mechanical ventilator. (Modified from https://aneskey.com/automated-weaning-modes/)

20.3.2 Clinical Evidence and Comparison of Automated Modes

The efficacy of automated modes in weaning has been validated by a significant number of clinical studies. A recent meta-analysis concluded that automated closed-loop weaning systems, such as IntelliVent-ASV®, not only reduce weaning time to mechanical ventilation but also reduce the incidence of tracheostomies and ICU length of stay [11]. However, this analysis also noted that no significant differences in hospital mortality and reintubation rates were observed compared to traditional weaning methods.

In specific studies, such as Rose et al. [10] IntelliVent-ASV® was shown to be safe and effective for long-term management of ventilation in patients with acute respiratory failure. This study highlights the potential for automated modes to become a standard tool in the ICU, especially in settings where staff are overburdened. However, the need for larger studies evaluating the application of these modes in different patient subgroups remains evident, as outcomes may vary significantly depending on the underlying pathology and respiratory dynamics of each patient [6].

On the other hand, a systematic review with meta-analysis published by Cochrane [5] compared the effectiveness of SmartCare® with nonautomated modes. The results were not favorable for this automated mode in terms of reduction of mechanical ventilation weaning time, all-cause mortality, ICU length of stay, and reintubation rate. In the subgroup analysis where they analyzed the prolongation of mechanical ventilation requirement (14 days and 21 days) between the use of SmartCare® and the control group, they also found no significant differences (RR, 0.76; 95% CI: 0.39–1.52 and RR, 0.88; 95% CI: 0.33–2.35, respectively).

Based on the studies included in the Cochrane systematic review [5], we performed a comparative subgroup analysis of nonautomated weaning modes versus the SmartCare ventilator mode with respect to mortality associated with prolonged mechanical ventilation. Using frequentist statistics, we performed a Cox regression model to estimate hazard by ventilator mode used for weaning. We found that the SmartCare mode was not associated with lower mortality compared to nonautomated modes (HR = 2.95; 95% CI: 0.75–11.68; p = 0.69 Long Rank Test) (Fig. 20.2).

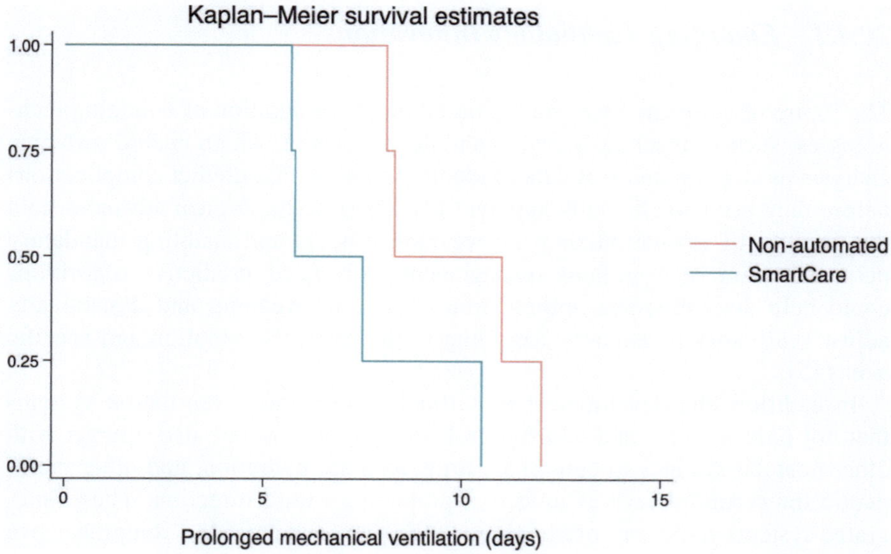

Fig. 20.2 Kaplan-Meier curves for mortality associated with prolongation of mechanical ventilation, according to the type of weaning mode (nonautomated and SmartCare)

20.3.3 Critical Considerations and Future Directions

As automated ventilation technology continues to evolve, it is critical that its implementation be undertaken in an informed and cautious manner. While these systems can provide valuable support in the management of ventilated patients, they should be viewed as adjuncts to clinical judgment rather than substitutes. Current evidence suggests that while automated modes may improve certain aspects of weaning, such as reducing the duration of mechanical ventilation and staff workload, their overall efficacy and safety are still highly dependent on the quality of human oversight and adaptation to individual patient needs [6, 11].

Future research should focus on validating these systems in larger studies that include a more heterogeneous diversity of populations, patients, and clinical scenarios. In addition, the integration of new advances in AI, such as machine learning, could improve the accuracy of these modes and allow for even greater personalization of ventilation therapy. However, there is also a need to address potential risks associated with excessive automation, such as loss of clinical skills among medical staff and overreliance on technology [6].

20.4 The Future of Weaning

20.4.1 Emerging Technology Innovations

The future of automated weaning is based on the integration of emerging technologies, such as machine learning and deep learning, which enable real-time analysis of large amounts of data to identify patterns that predict complications before they become clinically apparent [2]. These technological advances hold the promise of revolutionizing the weaning process and enabling mandatory personalization of ventilator management. Advanced predictive algorithms could help determine the optimal time to initiate weaning and dynamically adjust ventilatory parameters according to the patient's evolution and specific needs [5].

In addition, the development of virtually autonomous ventilation systems that not only monitor and adjust ventilatory parameters but also interact with other hospital systems to coordinate drug delivery, hydration, and other therapeutic interventions in real time is a promising future direction. These integrated systems could improve treatment efficiency and provide a comprehensive view of patient status, allowing for more informed and efficient decision making [6].

20.4.2 *Ethical Challenges and Considerations*

As technology advances, significant ethical and operational challenges arise. Excessive automation of ventilator weaning could lead to over-reliance on technology, which could undermine the most basic and essential clinical skills of medical staff [7]. Furthermore, the implementation of these systems will require rigorous clinical validation to ensure that they function appropriately in a variety of clinical settings and critically ill patient populations. The integration of AI into the mechanical ventilator weaning process also raises questions about accountability and decision-making, particularly in situations where algorithms may not be fully transparent or where actions and even outcomes may be unexpected [5].

Another important challenge is to ensure that all patients have access to these advanced technologies. Implementing automated systems can be costly, and not all ICUs have the same administrative capacity to integrate them, which could increase disparities in the quality of care between different institutions [8]. Furthermore, it is essential that automated systems respect patient autonomy and align with their values and wishes, which requires a careful balance between automation and human oversight.

20.4.3 *Future Prospects*

Despite these challenges, the future outlook for automated weaning is optimistic. The combination of AI with emerging technologies such as quantum computing and bioinformatics is expected to radically transform critical care in the not-too-distant future. The development of fully integrated ventilation systems that can adapt their operation not only to the physiological needs of the patient but also to their individual preferences and changing clinical conditions represents the next great leap in the care of critically ill patients from a ventilatory and mechanical weaning perspective [6].

In this context, the role of the intensivist is likely to evolve from a direct operator of mechanical ventilation to a supervisor of complex automated systems, where clinical judgment and experience will remain essential to interpret the data provided by these systems and make critical decisions in times of uncertainty.

20.5 Conclusions

Automated delivery of mechanical ventilation represents a significant advance in critical care medicine, with the potential to improve accuracy, efficiency, and clinical outcomes. Current algorithms, such as IntelliVent-ASV®, SmartCare/PS, and other automated modes, have been shown to be effective in reducing the time to need for mechanical ventilation and length of stay in the ICU, as well as reducing complications associated with prolonged ventilation [5, 6].

However, implementation of these systems is not without challenges. The need for robust clinical validation, consideration of ethical and operational implications, and the balance between automation and clinical judgment are critical issues that must be addressed as these technologies continue to evolve. The future of automated weaning is promising, but its success will depend on the ability to integrate these innovations in a way that complements, rather than replaces, clinical judgment and patient-centered care [2].

References

1. Boles JM, Bion J, Connors A, Herridge M, Marsh B, Melot C, et al. Weaning from mechanical ventilation. Eur Respir J. 2007;29(5):1033–56.
2. Grieco DL, Menga LS, Eleuteri D, Antonelli M, Conti G. Physiological comparison of three spontaneous breathing trials in difficult-to-wean patients. Intensive Care Med Exp. 2018;6(1):1–11.
3. Shimizu T, Yamaguchi S, Yamasaki Y. Successful automated weaning with IntelliVent-ASV in a spinal cord injury patient. Asian J Anesthesiol. 2018;56(2):92–6.
4. Rubulotta F, Soliman I, Franco F. Mechanical ventilation: past, present, and future. Intensive Care Med. 2020;46(6):1173–80.
5. Burns KE, Lellouche F, Lessard MR, Brochard LJ. Weaning from mechanical ventilation. Intensive Care Med. 2008;34(11):1757–65.
6. Ball L, Pelosi P. Automated mechanical ventilation modes in the intensive care unit: an obstacle course in building evidence. Minerva Anestesiol. 2016;82(6):621–4.
7. Neuschwander A, Bouneb R. Closed-loop systems for mechanical ventilation and weaning: a practical approach. J Clin Med. 2020;9(8):2685.
8. Bialais E, Rozé H, Ouattara A. Automated weaning from mechanical ventilation: reality or fantasy? Anesth Analg. 2016;123(4):986–93.
9. Morato M, Reis A, Silva C. Comparing ASV, MRV, and SmartCare modes for automated weaning: a simulation study. Respir Care. 2012;57(5):728–35.
10. Rose L, Schultz MJ, Cardwell CR, et al. Automated versus non-automated weaning for reducing the duration of mechanical ventilation for critically ill adults and children: a cochrane systematic review and meta-analysis. Crit Care 19. 2015;48. https://doi.org/10.1186/s13054-015-0755-6.
11. Max S. Meta-analysis on the efficacy of automated weaning modes. J Intensive Care Med. 2018;33(9):484–92.

Chapter 21
Nutrition and Weaning

Guilherme Duprat Ceniccola, Oellen Stuani Franzosi, Carina Rossoni, and Sandra R. Justino

Objectives of the Chapter
- Critical illness as a promoter of malnutrition and sarcopenia in the ICU.
- Strategies for identifying malnourished patients and maintaining their nutritional status during mechanical ventilation.
- The role of nutrition therapy in the rehabilitation of critically ill patients and weaning from MV.

21.1 Introduction

In critical illness, the patient is in a clinical state of fragility and is admitted to the ICU due to dysfunction of some organ or system and the threat of losing their life, thus requiring early and intensive clinical care [1–3]. This care is aimed at minimizing muscle wasting, myocardial fiber atrophy, and weakness, as the occurrence of these changes is associated with prolonged hospitalization and mechanical ventilation, the development of malnutrition, and increased hospital mortality [1, 2].

G. D. Ceniccola
Secretaria de Estado de Saúde do Distrito Federal, Brasília, Brazil

O. S. Franzosi
Nutrition and Dietetic Division, Hospital de Clínicas de Porto Alegre, Universidade Federal do Rio Grande do Sul, Porto Alegre, Brazil

C. Rossoni (✉)
Institute of Environmental Health (ISMAB) - Faculty of Medicine, University of Lisbon, Lisbon, Portugal

S. R. Justino
Federal University of Paraná (UFPR), Curitiba, Brazil

A. R. Baptistella et al. (eds.), *Weaning from Mechanical Ventilation*,
https://doi.org/10.1007/978-3-032-01145-9_21

Nutritional status has a notorious and direct impact on ICU outcomes [4], as the prevalence of malnutrition is significant and nutritional status tends to deteriorate throughout the hospital stay [5]. The literature shows that 45.5% of patients assessed in the first 48 h of admission to this unit are malnourished, of which 30% require mechanical ventilation, and in those assessed after 48 h, this prevalence increases to 70.3% [6]. Taking into account the different institutional protocols, in addition to the wide range of screening and nutritional assessment tools, this prevalence can reach 78% [6–11].

The compromised nutritional status of critically ill patients and the state of increased catabolic stress are associated with a systemic inflammatory response that is associated with complications due to infection, multiple organ dysfunction, prolonged hospitalization, and high mortality [12, 13]. In addition to high hospital costs, these patients have an increased burden of care, slower recovery, and lower quality of life [5, 8, 11, 14–19].

It should also be noted that patients identified as being at high nutritional risk on admission to the ICU are those at greater risk of complications [20, 21]. Furthermore, in critically ill elderly patients, frailty is considered one of the predictors of weaning failure, survival, and comorbidities in the short and medium term [22–25], compromising and prolonging functional outcomes [21, 26].

The result of these changes in body composition, such as unintentional weight loss, reduced muscle mass, and impaired muscle function, affects the overall condition of the critically ill patient, characterizing sarcopenia in critically ill patients [18, 27].

However, in the ICU, we are faced with a paradox of malnutrition, frailty, and sarcopenia on the one hand and obesity on the other. Currently, with the new concepts of malnutrition and sarcopenia, patients with obesity may also be malnourished or already sarcopenic, known as sarcopenic obesity. Approximately 28%–36% of admissions to intensive care units worldwide are patients living with obesity, which is considered a chronic disease characterized by qualitative malnutrition due to micronutrient deficiencies and may also have a low amount of lean mass [18, 24, 28–33]. This disease significantly affects multiple organs and systems, predisposing to a state of chronic low-grade inflammation, procoagulant tendencies, and insulin resistance. This shows a strong correlation with the development of cardiometabolic diseases, a high incidence of morbidity and mortality, and a significant reduction in quality of life [24, 34].

These are the challenges posed by the heterogeneity characteristic of critically ill patients, which requires us to be assertive in nutritional intervention in order to develop short- and medium-term results. This nutritional care must be early, systematic, and individualized, as it is known to directly contribute to the reduction of MV time, shorter hospital stays ([21, 24, 35, 36];), lower complication rates [37, 38], mortality, and improved quality of life [21, 24, 35, 36].

Given the recognition of the fundamental contribution of adequate nutrition to the prognosis of critically ill patients, this chapter, “Nutrition and Weaning”, represents this very important work.

21.2 Malnutrition and Sarcopenia in Critically Ill Patients

In critical illness, the inflammatory process associated with the catabolic stress in which the critically ill patient finds himself is characterized by various physiological changes in an attempt to adapt the body to the lack of nutrients, thus promoting a compromised nutritional status. However, it should be noted that a pre-existing compromised nutritional status, such as malnutrition, fatigue, dynapenia, sarcopenia, obesity, and/or sarcopenic obesity, on admission to the ICU contributes to unfavorable outcomes that affect the patient's prognosis: duration of mechanical ventilation, prolonged hospital stay, and increased mortality [39].

Malnutrition is characterized by a pathological condition resulting from a relative or absolute deficiency or excess of one or more essential nutrients, which may be clinically manifested or detected by biochemical, anthropometric, topographical, or physiological tests [40]. Higher rates of malnutrition are often observed in specialized areas such as geriatrics, oncology, and intensive care, where patients are more susceptible to nutritional deficiencies, involuntary weight loss, and reduced muscle mass [18, 41–43]. These, combined with impaired physical function, cognitive aspects, and social isolation, contribute to the development of fatigue and directly to the presence of frailty. This is characterized by a lack of energy or exhaustion proportional to physical exertion that limits daily activities and is not relieved by rest [44], a characteristic of age-related sarcopenia [45]. However, the sarcopenia that affects the critically ill is much broader, encompassing both malnutrition and cachexia, i.e., it is characterized as a syndrome by the generalized and progressive loss of muscle mass and strength, with a risk of adverse outcomes, affecting them physically as well as their quality of life and increasing the risk of death [46]. In critically ill patients, sarcopenia has an interface with ICU-acquired weakness and frailty, and critical illness-related malnutrition encompasses all of these concepts [47]. The clinical condition is also present in sarcopenic obesity, reduced muscle functionality, altered body composition, but high presence of fat mass [18, 48].

When analyzing body mass index (BMI) categories and mortality risk in hospitalized patients, weight loss was found to increase mortality risk in all categories. However, in patients with a BMI $\geq$ 30 kg/m2, this result was only obtained when there was a loss of more than 12.6% [18], suggesting that this percentage of weight loss in hospitalized patients living with obesity may indicate a risk of malnutrition [18, 49].

During weight loss, it is important to distinguish whether this reduction is at the expense of fat or muscle mass, because if it is muscle mass, the risk of sarcopenia is greatly increased [50], as well as its deleterious consequences. This difficulty in assessing changes in body composition becomes even more apparent when identifying malnutrition in critically ill patients with obesity [51].

Noninvasive methods of assessing body composition in the ICU are increasingly being used, including ultrasound, tomography, and bioimpedance. These have the potential to be widely used in clinical practice in the critically ill, depending on the realities of each institution and cost benefits, as each method has advantages and disadvantages that need to be considered in each context [8, 52].

Assessing and monitoring changes in lean mass will allow for more precise nutritional intervention, as the determination of daily protein intake today is based on total body weight, so we may induce an overdose in the context of sarcopenic obesity and an underdose in non-sarcopenic obesity [53, 54]. Chapple and Cols [55] showed that critically ill patients have 60% less muscle protein synthesis than healthy individuals, despite normal protein absorption from the gut. In other populations, the use of specific anabolic nutrients, such as hydroxymethylbutyrate (HMB), creatine, and leucine, has shown promise and appears to improve muscle strength/mass, but it merits future study because in addition to our population being characterized by heterogeneity, the dose used in the studies also has the same profile [54]. Identifying the risk and/or presence of malnutrition and sarcopenia will also be crucial in the decision-making process for nutritional intervention, as critically ill patients with severe malnutrition are at potential risk of refeeding syndrome [56–58].

21.3 Systemizing Nutrition Care in the ICU

The systematization of nutritional care (SAN) for critically ill patients and weaning from mechanical ventilation are highly relevant topics in clinical practice, especially in the ICU, where integration and interdisciplinary management are fundamental for recovery and minimization of complications. In ICU patients, the interaction between nutritional therapy and respiratory mechanisms is fundamental, considering that nutritional deficits can negatively affect muscle strength, including the diaphragm, and prolong dependence on ventilatory support.

SAN is a process that defines nutrition interventions across a continuum of care. The model is based on stages that include screening, assessment, intervention, and monitoring [59, 60].

21.3.1 Nutritional Screening

Nutritional screening is the first step in identifying patients at nutritional risk, i.e., those who would benefit from individualized nutritional therapy. Tools such as the NRS-2002 (Nutrition Risk Screening) and the NUTRIC score are widely used for this purpose. Admission screening allows identification of patients who will benefit most from early nutritional interventions, such as gradual and controlled initiation of NT to avoid refeeding syndrome and other harms associated with hyperalimentation, while promoting continuous nutrient delivery [61].

21.3.2 Nutritional Assessment

After screening, a detailed nutritional assessment is performed, including dietary history, anthropometry, biochemistry, and physical examination. This allows a nutritional diagnosis to be made and an individualized nutritional intervention plan to be developed. The assessment is critical for adjusting NT according to the patient's clinical evolution. Among the options for nutritional assessment protocols is the GLIM malnutrition detection initiative [61].

21.3.3 Intervention and Monitoring

Patients at high nutritional risk should receive early NT. The initial approach usually involves a hypocaloric and hyperproteic diet on day 4 of nutritional therapy, with targets adjusted according to the patient's tolerance and evolution. Daily monitoring of parameters such as caloric intake, protein, electrolytes, and signs of gastrointestinal intolerance is essential. Studies show that achieving 100% of the protein target is associated with greater preservation of lean mass and a reduction in complications such as infections and healing difficulties [62, 63].

21.4 Refeeding Syndrome in the ICU

Refeeding syndrome (RS) is a potentially serious condition that is often unrecognized or neglected [64, 65]. The fact that it presents with nonspecific symptoms contributes to its under-recognition [65]. On the other hand, there is heterogeneity between published definitions; this lack of a universally accepted definition makes it difficult to obtain estimates of its incidence ([66]), which varies from 0% to 80% depending on the definition and the population studied, being described in 34% of ICU patients [65]. The most severe cases of RS can be fatal or even cause ICU admission [64].

Definitions of RS range from hypophosphatemia alone to the presence of other electrolytes reduced to severe levels along with fluid balance abnormalities and/or organ dysfunction [65]. Hypophosphatemia is most often considered the defining feature of RS because phosphate is a vital component of ATP, the primary form of energy storage in the human body [64]. Its depletion can lead to respiratory muscle dysfunction, cardiac arrhythmias, and tissue hypoxia, among other consequences [64]. Hypophosphatemia has been associated with acute respiratory failure and failure to wean from mechanical ventilation [62]. However, the extent of the decrease in serum levels of one or more electrolytes (hypophosphatemia and/or hypokalemia and/or hypomagnesemia) qualifies the presence of RS [66, 67]. RS is a set of metabolic and electrolytic changes related to the NT supply when it is initiated or resumed after periods of fasting, low caloric intake, or when the caloric supply is rapidly increased by means of nutrition (oral, enteral, parenteral) or intravenous (IV) glucose solutions and drugs with lipid composition (propofol), especially in previously malnourished individuals and/or those in a catabolic state, such as critically ill patients [65, 66, 68–71].

21.4.1 Diagnosis of RS

Although RS has been identified as an ongoing problem in critically ill patients, there is no "gold standard" nutritional assessment tool for this patient population [70]. The National Institute for Health and Clinical Excellence (NICE) criteria (www.nice.org.uk/guidance/cg32) are considered an important clinical assessment tool for identifying risk factors for RS because of their practical application for bedside use [72]. Recently, the American Society for Parenteral and Enteral Nutrition and Society of Critical Care Medicine)/ASPEN (2020), based on the analysis of different tools, published a consensus on RS, in which there are some additional criteria and with some differences from the NICE criteria, but the focus is on variations in BMI, time and degree of weight loss, the presence of fasting or reduced food intake, and changes in phosphorus, potassium, and magnesium [66].

ASPEN [66] established that the diagnostic criteria for RS should be stratified in terms of serum levels of reduction in one or more of the electrolytes (phosphorus, potassium and magnesium) from baseline to classify the severity of the risk of RS as: mild: 10%–20%, moderate: 20%–30% or >30% and/or organ dysfunction resulting from the reduction in one of these electrolytes and/or severe vitamin B1 (thiamine) deficiency occurring within 5 days of caloric repletion.

A recent prospective cohort study [73] of 327 critically ill Covid-19 patients who were assessed for risk of developing RS according to the ASPEN consensus [66, 74] found that 268 (82%) were at risk of RS, with 36% developing the syndrome. After accounting for the ASPEN suggested decrease in baseline electrolyte levels [66], the study found no association with death, but serum phosphorus levels before feeding were strongly predictive of severe RS [75].

Symptoms of RS generally appear within 2–5 days of refeeding and can range from absent/mild to a severe, life-threatening clinical syndrome, depending on the degree of pre-existing malnutrition and comorbidity [65]. As a result, all organs of the body may be affected, resulting in cardiac, respiratory, hematologic, gastrointestinal, neurologic, and musculoskeletal manifestations, including death [65, 66].

21.4.2 Prevention, Treatment, and Recommendations for SR

There are numerous and diverse recommendations for the prevention and treatment of RS [66]. However, as they are not specific to critically ill patients, they need to be adapted to the clinical conditions of the individual patient. Table 21.1 shows the consensus-based ASPEN recommendations [66], and Table 21.2 shows the ESPEN recommendations and comments for critically ill patients [76, 77].

Considering that the population of critically ill patients is susceptible to RS, a multidisciplinary approach, established in a protocol that includes nutritional assessment, monitoring of key minerals, and supported by risk classification tools for the syndrome, is essential for early and individualized identification and treatment from admission throughout the ICU stay.

Table 21.1 ASPEN Consensus Recommendations (2020) for the prevention and management of RS in adults at risk

Electrolytes and vitamins	Before starting NT, check serum levels: Phosphate (PO4), potassium (K), magnesium (Mg) Vitamin B1 (administration of 100 mg intravenously or orally); if there are signs of deficiencies (e.g., alcohol abuse or prolonged abstinence), replacement will be for 5–7 days or longer according to the degree of deficiency	Monitor electrolytes every 12 h for the first 3 days in high-risk patients May be more frequently depending on clinical condition Reset low electrolytes according to treatment standards No prophylactic recommendations can be made if preload is normal	Patients at moderate to high risk of RS with low electrolyte levels: consider discontinuing initiation or increasing calories until electrolytes are replenished and/or normalized Seriously low and/or life-threatening levels or rapidly declining: Suspend NT
Caloric intake	*Start:* Patient at risk: 10–20 kcal/kg/day or 100–150 g dextrose High-risk patient: 5 kcal/kg/day *Progress*: Progress 33% of goal every 1–2 days	Calories from IV dextrose solutions and dextrose-infused drugs should be considered within established limits and/or initiated with caution in patients at moderate to severe risk for RS Include enteral or parenteral glucose	
Monitoring and long-term care	Vital signs every 4 h for the first 24 h after starting calories in at-risk patients Cardiorespiratory monitoring is recommended for unstable or severely compromised patients based on established standards of care Monitor daily weights with intake and output Evaluate nutrition therapy goals daily until the patient is stabilized (e.g., no need for electrolyte supplementation for 2 days, based on institutional standards of care)		

Adapted from da Silva et al. [66]

Table 21.2 ESPEN (2023) recommendations and comments on the prevention and treatment of RS in critically ill patients

Recommendations		Comments and considerations
Onset and progression of NT	Cautious and progressive Slow progression within the first 72 h should be considered to facilitate control of electrolyte disturbances when RS is anticipated or detected	Especially in severely malnourished patients or those who have fasted prior to admission In the event of hypophosphatemia on refeeding, energy intake should be restricted for 48 h and then gradually increased Electrolyte alterations have been shown to be less likely with cautious feeding
Monitoring Phosphorus Potassium Magnesium	Include at admission, along with nutritional assessment Measure at least once daily for the first week In patients with feedback hypophosphatemia (<0.65 mmol/L or a drop of >0.16 mmol/L), electrolytes should be measured 2 to 3 times daily and replenished as needed	Important for prevention and detection of serious complications of RS Repeat measurements at the start of feeding are important to detect refeeding syndrome Remember that in critically ill patients, electrolyte disturbances after refeeding are not limited to those with obvious malnutrition The occurrence of refeeding hypophosphatemia can be considered a warning sign. Its rapid progression to a severe form, if unrecognized, can lead to death after the start of feeding. This is because malnutrition may be present before or during hospitalization

Adapted from Singer et al. [76, 77]

21.5 Strategies for Feeding the Critically Ill Patient at Different Stages of Critical Illness

It is believed that a nutritional therapy strategy that is implemented in a timely manner and ensures adequate nutritional intake according to the patient's stage of critical illness is the best strategy to prevent malnutrition and minimize lean mass loss in critically ill patients [37].

Estimating nutritional requirements is a fundamental step in planning nutritional therapy. The methods available for estimating energy requirements are: indirect calorimetry, predictive equations, and pocket formulas. Indirect calorimetry is the gold standard for estimating energy expenditure. If indirect calorimetry is not available, predictive equations and pocket equations can be used. Table 21.3 summarizes the methods for determining energy expenditure and caloric goals as recommended by nutrition therapy societies for critically ill patients [13, 76–80]. The provision of energy should be progressive, taking into account the stage of the patient's illness. It is believed that providing 100% of the estimated nutritional needs in the acute phase of the disease may lead to overfeeding, considering that endogenous energy synthesis is substantial in this phase of the disease.

Table 21.3 Nutritional therapy strategies for the critically ill patient

	Acute phase (day 1–4)	Post-acute phase (> day 5)	Post-ICU phase—rehabilitation	Critically ill patient with obesity
Determine energy expenditure (EE)	Indirect calorimetry (IC)	Indirect calorimetry (IC)	Indirect calorimetry (IC)	Indirect calorimetry (IC)
Calorie targets[a]	50%–70% EE estimated by IC Or 12–20 Kcal/kg/day	80%–100% EE estimated by IC Or 20 Kcal/kg/day and progress to 25 kcal/kg or more	125% EE estimated by IC Or 30–35 kcal/kg/day	Not exceed 60%–70% EE estimated by IC Or BMI:30–50 Kg/m^2 (11–14 kcal/kg of current weight) and BMI > 50 kg/m^2 (22–25 kcal/kg of ideal weight)
Protein targets[a]	0.8 g/kg (days 1–2) 0.8–1.2 g/kg (days 3–5)	>1.2–2.0 g/kg	1.5–2.0 g/kg Progress to 2.0–2.5 g/kg	1.2–2.0 g/kg (from day 5) of predicted weight calculated for BMI 25 kg/m^2

Compher et al. (ASPEN [4]) recommend reaching 12–25 Kcal/kg/day in the first 7–10 days (patients who met this recommendation were in the overweight or obese range)
[a]Energy and protein prescriptions should be progressive according to the patient's clinical evolution

Critically ill patients exhibit protein catabolism and anabolic resistance [55, 81], physiological responses that highlight the importance of protein intake in this population. Current evidence suggests that protein intake should be 1.2–2.0 g/kg of protein, with a staged progression associated with physical activity, to achieve better clinical and functional outcomes [82]. It is recommended to provide protein in a progressive amount of 0.8 g/kg on days 1–2, 0.8–1.2 g/kg on days 3–5, and > 1.2–2.0 g/kg from day 5 [83]. Table 21.3 summarizes protein supplementation recommendations for critically ill patients [13, 76–80].

Regarding the timing of initiation of nutrition therapy, evidence from randomized clinical trials suggests that enteral nutrition initiated in the first 48 h after adequate volume resuscitation with improved perfusion parameters correlates with favorable clinical outcomes in critically ill patients [37]. In severely burned patients, the indication for starting enteral nutrition is even earlier, within 12 h of injury [84].

It is recommended to delay the initiation of enteral nutrition if shock is not controlled and hemodynamic, tissue perfusion, and metabolic goals are not met, and to initiate low-dose enteral nutrition as soon as shock is controlled with fluids and vasopressors/inotropes [85]. It is essential to proactively assess hemodynamic and perfusion parameters at the bedside when implementing nutrition therapy in the ICU. Improved hemodynamic and skin perfusion parameters during hemodynamic resuscitation are associated with successful nutrition therapy in patients with septic shock [86].

21.6 Challenges of Nutritional Therapy in MV Patients

Mechanical ventilation is associated with decreased splanchnic blood flow and increased inflammatory mediators, which may limit tolerance to enteral nutrition. A study by Blaser et al. [87] found a significant prevalence of gastrointestinal symptoms, >35% prevalence, such as increased gastric residual volume (GRV), which can affect nutrient infusion [87].

Recommendations include starting NT with low volumes and gradual progression, monitoring tolerance, and adjusting goals according to clinical response. In addition, interruption of enteral nutrition during pronation or extubation maneuvers should follow specific protocols to minimize risk and be performed according to locally validated protocols [87, 88].

21.6.1 Weaning from MV

The transition from MV requires a multidisciplinary approach that integrates nutritional support to prevent energy and protein deficits that can impair muscle strength and respiratory recovery. Studies show that patients with energy and protein deficits after extubation often experience clinical deterioration and longer hospital stays [89, 90].

During weaning, NT should be adjusted to avoid overfeeding, which can increase CO_2 production, hindering the process of spontaneous ventilation. Frequent assessments, including nitrogen balance and arterial blood gas, help guide nutritional adequacy [89].

21.6.2 Synergy Between Nutrition and Rehabilitation

Nutritional rehabilitation of critically ill patients extends beyond discharge from the ICU. Early mobilization and protein supplementation are effective strategies to minimize lean mass loss and promote functional recovery. Integrated programs that include physical, occupational, and nutritional therapy should be considered as part of post-ICU rehabilitation [91].

21.7 Final Considerations

Nutrition management during mechanical ventilation is one of the cornerstones for improving clinical outcomes in critically ill patients, as it supports the rehabilitation of the patient through the various stages of treatment. The implementation of evidence-based protocols, continuous monitoring, and frequent reassessment is essential to ensure a personalized and effective approach. The integration of multidisciplinary teams is also critical to optimizing the recovery of these patients, underscoring the importance of coordinated, patient-centered care.

References

1. Griffiths RD, Bongers T. Nutrition support for patients in the intensive care unit. Postgrad Med J. 2005;81(960):629–36. https://doi.org/10.1136/pgmj.2005.033399. PMID: 16210458; PMCID: PMC1743378
2. Langhans C, Weber-Carstens S, Schmidt F, Hamati J, Kny M, Zhu X, et al. Inflammation-induced acute phase response in skeletal muscle and critical illness myopathy. PLoS One. 2014;9(3):e92048. https://doi.org/10.1371/journal.pone.0092048. PMID: 24651840; PMCID: PMC3961297
3. Paz LSC, Couto AV. Nutritional assessment in critically ill patients: literature review. BRASPEN J, vol.31, n 3, p.269–277, 2016. https://doi.org/10.37111/braspenj.2016.31.3.16.
4. Compher C, Bingham AL, McCall M, Patel J, Rice TW, Braunschweig C, et al. Guidelines for the provision of nutrition support therapy in the adult critically ill patient: the American Society for Parenteral and Enteral Nutrition. J Parenter Enteral Nutr. 2022, 46;(1):12–41. https://doi.org/10.1002/jpen.2267. Epub 2022 Jan 3. Erratum in: JPEN J Parenter Enteral Nutr 2022 Aug;46(6):1458–1459. 10.1002/jpen.2419
5. Correia MITD, Perman MI, Waitzberg DL. Hospital malnutrition in Latin America: a systematic review. Clin Nutr. 2017;36(4):958–67. https://doi.org/10.1016/j.clnu.2016.06.025. Epub 2016 Jul 19
6. Fontes D, Simone de Vasconcelos Generoso, Toulson Davisson Correia MI. Subjective global assessment: a reliable nutritional assessment tool to predict outcomes in critically ill patients. Clin Nutr 2014 Apr;33(2):291–295. doi: https://doi.org/10.1016/j.clnu.2013.05.004. Epub 2013 May 13.
7. Atalay BG, Yagmur C, Nursal TZ, Atalay H, Noyan T. Use of subjective global assessment and clinical outcomes in critically ill geriatric patients receiving nutrition support. JPEN J Parenter Enteral Nutr. 2008;32(4):454–9. https://doi.org/10.1177/0148607108314369.
8. Ceniccola GD, Holanda TP, Pequeno RSF, Mendonça VS, Oliveira ABM, Carvalho LSF, et al. Relevance of AND-ASPEN criteria of malnutrition to predict hospital mortality in critically ill patients: a prospective study. J Crit Care. 2018;44:398–403. https://doi.org/10.1016/j.jcrc.2017.12.013. Epub 2017 Dec 21
9. Facin BV. Caracterização do estado nutricional dos pacientes internados em unidade de terapia intensiva através da espessura do músculo adutor do polegar [monografia para conclusão de curso]. São Paulo: Instituto de Infectologia Emílio Ribas; 2013.
10. Lew CCH, Yandell R, Fraser RJL, Chua AP, Chong MFF, Miller M. Association between malnutrition and clinical outcomes in the intensive care unit: a systematic review [formula: see text]. JPEN J Parenter Enteral Nutr. 2017;41(5):744–58. https://doi.org/10.1177/0148607115625638. Epub 2016 Feb 2
11. Mogensen KM, Robinson MK, Casey JD, Gunasekera NS, Moromizato T, Rawn JD, et al. Nutritional status and mortality in the critically ill. Crit Care Med. 2015;43(12):2605–15. https://doi.org/10.1097/CCM.0000000000001306.
12. Brasil. Ministério da Saúde. Portaria n° 2.338, de 3 de Outubro de 2011. Política Nacional de Atenção às Urgências e institui a Rede de Atenção às Urgências no SUS, estabelecendo as diretrizes e criando mecanismos para a implantação do componente Sala de Estabilização (SE) da Rede de Atenção às Urgências [Internet]. Brasília, DF; 2011. [citado 2015 Jun 20]. Available at: http://bvsms.saude.gov.br/bvs/saudelegis/gm/2011/prt2338_03_10_2011.html.

13. McClave SA, Taylor BE, Martindale RG, Warren MM, Johnson DR, Braunschweig C, et al. Society of Critical Care Medicine; American Society for Parenteral and Enteral Nutrition. Guidelines for the Provision and Assessment of Nutrition Support Therapy in the Adult Critically Ill Patient: Society of Critical Care Medicine (SCCM) and American Society for Parenteral and Enteral Nutrition (A.S.P.E.N.). J Parenter Enteral Nutr. 2016;40(2):159–211. https://doi.org/10.1177/0148607115621863. Erratum in: JPEN J Parenter Enteral Nutr. 2016 Nov;40(8):1200. 10.1177/0148607116670155.
14. Barker LA, Gout BS, Crowe TC. Hospital malnutrition: prevalence, identification and impact on patients and the healthcare system. Int J Environ Res Public Health. 2011;8(2):514–27. https://doi.org/10.3390/ijerph8020514. Epub 2011 Feb 16. PMID: 21556200; PMCID: PMC3084475
15. Freijer K, Tan SS, Koopmanschap MA, Meijers JM, Halfens RJ, Nuijten MJ. The economic costs of disease related malnutrition. Clin Nutr. 2013;32(1):136–41. https://doi.org/10.1016/j.clnu.2012.06.009. Epub 2012 Jul 10
16. Guerra RS, Sousa AS, Fonseca I, Pichel F, Restivo MT, Ferreira S, et al. Comparative analysis of undernutrition screening and diagnostic tools as predictors of hospitalisation costs. J Hum Nutr Diet. 2016;29(2):165–73. https://doi.org/10.1111/jhn.12288. Epub 2014 Dec 23
17. Kruizenga H, van Keeken S, Weijs P, Bastiaanse L, Beijer S, Huisman-de Waal G, et al. Undernutrition screening survey in 564,063 patients: patients with a positive undernutrition screening score stay in hospital 1.4 d longer. Am J Clin Nutr. 2016;103(4):1026–32. https://doi.org/10.3945/ajcn.115.126615.
18. Mwala NN, Borkent JW, van der Meij BS, de van der Schueren MAE. Challenges in identifying malnutrition in obesity; an overview of the state of the art and directions for future research. Nutr Res Rev. 2024;5:1–10. https://doi.org/10.1017/S095442242400012X. Epub ahead of print. PMID: 38576127; PMCID: PMC7616526.
19. White JV, Stotts N, Jones SW, Granieri E. Managing postacute malnutrition (undernutrition) risk. JPEN J Parenter Enteral Nutr. 2013;37(6):816–23. https://doi.org/10.1177/0148607113492339. Epub 2013 Aug 22
20. Jeong DH, Hong SB, Lim CM, Koh Y, Seo J, Kim Y, et al. Relationship between nutrition intake and 28-day mortality using modified NUTRIC score in patients with sepsis. Nutrients. 2019;11(8):1906. https://doi.org/10.3390/nu11081906. PMID: 31443186; PMCID: PMC6723508
21. Pardo E, Lescot T, Preiser JC, Massanet P, Pons A, Jaber S, et al. FRANS study group. Association between early nutrition support and 28-day mortality in critically ill patients: the FRANS prospective nutrition cohort study. Crit Care. 2023;27(1):7. https://doi.org/10.1186/s13054-022-04298-1. PMID: 36611211; PMCID: PMC9826592
22. Er B, Mızrak B, Aydemir A, Binay S, Doğu C, Kazancı D, Turan S. Association of nutritional status, frailty, and rectus femoris muscle thickness measured by ultrasound and weaning in critically ill elderly patients. Tuberk Toraks. 2023;71(1):1–6. https://doi.org/10.5578/tt.20239901. PMID: 36912403; PMCID: PMC10795233
23. Mart MF, Ely EW, Tolle JJ, Patel MB, Brummel NE. Physiologic responses to exercise in survivors of critical illness: an exploratory pilot study. Intensive Care Med Exp. 2022;10(1):35. https://doi.org/10.1186/s40635-022-00461-8. PMID: 36008625; PMCID: PMC9410741
24. Martínez-Camacho MÁ, Jones-Baro RA, Gómez-González A, Morales-Hernández D, Lugo-García DS, Melo-Villalobos A, et al. Physical and respiratory therapy in the critically ill patient with obesity: a narrative review. Front Med (Lausanne). 2024;11:1321692. https://doi.org/10.3389/fmed.2024.1321692. PMID: 38455478; PMCID: PMC10918845
25. Singer P. Protein metabolism and requirements in the ICU. Clin Nutr ESPEN. 2020;38:3–8. https://doi.org/10.1016/j.clnesp.2020.03.026. Epub 2020 May 31. PMID: 32690175
26. Herridge MS, Tansey CM, Matté A, Tomlinson G, Diaz-Granados N, Cooper A, et al. Canadian critical care trials group. Functional disability 5 years after acute respiratory distress syndrome. N Engl J Med. 2011;364(14):1293–304. https://doi.org/10.1056/NEJMoa1011802.

27. Landi F, Camprubi-Robles M, Bear DE, Cederholm T, Malafarina V, Welch AA, et al. Muscle loss: the new malnutrition challenge in clinical practice. Clin Nutr. 2019;38(5):2113–20. https://doi.org/10.1016/j.clnu.2018.11.021. Epub 2018 Nov 30
28. Abhyankar S, Leishear K, Callaghan FM, Demner-Fushman D, McDonald CJ. Lower short- and long-term mortality associated with overweight and obesity in a large cohort study of adult intensive care unit patients. Crit Care. 2012;16(6):R235. https://doi.org/10.1186/cc11903. PMID: 23249446; PMCID: PMC3672624
29. Alexopoulos AS, Fayfman M, Zhao L, Weaver J, Buehler L, Smiley D, et al. Impact of obesity on hospital complications and mortality in hospitalized patients with hyperglycemia and diabetes. BMJ Open Diabetes Res Care. 2016;4(1):e000200. https://doi.org/10.1136/bmjdrc-2016-000200. PMID: 27486518; PMCID: PMC4947725
30. De Jong A, Verzilli D, Sebbane M, Monnin M, Belafia F, Cisse M, Conseil M, Carr J, Jung B, Chanques G, Molinari N, Jaber S. Medical versus surgical ICU obese patient outcome: a propensity-matched analysis to resolve clinical trial controversies. Crit Care Med. 2018;46(4):e294–301. https://doi.org/10.1097/CCM.0000000000002954.
31. Finkielman JD, Gajic O, Afessa B. Underweight is independently associated with mortality in post-operative and non-operative patients admitted to the intensive care unit: a retrospective study. BMC Emerg Med. 2004;4(1):3. https://doi.org/10.1186/1471-227X-4-3. PMID: 15462681; PMCID: PMC535928
32. Sakr Y, Alhussami I, Nanchal R, Wunderink RG, Pellis T, Wittebole X, et al. Intensive care over nations investigators. Being overweight is associated with greater survival in ICU patients: results from the intensive care over nations audit. Crit Care Med. 2015;43(12):2623–32. https://doi.org/10.1097/CCM.0000000000001310.
33. Van der Pols-Vijlbrief R, Wijnhoven HA, Schaap LA, Terwee CB, Visser M. Determinants of protein-energy malnutrition in community-dwelling older adults: a systematic review of observational studies. Ageing Res Rev. 2014;18:112–31. https://doi.org/10.1016/j.arr.2014.09.001. Epub 2014 Sep 22
34. Heymsfield SB, Wadden TA. Mechanisms, pathophysiology, and Management of Obesity. N Engl J Med. 2017;376(15):1492. https://doi.org/10.1056/NEJMc1701944.
35. Reintam Blaser A, Starkopf J, Alhazzani W, Berger MM, Casaer MP, Deane AM, ESICM Working Group on Gastrointestinal Function, et al. Early enteral nutrition in critically ill patients: ESICM clinical practice guidelines. Intensive Care Med. 2017;43(3):380–98. https://doi.org/10.1007/s00134-016-4665-0. Epub 2017 Feb 6. PMID: 28168570; PMCID: PMC5323492.
36. Singer P, Blaser A, Berger M, Alhazzani W, Calder P, Casaer M, et al. ESPEN guideline on clinical nutrition in the intensive care unit. Clin Nutr. 2019;38:48–79.
37. Heyland DK, Lee Z-Y, Lew CCH, Ortiz LA, Patel J, Stoppe C. Early vs. delayed enteral. Nutrition. 2021; Critical Care Nutrition.com [December 26, 2024]
38. Stumpf F, Keller B, Gressies C, Schuetz P. Inflammation and nutrition: friend or foe? Nutrients. 2023;15(5):1159. https://doi.org/10.3390/nu15051159. PMID: 36904164; PMCID: PMC10005147
39. Lawson CM, Daley BJ, Sams VG, Martindale R, Kudsk KA, Miller KR. Factors that impact patient outcome: nutrition assessment. JPEN J Parenter Enteral Nutr. 2013;37(5 Suppl):30S–8S. https://doi.org/10.1177/0148607113499372.
40. Sarni RO, Munekata RV. Terapia nutricional na desnutrição energético-proteíca grave. In: Lopez FA, Sigulem DM, Taddei JA, editores. Fundamentos da terapia nutricional em pediatria. São Paulo: Sarvier; 2002. p. 115–132.
41. Böhne SEJ, Hiesmayr M, Sulz I, Tarantino S, Wirth R, Volkert D. Recent and current low food intake – prevalence and associated factors in hospital patients from different medical specialities. Eur J Clin Nutr. 2022;76(10):1440–8. https://doi.org/10.1038/s41430-022-01129-y. Epub 2022 Apr 11. PMID: 35411028; PMCID: PMC9550619

42. De van der Schueren MAE, Borkent JW, Spaans GW, Nijhof A, Manders M. GLIM in nursing homes; practical implications. Clin Nutr. 2022;41(11):2442–5. https://doi.org/10.1016/j.clnu.2022.09.003. Epub 2022 Sep 10
43. Santarpia L, Contaldo F, Pasanisi F. Nutritional screening and early treatment of malnutrition in cancer patients. J Cachexia Sarcopenia Muscle. 2011;2(1):27–35. https://doi.org/10.1007/s13539-011-0022-x. Epub 2011 Feb 22. PMID: 21475618; PMCID: PMC3063880
44. Barsevick AM, Cleeland CS, Manning DC, O'Mara AM, Reeve BB, Scott JA, Sloan JA. ASCPRO (Assessing symptoms of cancer using patient-reported outcomes). ASCPRO recommendations for the assessment of fatigue as an outcome in clinical trials. J Pain Symptom Manag. 2010;39(6):1086–99. https://doi.org/10.1016/j.jpainsymman.2010.02.006. PMID: 20538190; PMCID: PMC2909842
45. Rosenberg IH. Sarcopenia: origins and clinical relevance. J Nutr. 1997;127(5 Suppl):990S–1S. https://doi.org/10.1093/jn/127.5.990S.
46. Cruz-Jentoft AJ, Baeyens JP, Bauer JM, Boirie Y, Cederholm T, Landi F, Martin FC, Michel JP, Rolland Y, Schneider SM, Topinková E, Vandewoude M, Zamboni M, European Working Group on Sarcopenia in Older People. Sarcopenia: European consensus on definition and diagnosis: report of the European working group on sarcopenia in older people. Age Ageing. 2010;39(4):412–23. https://doi.org/10.1093/ageing/afq034. Epub 2010 Apr 13. PMID: 20392703; PMCID: PMC2886201
47. Cesari M, Landi F, Vellas B, Bernabei R, Marzetti E. Sarcopenia and physical frailty: two sides of the same coin. Front Aging Neurosci. 2014;6:192. https://doi.org/10.3389/fnagi.2014.00192. PMID: 25120482; PMCID: PMC4112807
48. Donini LM, Busetto L, Bischoff SC, Cederholm T, Ballesteros-Pomar MD, Batsis JA, et al. Definition and diagnostic criteria for sarcopenic obesity: ESPEN and EASO consensus statement. Clin Nutr. 2022;41(4):990–1000. https://doi.org/10.1016/j.clnu.2021.11.014. Epub 2022 Feb 22
49. Aldahhan RA, Motawei KH, Al-Hariri MT. Lipotoxicity-related sarcopenia: a review. J Med Life. 2022;15(11):1334–9. https://doi.org/10.25122/jml-2022-0157. PMID: 36567835; PMCID: PMC9762358
50. Cava E, Yeat NC, Mittendorfer B. Preserving healthy muscle during weight Loss. Adv Nutr. 2017;8(3):511–9. https://doi.org/10.3945/an.116.014506. PMID: 28507015; PMCID: PMC5421125
51. Dickerson RN, Andromalos L, Brown JC, Correia MITD, Pritts W, Ridley EJ, Robinson, et al. Obesity and critical care nutrition: current practice gaps and directions for future research. Crit Care. 2022;26(1):283. https://doi.org/10.1186/s13054-022-04148-0. Erratum in: Crit Care. 2023 May 8;27(1):177. 10.1186/s13054-023-04456-z. PMID: 36127715; PMCID: PMC9486775.
52. Ceniccola GD, Castro MG, Piovacari SMF, Horie LM, Corrêa FG, Barrere APN, Toledo DO. Current technologies in body composition assessment: advantages and disadvantages. Nutrition. 2019;62:25–31. https://doi.org/10.1016/j.nut.2018.11.028. Epub 2018 Dec 6.
53. Moonen HPFX, Beckers KJH, van Zanten ARH. Energy expenditure and indirect calorimetry in critical illness and convalescence: current evidence and practical considerations. J Intensive Care. 2021;9:8. https://doi.org/10.1186/s40560-021-00524-0.
54. Wischmeyer PE, Bear DE, Berger MM, De Waele E, Gunst J, McClave SA, et al. Personalized nutrition therapy in critical care: 10 expert recommendations. Crit Care. 2023;27(1):261. https://doi.org/10.1186/s13054-023-04539-x. PMID: 37403125; PMCID: PMC10318839
55. Chapple LS, Kouw IWK, Summers MJ, Weinel LM, Gluck S, Raith E, Slobodian P, et al. Muscle protein synthesis after protein administration in critical illness. Am J Respir Crit Care Med. 2022a;206(6):740–9. https://doi.org/10.1164/rccm.202112-2780OC.
56. Koekkoek WACK, Van Zanten ARH. Is refeeding syndrome relevant for critically ill patients? Curr Opin Clin Nutr Metab Care. 2018;21(2):130–7. https://doi.org/10.1097/MCO.0000000000000449.

57. Van Zanten AR. Nutritional support and refeeding syndrome in critical illness. Lancet Respir Med. 2015;3(12):904–5. https://doi.org/10.1016/S2213-2600(15)00433-6. Epub 2015 Nov 18
58. Yébenes JC, Bordeje-Laguna ML, Lopez-Delgado JC, Lorencio-Cardenas C, De Lagran Zurbano IM, et al. Smartfeeding: a dynamic strategy to increase nutritional efficiency in critically ill patients-positioning document of the metabolism and nutrition working group and the early mobilization Working Group of the Catalan Society of Intensive and Critical Care Medicine (SOCMiC). Nutrients. 2024;16(8):1157. https://doi.org/10.3390/nu16081157. PMID: 38674847; PMCID: PMC11054493.
59. Border K, Endrizal C, Cecil M. Academy of nutrition and dietetics: revised 2018 standards of professional performance for registered dietitian nutritionists (competent, proficient, and expert) in education of nutrition and dietetics practitioners. J Acad Nutr Diet. 2019;119(1):124–136.e29. https://doi.org/10.1016/j.jand.2018.10.014.
60. Tappenden KA, Quatrara B, Parkhurst ML, Malone AM, Fanjiang G, Ziegler TR. Critical role of nutrition in improving quality of care: an interdisciplinary call to action to address adult hospital malnutrition. JPEN J Parenter Enteral Nutr. 2013;37(4):482–97. https://doi.org/10.1177/0148607113484066.
61. Field LB, Hand RK. Differentiating malnutrition screening and assessment: a nutrition care process perspective. J Acad Nutr Diet. 2015;115(5):824–8. https://doi.org/10.1016/j.jand.2014.11.010.
62. Allen K, Hoffman L. Enteral nutrition in the mechanically ventilated patient. Nutr Clin Pract. 2019;34(4):540–57. https://doi.org/10.1002/ncp.10242.Epub.
63. Sundström Rehal M, Liebau F, Wernerman J, Rooyackers O. Whole-body protein kinetics in critically ill patients during 50 or 100% energy provision by enteral nutrition: a randomized cross-over study. PLoS One. 2020;15(10):e0240045. https://doi.org/10.1371/journal.pone.0240045. PMID: 33017434; PMCID: PMC7535026
64. Heuft L, Voigt J, Selig L, Stumvoll M, Schlögl H, Kaiser T. Refeeding syndrome. Dtsch Arztebl Int. 2023;120:107–14. https://doi.org/10.3238/arztebl.m2022.0381.
65. Ponzo V, Pellegrini M, Cioffi I, Scaglione L, Bo S. The refeeding syndrome: a neglected but potentially serious condition for inpatients. A narrative review. Intern Emerg Med. 2020;16(1):49–60. https://doi.org/10.1007/s11739-020-02525-7.
66. Da Silva JSV, Seres D, Sabino K, Adams SC, Berdahl GJ, Citty SW, et al. ASPEN consensus recommendations for refeeding syndrome. Nutr Clin Pract. 2020;00:1–18.
67. NICE. www.nice.org.uk/guidance/cg32. Nutrition support for adults: oral nutrition support, enteral tube feeding and parenteral nutrition Clinical Guideline. Published: 22 February. 2006. Last updated: 04 august. 2017.
68. Cioffi I, Ponzo V, Pellegrini M, Evangelista A, Bioletto F, Ciccone G, et al. The incidence of the refeeding syndrome. A systematic review and meta-analyses of literature. Clin Nutr. 2021;40:3688–701.
69. De Man AME, Gunst J, Blaser AR. Nutrition in the intensive care unit: from the acute phase to beyond. Intensive Care Med. 2024;50:1035–48. https://doi.org/10.3389/fnut.2022.830457.
70. McKnigh CL, Newberry C, Sarav M, Martindale R, Hurt R, Daley B. Refeeding syndrome in the critically ill: a literature review and clinicians guide. Curr Gastroenterol Rep. 2019;21:58. https://doi.org/10.1007/s11894-019-0724-3.
71. Nunes G, Brito M, Santos CA, Fonseca J. Refeeding syndrome in the gastroenterology practice: how concerned should we be? Eur J Gastroenterol Hepatol. 2019;21:1270–6.
72. Sakai AF, Costa NC. Síndrome de realimentação: da fisiopatologia ao manejo. Rev Fac Ciênc Méd Sorocaba. 2018;20(2):70–2.
73. Shariatpanahi ZV, Shariatpanahi MV, Shahbazi E, Shahbazi S. Refeeding syndrome and its related factors in critically ill coronavirus disease 2019 patients: a prospective cohort study. Front Nutr. 2022;11(9):830457.
74. Da Silva JSV. Erratum. ASPEN consensus recommendations for refeeding syndrome. Nutr Clin Pract. 2020;35(3):584–5.

75. Adika E, Jia R, Li J, Seres D, Freedberg DE. Evaluation of the ASPEN guidelines for refeeding syndrome among hospitalized patients receiving enteral nutrition: a retrospective Cohort study. J Parenter Enteral Nutr. 2022;46(8):1859–66. https://doi.org/10.1002/jpen.2368.
76. Singer P, Blaser AR, Berger MM, Calder PC, Casaer M, Hiesmayr M, et al. ESPEN practical and partially revised guideline: clinical nutrition in the intensive care unit. Clin Nutr. 2023a;42:1671–89. https://doi.org/10.1016/j.clnu.2023.07.011.
77. Singer P, Blaser AR, Berger MM, Calder PC, Casaer M, Hiesmayr M, Mayer K, Montejo-Gonzalez JC, Pichard C, et al. ESPEN practical and partially revised guideline: clinical nutrition in the intensive care unit. Clin Nutr. 2023b;42:1671–89.
78. Associação de Medicina Intensiva e Sociedade Brasileira de Pneumologia e Tisiologia. Orientações Práticas em Ventilação Mecânica AMIB e SBPT, 2024. [Internet]. [citado 2025 Jan 28]. Available at: https://d1xe7tfg0uwul9.cloudfront.net/amib-portal/wp-content/uploads/2024/09/18120131/Orientacoes-Praticas-de-Ventilacao-Mecanica-Interativo-SET-17.pdf.
79. Castro MV, Ribeiro PC, Souza IAO, Cunha HFR, Silva MHN, Rocha EEM, et al. Diretriz Brasileira de Terapia Nutricional no Paciente Grave. BRASPEN J. 2018;33(Supl 1):2–36.
80. van Zanten ARH, De Waele E, Wischmeyer PE. Nutrition therapy and critical illness: practical guidance for the ICU, post-ICU, and long-term convalescence phases. Crit Care. 2019;23(1):368. https://doi.org/10.1186/s13054-019-2657-5. PMID: 31752979
81. Chapple LS, Kouw IWK, Summers MJ, Weinel LM, Gluck S, Raith E, Slobodian P, Soenen S, Deane AM, van Loon LJC, Chapman MJ. Muscle protein synthesis after protein Administration in Critical Illness. Am J Respir Crit Care Med. 2022b;206(6):740–9.
82. De Azevedo JRA, Lima HCM, Frota PHDB, Nogueira IROM, de Souza SC, Fernandes EAA, Cruz AM. High-protein intake and early exercise in adult intensive care patients: a prospective, randomized controlled trial to evaluate the impact on functional outcomes. BMC Anesthesiol. 2021;21(1):283.
83. Koekkoek WACK, van Setten CHC, Olthof LE, Kars JCNH, van Zanten ARH. Timing of PROTein INtake and clinical outcomes of adult critically ill patients on prolonged mechanical VENTilation: the PROTINVENT retrospective study. Clin Nutr. 2019;38(2):883–90.
84. Rousseau AF, Losser MR, Ichai C, Berger MM. ESPEN endorsed recommendations: nutritional therapy in major burns. Clin Nutr. 2013;32(4):497–502. https://doi.org/10.1016/j.clnu.2013.02.012. Epub 2013 Mar 14. Erratum in: Clin Nutr. 2013 Dec;32(6):1083.
85. Blaser AR, Starkopf J, Alhazzani W, Berger MM, Casaer MP, Deane AM, et al. Early enteral nutrition in critically ill patients: ESICM clinical practice guidelines. Intensive Care Med. 2017;43:380–98.
86. Franzosi OS, Nunes DSL, Klanovicz TM, Loss SH, Batassini É, Turra EE, Teixeira C, Vieira SRR. Hemodynamic and skin perfusion is associated with successful enteral nutrition therapy in septic shock patients. Clin Nutr. 2020;39(12):3721–9. https://doi.org/10.1016/j.clnu.2020.03.033.
87. Blaser AR, Starkopf J, Kirsimägi Ü, Deane AM. Definition, prevalence, and outcome of feeding intolerance in intensive care: a systematic review and meta-analysis. Acta Anaesthesiol Scand. 2014;58(8):914–22. https://doi.org/10.1111/aas.12302. Epub 2014 Mar 11
88. de la Fuente IS, de la Fuente JS, Quintana Estelles MD, Garcia Gigorro R, Terceros Almanza LJ, Sanchez Izquierdo JA, Montejo Gonzalez JC. Enteral nutrition in patients receiving mechanical ventilation in a prone position. JPEN J Parenter Enteral Nutr. 2016;40(2):250–5. https://doi.org/10.1177/0148607114553232.
89. Campos L.F, Barreto AP, Ceniccola DG, Gonçalves CR, De Matos BNL, Zambelli CMSF, Castro MG. Review of the BRASPEN technical report on nutritional therapy in patients hospitalized with COVID-19, BRASPEN J, vol.36, n 1, 122-126, 2021. https://doi.org/10.37111/braspenj.COVID2021

90. Peterson SJ, Tsai AA, Scala CM, Sowa DC, Sheean PM, Braunschweig CL. Adequacy of oral intake in critically ill patients 1 week after extubation. J Am Diet Assoc. 2010;110(3):427–33. https://doi.org/10.1016/j.jada.2009.11.020.
91. Jones C, Eddleston J, McCairn A, Dowling S, McWilliams D, Coughlan E, Griffiths RD. Improving rehabilitation after critical illness through outpatient physiotherapy classes and essential amino acid supplement: a randomized controlled trial. J Crit Care. 2015;30(5):901–7. https://doi.org/10.1016/j.jcrc.2015.05.002.

Chapter 22
Sleep Disorders, Delirium, and Weaning

Leonardo Pamponet Simões, Emanuele da Silva Passos Damázio, and Darlan Nitz

22.1 Introduction

Sleep is a vital physiological process during which the body rests and recovers normal functions, and total sleep time and sleep quality are essential to ensure this process. Sleep is a phase of the circadian rhythm or cycle, a variation in the biological functions of different living beings that repeats itself regularly over approximately 24 h. The circadian cycle, controlled by the hypothalamus through the suprachiasmatic nucleus, promotes the normal functioning and maintenance of the sleep-wake state [1]. During the night, melatonin, a biological clock agent synthesized by the pineal gland, begins to be released around 10 pm in the absence of light, peaks around 3 am, and serum levels return to minimum levels around 9 am. The ICU environment inherently poses risks to the normal functioning of the circadian cycle, including low daytime light levels and high nighttime light levels [2].

According to the Rechtschaffen and Kales' (1968) classification [3], sleep can be divided into two states: non-rapid eye movement (NREM) sleep and rapid eye movement (REM) sleep. NREM sleep is divided into three stages and accounts for approximately 75%–80% of total sleep time. Stages 1 and 2 are considered lighter sleep, while stage 3 is deep sleep, characterized by slow waves on the electroencephalogram (EEG). REM sleep accounts for about 20%–25% of total

L. P. Simões (✉)
Hospital da Mulher, Salvador, Bahia, Brazil

Aliviare Saúde, Salvador, Bahia, Brazil
e-mail: leonardo@aliviare.com.br

E. da Silva Passos Damázio
Liga de Medicina Intensiva, UESB, Jequié, Bahia, Brazil

D. Nitz
Intensiphysio Fisioterapia Intensiva, Curitiba, Paraná, Brazil

A. R. Baptistella et al. (eds.), *Weaning from Mechanical Ventilation*, https://doi.org/10.1007/978-3-032-01145-9_22

sleep time and is characterized by low-voltage EEG activity, rapid eye movements, and peripheral muscle atonia [3].

Drouot et al. [4] showed that patients on mechanical ventilation (MV) could not be classified according to the classical sleep disorder criteria of Rechtschaffen and Kales and proposed a new classification for sleep analysis, adding two new states: atypical sleep and pathological wakefulness. Patients in this study had been weaned from sedation for at least 48 h and were undergoing ventilatory weaning.

Atypical sleep is characterized by prolonged periods of high amplitude (50–100 μV) continuous and irregular delta activity without fast frequencies or rapid eye movements and with low submental muscle tone. It has similarities to slow-wave sleep but lacks K-complexes and sleep spindles.

Pathological wakefulness is characterized by periods suggestive of wakefulness with rapid eye movements and sustained submental muscle activity with behavioral correlates of wakefulness, but not meeting Rechtschaffen and Kales' criteria for wakefulness due to very slow background EEG activity (at or below 6 Hz).

Physiological changes occur during sleep that may affect the process of weaning from mechanical ventilation. These changes include a reduction in airway muscle tone, altered ventilatory response to hypercapnia and hypoxemia, and changes in breathing patterns. These changes can lead to apnea and hypopnea, particularly during REM sleep when neuromuscular control of breathing is less stable [5].

Polysomnography (PSG) is the gold standard for comprehensive sleep assessment. However, its use in the ICU is hampered by several factors, including unreliable signals due to electrical interference from ICU equipment, sedation, renal failure, or liver dysfunction [2].

ICU patients, especially those on MV, experience poor sleep quality and quantity with disrupted circadian cycles, irregular daytime and nighttime sleep periods, increased proportions of NREM stages 1 and 2, reduced slow-wave sleep (stage 3), and significant reductions in REM sleep, with fragmented sleep and low efficiency [2]. These findings result in excessive daytime sleepiness, which can impair patient performance during ventilator weaning.

In critically ill patients, the sleep fragmentation index, defined by the number of arousals per hour, is similar to that of patients with severe obstructive sleep apnea (OSA) with an apnea-hypopnea index (AHI) greater than 30 events per hour [5, 6].

There are several causes in the ICU that can contribute to sleep disturbances in MV patients, especially during ventilator weaning. These include:

- Noise: Various noises are present in the ICU, primarily alarms from devices such as mechanical ventilators, infusion pumps, and multiparameter monitors. Other common noises come from members of the multidisciplinary team, such as loud conversations in corridors and nursing stations during the day and night [1].
- Light: Maintaining light levels in the ICU throughout the day and night may contribute to circadian disruption. Melatonin production depends on darkness and is affected by excessive light exposure [1].
- Testing routines: It is common for laboratory and imaging tests to be performed in the middle of the night, contributing to sleep fragmentation [1].

- Inadequate ventilatory adjustments: Over-assistance can lead to hyperventilation and induce central apnea. Under-assistance leads to excessive effort and patient-ventilator asynchrony, contributing to sleep fragmentation [7].
- Sedatives and analgesics: Some drugs, such as benzodiazepines, decrease slow-wave sleep and REM sleep; anti-inflammatory drugs decrease sleep efficiency and promote fragmentation; opioids decrease upper airway muscle tone during sleep, leading to obstruction, apnea, and sleep fragmentation [1].
- Patient's clinical condition: Patients with lung disease, heart disease, associated comorbidities such as hypertension, diabetes, obesity, presence of OSA, and organ dysfunction are more prone to worsening sleep quality.

Studies show that pressure support ventilation (PSV) mode, predominantly used during ventilator weaning, especially during the spontaneous breathing test (SBT) with lower levels such as PSV = 7 cm H_2O, provides inferior sleep quality compared to assisted controlled ventilation (ACV) modes. Toublanc et al. [8] compared sleep quality in 20 mechanically ventilated patients between ACV mode and low-level support (PSV=6 cm H_2O). The results showed better sleep efficiency and patient-perceived sleep quality in ACV mode. In the first part of the study, between 10 pm and 2 am, there was a greater reduction in wakefulness and an increase in NREM stages 1 and 2 with ACV compared to PSV = 6 cm H_2O. In the second part, between 2 am and 6 am, the duration of stage 3 was also longer in ACV patients. Andréjak et al. [9] compared nocturnal ventilation in 26 patients with chronic obstructive pulmonary disease (COPD) between pressure-controlled ventilation (PCV) and PSV = 6 cm H_2O and showed better muscle relaxation, sleep efficiency, slow-wave sleep, and REM sleep in PCV.

Bosma et al. [10] compared ventilation in 13 patients starting daily sedation interruption for ventilatory weaning. One group used PSV and the other proportional assist ventilation (PAV). PAV patients had better sleep quality and higher proportions of slow-wave and REM sleep compared to PSV. PAV reduced patient-ventilator asynchrony, which may contribute to better sleep quality.

Dress et al. [11] conducted a prospective, randomized physiological study in three French ICU centers, evaluating weaning patients eligible for SBT based on clinical criteria. Polysomnograms were performed for 15 h the day before SBT to assess atypical sleep and pathological wakefulness. Of the 37 study patients, 19 passed the SBT, but only 11 were extubated; the remaining 8 remained intubated based on clinical decisions, and 18 failed the SBT. Pathologic wakefulness and atypical sleep patterns were found in 39% and 55% of patients who failed the SBT, respectively, higher than those who passed. Approximately 50% of those who passed the SBT but were not extubated had pathologic wakefulness and atypical sleep, whereas only 27% of those who passed and were extubated had these patterns, suggesting that patients with predominant atypical sleep and pathologic wakefulness are more prone to weaning failure.

Another study used PSG to evaluate sleep disturbances in patients with difficult weaning. Twenty-seven patients in the difficult weaning phase, defined as three or more failed weaning attempts, underwent 24-h PSG. The study showed that patients in this phase had a high frequency of sleep disturbances, with reduced sleep efficiency, reduced slow-wave sleep, and reduced REM sleep. There was a significant correlation between sleep fragmentation and weaning difficulty, suggesting that sleep disturbance may be an independent risk factor for weaning failure [7].

In light of the above, it is necessary to provide a more conducive sleep environment for patients undergoing ventilator weaning in order to reduce sleep disturbance and improve weaning success rates. Measures such as appropriate lighting, noise level control in the unit, reduction in the use of sedoanalgesia when possible, and well-designed ventilator settings or new ventilator modes that reduce patient-ventilator asynchrony and promote adequate ventilation without over- or under-assistance will contribute to better patient performance throughout the weaning process.

For those patients who pass the SBT and are extubated, it is extremely important to identify the presence of sleep disorders such as OSA and central apnea. Treatment with positive pressure, such as continuous positive airway pressure (CPAP) or bilevel positive airway pressure (BiPAP), should be initiated early to avoid potential weaning failures and promote rapid patient recovery [2].

22.2 The Impact of Delirium on Weaning

Intensive care units are areas of uncertainty. The complexity of their interventions—intensified, dense, and sophisticated care—is available in a tumultuous environment for the harmonious exercise of basic physiological functions. These units have a hectic routine: lights, noises, procedures, stressors, and potentially traumatic factors that affect the patient during their illness and the lack of autonomy experienced by critically ill patients. In this scenario, organic insults mix with psycho-emotional suffering, making the experience of the multidisciplinary team challenging.

In the ICU, delirium and ventilator weaning receive specific and combined attention and management, as both conditions, when combined, lead to unfavorable outcomes for critically ill patients. Delirium is a condition with a variable prevalence in the medical literature, estimated to occur in 60%–80% of mechanically ventilated patients [12]. In addition, it is a predictor of adverse outcomes [13], being an independent risk factor for higher 6-month mortality and higher rates of ICU and hospital stay [12, 13].

Delirium is defined as an acute cognitive disorder characterized by fluctuations in the level of consciousness and higher mental functions, particularly attention, that are not related to other organic causes, intoxication, or a pre-existing, existing, or developing neurocognitive disorder [14].

The pathophysiology of delirium is complex and remains difficult to elucidate. It is known that through a complex interaction of precipitating factors provided by the environment and predisposing factors of the individual, added to the vulnerability created by critical illness, delirium manifests as a disconnection syndrome [15].

This is due to a disruption of neural networks leading to a fluctuating state of consciousness [16] (Fig. 22.1).

Experimental studies measuring neuroinflammation after mechanical ventilation have found elevated levels of reactive astrocytes and inflammatory markers, in addition to the presence of apoptosis biomarkers [18, 19]. In addition, hypoxia may lead to increased brain dysfunction in critically ill patients, ultimately contributing to long-term cognitive deficits [20].

Delirium is subclassified according to symptom presentation. In hypoactive delirium, symptoms of reduced motor activity predominate; these patients are the most lethargic and inattentive. In hyperactive delirium, psychomotor agitation predominates. Mixed delirium presents with symptoms of the other two subtypes and may change over the course of the illness [21].

Patients with delirium exhibit features such as disorganized thinking, memory deficits, anxiety, sadness, and irritability. In addition, autonomic demands such as tachycardia and hyperventilation are common, which can overwhelm the cardiovascular and respiratory systems [15].

Given its common occurrence in the hospital setting, knowledge of risk factors may aid in the early diagnosis of delirium. These factors include duration of mechanical ventilation, high doses of sedation, age > 65 years, physical immobility, muscle weakness, Acute Physiology and Chronic Health Evaluation II (APACHE II) score, sepsis, systemic arterial hypertension, low hemoglobin levels on hospital

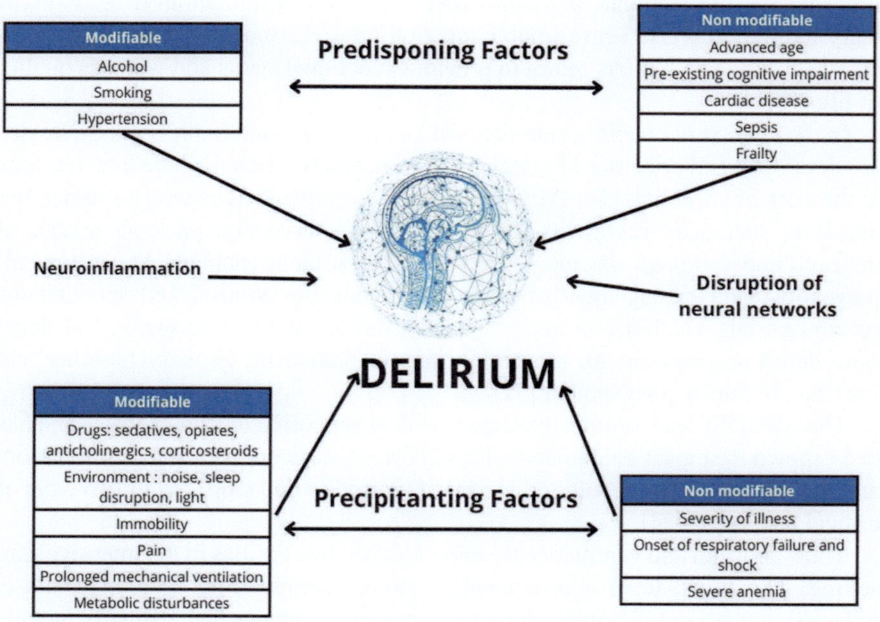

Fig. 22.1 Factors for developing ICU delirium. Predisposing factors—related to the individual. They can be modifiable or non-modifiable. Precipitating factors—related to the environment, critical illness, and procedures. They can be modifiable or non-modifiable. (Adapted from [17])

admission, smoking, alcohol consumption (>2 drinks per day), and low albumin levels on ICU admission [15].

When delirium is present at the onset of ventilator weaning, there are higher rates of complications: return to controlled modes, ventilator-associated pneumonia, and prolonged use of sedation or analgesia [22]. In addition, rates of extubation failure, difficult weaning, and tracheostomy are higher in patients with delirium [13, 22, 23].

One factor contributing to delirium is sleep deprivation or poor sleep quality, both of which are common in the hospital setting and are caused by changes in the circadian cycle [24].

In this sense, changes in circadian rhythms, sleep architecture, and quality are common adverse effects of ICU admission [22, 25] and not only favor delirium but also alter sleep patterns and quality [6]. The severity of critical illness and excessive medication also favor sleep deprivation and changes in its architecture [26]. Atypical sleep has been reported in patients who have had more hours of mechanical ventilation, with a significant reduction in the frequency of deep sleep and REM sleep [6, 27, 28]. In addition, patients with delirium have a lower rate of melatonin secretion [22]. Thus, poor sleep quality, delirium, and prolonged weaning are pathways that feed into each other and lead to long-term functional and cognitive impairment [27, 29, 30].

ICUs have evolved from obscure places to environments where technology and science work together to save more and more lives. In this context, return to social functioning is essential to ensure quality of life after critical illness. Studies measuring outcomes of functional limitations have found greater limitations in activities of daily living and worse sensorimotor function up to 12 months after hospital discharge [29], which hinders return to previous functional status and worsens quality of life [17].

In the context of enabling care focused on humanized attention, some strategies are developed and prioritized in intensive care routines. These include interventions in the form of checklists. The ABCDEF strategy, organized as an easy-to-remember acronym, succinctly represents the high-impact intervention package related to delirium and ventilator weaning outcomes. This strategy includes A: assessment, prevention, and management of pain; B: spontaneous arousal and spontaneous breathing trials; C: choice of analgesia and sedation; and D: management of delirium: delirium—assessment, prevention, and management; E: early mobility and exercise; F: family involvement [31].

The ABCDEF intervention package is widely supported by clinical trials and has been shown to impact outcomes such as delirium, days on mechanical ventilation, and ICU readmissions, resulting in reduced morbidity and mortality in survivors of critical illness [32–34].

Thus, delirium and ventilatory weaning are dynamic entities in the intensive care setting. The broad team commitment to saving people from critical insults is reflected in modern ICUs through multicomponent strategies that primarily include non-pharmacological, safe, cost-effective, and feasible strategies within the units, such as early mobilization, paving the way for other strategies beyond pharmacological ones.

22.3 The Use of Virtual Reality, Delirium, and Weaning

ICU admission is associated with many causes of distress related to illness or intensive therapies [32, 35]. The consequences can be severe, ranging from the development of an adrenergic stress response that interferes with critical illness (tachycardia, tachypnea, patient-ventilator asynchrony, agitation, immunosuppression, etc.) to the development of the post-intensive care syndrome (PICS), including neuropsychological disorders (anxiety, depression, post-traumatic stress syndrome) and chronic pain that delay the return to normal social and occupational life [36, 37].

The link between suffering in the ICU and the development of PICS has long been highlighted [38], leading to the concept of modern intensive care as being as humane as possible [39, 40]. For all these reasons, supportive care has become part of intensive care, along with the treatment of organic dysfunction. To prevent drug-related side effects, which can be severe in critically ill patients [41], current guidelines for the management of pain, agitation, delirium, immobility, and sleep disturbance (PADIS) suggest the development of non-pharmacological therapies.

Patients often experience the ICU as a "hostile" environment due to several factors, including excessive noise, loss of autonomy, and lack of information. This is exacerbated by stress and anxiety, both of which are considered significant risk factors for the development of delirium. As pharmacological interventions often have undesirable and serious side effects, non-pharmacological options are extremely important for the prevention and treatment of delirium [42].

Innovative electronic technologies, such as immersive virtual reality (VR), have been developed in medical settings to provide non-pharmacological treatment for pain, anxiety, and delirium in the ICU [43] (Fig. 22.2).

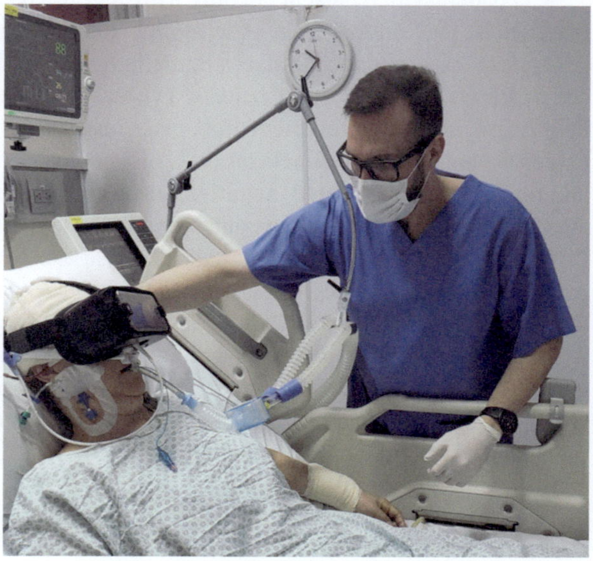

Fig. 22.2 Photo from the author's personal collection

VR applications are gaining momentum in critical care medicine. Recently, the E-CHOISIR (Electronic-CHOIce of a System for Intensive care Relaxation) study published in *Critical Care* was the first randomized controlled trial to demonstrate the benefits of VR in alleviating symptoms of stress, discomfort, and pain in critically ill patients [44]. The authors compared several VR devices with standard relaxation and music therapy and found that VR with computer-generated imagery was most effective in improving overall discomfort and reducing the physiological stress response in ICU patients.

From the patient's perspective, in addition to minimizing emotional discomfort and pain, VR can promote coordination, mobilization, and physical and mental rehabilitation [45]. Furthermore, the type of virtual world and music therapy may have different effects: the beneficial effects of these new therapies depend on the characteristics of the device and the targeted symptoms [44].

In a pilot study evaluating 5-min VR sessions in ten mechanically ventilated patients, VR therapy proved to be a potential means of controlling anxiety without the occurrence of predefined safety events or cyber sickness [46]. Sleep quality may also be positively affected by VR use. In a study of 100 patients, VR use was shown to significantly improve sleep quality, although total sleep time and light sleep time did not differ between groups [47].

Jawed et al. [48] investigated the usefulness of VR in reducing overload and sensory deprivation in the ICU. The study used virtual reality goggles on 15 ICU patients for 15 min to expose them to relaxing beach videos with natural sound effects. Most patients tolerated the headphones well and reported positive effects of VR therapy on anxiety and stress [48]. Naef et al. [49] investigated how long visual and auditory stimuli should be provided to ICU patients. Visual stimuli should not exceed 10–15 min, while auditory stimuli should not exceed 1 h to avoid adverse effects.

ICU patients often present not only with delirium but also with other neurocognitive deficits [50]. In this context, in a pilot study, Turon et al. [51] investigated the benefits of early neurocognitive stimulation supported by VR in 20 critically ill adult patients. The simulation includes a virtual avatar that accompanies the patients, helps them with temporal orientation, gives instructions, motivates them to perform exercises, and encourages relaxation. This application proved to be feasible, safe and reliable, and stimulated cognitive functions. Navarra-Ventura et al. also evaluated a VR-based neurocognitive intervention during ICU admission in 34 critically ill patients. A 1-month follow-up showed that these patients had better working memory scores and up to 50% less nonspecific anxiety and depression compared to the control group [52].

ICU stays are a significant psychological burden for patients. Vlake et al. [53] investigated the effects of ICU-specific virtual reality on mental health. The study, which included 104 patients, assessed the group three and 6 months after ICU treatment, and the repetition of 14-min VR modules about ICU treatment improved subjective well-being and quality of life. VR led to a reduction in post-traumatic stress disorder and depression scores, and the effect was still present 6 months after exposure.

Here we want to show that VR offers new possibilities for many aspects of intensive care medicine, including ventilator weaning. They provide a safe environment to practice critical care procedures without risk of harm to the patient. In addition, VR technologies can positively impact delirium control and stress levels, promoting a patient experience that facilitates the ventilator weaning process.

Attention should be paid to the duration of use of these technologies, as overstimulation can negatively affect patient outcomes [49]. In addition, cyber sickness may occur during application [44]. Finally, the implementation of these technologies in clinical practice requires a significant time commitment from the ICU team, which may also reduce availability for their use.

Overall, VR will not replace established therapies, but it can be a useful tool in combination with other therapies to improve patient stay in the ICU. Virtual reality is no longer the realm of science fiction. We are on the verge of making VR a dominant trend in medicine and critical care with the potential to lead this evolution. However, it is important to remember that VR is not intended to distract the patient. VR will be used to complement and enhance the healthcare provider-patient relationship, not replace it. And it is still in the research and development phase. Our involvement in this process is important to ensure that these technological developments are made in the best interest of our patients. This allows us to provide the best care and improve the quality of the ICU experience.

Finally, to say that VR works is like saying that a syringe works; it's what's in the syringe and its specificity that really matters. VR is just a headset; it's the software, the latency, the application time, the quality, the imagery, and the indication of this digital therapy that matters, and that's what differentiates it from a game to digital medicine.

VR can improve sleep quality, reduce the incidence of delirium, and improve the patient's physical functioning. These three potential effects of VR can improve the process and impact on better weaning outcomes for critically ill patients.

References

1. Simões LP, Cordeiro ALL, Soares LO. Distúrbios do sono na unidade de terapia intensiva. In: Martins JA, Andrade FMD, Reis LLF, editors. PROFISIO Programa de Atualização em Fisioterapia em Terapia Intensiva Adulto: Ciclo 13; 2022. p. 105–34.
2. Rittayamai N, Wilcox E, Drout X, Mehta S, Goffi A. Brochard L positive and negative effects of mechanical ventilation on sleep in the ICU: a review with clinical recommendations. Intensive Care Med. 2006;42:531–41.
3. Hori T, Sugita Y, Koga E, Shirakawa S, Inoue K, Uchida S, et al. Proposed supplements and amendments to '*a manual of standardized terminology, techniques and scoring system for sleep stages of human subjects*', the Rechtschaffen & Kales (1968) standard. Psychiatry Clin Neurosci. 2001;55:305–10.
4. Drout X, Roche-Campo F, Thille AW, Cabello B, Galia F, Margarit L, et al. A new classification for sleep analysis in critically ill patients. Sleep Med. 2012;13:7–14.
5. Parthasarathy S, Tobin MJ. Effect of ventilator mode on sleep quality in critically ill patients. Am J Respir Crit Care Med. 2002;166:1423–9.

6. Pisani MA, Friese RS, Gehlbach BK, Schwab RJ, Weinhouse GL, Jones SF. Sleep in the intensive care unit. Am J Respir Crit Care Med. 2015;191(7):731–8. https://doi.org/10.1164/rccm.201411-2099CI.
7. Cabello B, Parthasarathy S, Mancebo J. Mechanical ventilation: let us minimize sleep disturbance. Curr Opin Crit Care. 2007;13:20–6.
8. Toublanc B, Rose D, Glérant JC, Francois G, Mayeux I, Rodenstein D, et al. Assist-control ventilation vs. low levels of pressure support ventilation on sleep quality in intubated ICU patients. Intensive Care Med. 2007;33:1148–54.
9. Andréjak C, Monconduit J, Rose D, Toublanc B, Mayeux I, Rodenstein D, et al. Does using pressure-controlled ventilation to rest respiratory muscles improve sleep in ICU patients? Respir Med. 2013;107:534–41.
10. Bosma K, Ferreyra G, Ambrogio C, Pasero D, Mirabella L, Braghiroli A, et al. Patient-ventilator interaction and sleep in mechanically ventilated patients: pressure support versus proportional assist ventilation. Crit Care Med. 2007;35(4):1048–54.
11. Dres M, Younes M, Rittayamai N, Kendzerska T, Telias I, Grieco DL, et al. Sleep and pathological wakefulness ate the time of liberation from mechanical ventilation (SLEEWE) – a prospective multicenter physiological study. Am J Respir Crit Care Med. 2019;199(9):1106–15.
12. Ely EW, Shintani A, Truman B, Speroff T, Gordon SM, Harrell FE Jr, et al. Delirium as a predictor of mortality in mechanically ventilated patients in the intensive care unit. JAMA. 2004;291(14):1753–62. https://doi.org/10.1001/jama.291.14.1753. PMID: 15082703.7
13. Jeon K, Jeong BH, Ko MG, Nam J, Yoo H, Chung CR, et al. Impact of delirium on weaning from mechanical ventilation in medical patients. Respirology. 2016;21(2):313–20. https://doi.org/10.1111/resp.12673. Epub 2015 Nov 4. PMID: 26534738
14. American Psychiatric Association, DSMTF, et al. Diagnostic and statistical manual of mental disorders: DSM-5. Washington, DC: American psychiatric association; 2013.
15. Slooter AJ, Van De Leur RR, Zaal IJ. Delirium in critically ill patients. Handb Clin Neurol. 2017;141:449–66. https://doi.org/10.1016/B978-0-444-63599-0.00025-9. PMID: 28190430
16. Choi SH, Lee H, Chung TS, Park KM, Jung YC, Kim SI, et al. Neural network functional connectivity during and after an episode of delirium. Am J Psychiatry. 2012;169(5):498–507. https://doi.org/10.1176/appi.ajp.2012.11060976. PMID: 22549209
17. Mart MF, Williams Roberson S, Salas B, Pandharipande PP, Ely EW. Prevention and management of delirium in the intensive care unit. Semin Respir Crit Care Med. 2021;42(1):112–26. https://doi.org/10.1055/s-0040-1710572. Epub 2020 Aug 3. PMID: 32746469; PMCID: PMC7855536
18. Chen T, Chen C, Zhang Z, Zou Y, Peng M, Wang Y. Toll-like receptor 4 knockout ameliorates neuroinflammation due to lung-brain interaction in mechanically ventilated mice. Brain Behav Immun. 2016;56:42–55. https://doi.org/10.1016/j.bbi.2016.04.004.
19. Varatharaj A, Galea I. The blood-brain barrier in systemic inflammation. Brain Behav Immun. 2017;60:1–12. https://doi.org/10.1016/j.bbi.2016.03.010. Epub 2016 Mar 16. PMID: 26995317
20. Turon M, Fernández-Gonzalo S, de Haro C, Magrans R, López-Aguilar J, Blanch L. Mechanisms involved in brain dysfunction in mechanically ventilated critically ill patients: implications and therapeutics. Annal Transl Med. 2018;6(02):30–95.
21. Peterson JF, Pun BT, Dittus RS, Thomason JWW, Jackson JC, Shintani AK, et al. Delirium and its motoric subtypes: a study of 614 critically ill patients. J Am Geriatr Soc. 2006;54(03):479–84.
22. Dessap AM, Roche-Campo F, Launay JM, Charles-Nelson A, Katsahian S, Brun-Buisson C, a. Delirium and circadian rhythm of melatonin during weaning from mechanical ventilation: an ancillary study of a weaning trial. Chest. 2015;148(5):1231–41. https://doi.org/10.1378/chest.15-0525. PMID: 26158245
23. Shehabi Y, Riker RR, Bokesch PM, Wisemandle W, Shintani A, Ely EW. Delirium duration and mortality in lightly sedated, mechanically ventilated intensive care patients. Crit Care Med. 2010;38(12):2311–8. https://doi.org/10.1097/CCM.0b013e3181f85759.
24. Borbély AA. A two process model of sleep regulation. Hum Neurobiol. 1982;1(3):195–204.

25. Tembo AC, Parker V, Higgins I. The experience of sleep deprivation in intensive care patients: findings from a larger hermeneutic phenomenological study. Intensive Crit Care Nurs. 2013;29(6):310–6.
26. Drouot X, Cabello B, d'Ortho MP, Brochard L. Sleep in the intensive care unit. Sleep Med Rev. 2008;12:391–403.
27. Thille AW, Reynaud F, Marie D, Barrau S, Rousseau L, Rault C, et al. Impact of sleep alterations on weaning duration in mechanically ventilated patients: a prospective study. Eur Respir J. 2018;51:1–10.
28. Jean R, Shah P, Yudelevich E, Genese F, Gershner K, Levendowski D, et al. Effects of deep sedation on sleep in critically ill medical patients on mechanical ventilation. J Sleep Res. 2020;29:e12894. https://doi.org/10.1111/jsr.12894.
29. Brummel NE, Jackson JC, Pandharipande PP, Thompson JL, Shintani AK, Dittus RS, et al. Delirium in the ICU and subsequent long-term disability among survivors of mechanical ventilation. Crit Care Med. 2014;42(02):369–77.
30. Girard TD, Jackson JC, Pandharipande PP, Pun BT, Thompson JL, Shintani AK, et al. Delirium as a predictor of long-term cognitive impairment in survivors of critical illness. Crit Care Med. 2010;38(7):1513–20. https://doi.org/10.1097/CCM.0b013e3181e47be1. PMID: 20473145
31. Ely EW. The ABCDEF bundle: science and philosophy of how ICU liberation serves patients and families. Crit Care Med. 2017;45(2):321–30. https://doi.org/10.1097/CCM.0000000000002175. PMID: 28098628
32. Devlin JW, Skrobik Y, Gelinas C, Needham DM, Slooter AJC, Pandhariÿ PP, et al. Clinical practice guidelines for the prevention and management of pain, agitation/sedation, delirium, immobility, and sleep disruption in adult patients in the ICU. Crit Care Med. 2018;46(9):e825–73.
33. Pun BT, Balas MC, Barnes-Daly MA, Thompson JL, Aldrich JM, Barr J, et al. Caring for critically ill patients with the ABCDEF bundle: results of the ICU liberation collaborative in over 15,000 adults. Crit Care Med. 2019;47(1):3–14. https://doi.org/10.1097/CCM.0000000000003482. PMID: 30339549
34. Barr J, Downs B, Ferrell K, Talebian M, Robinson S, Kolodisner L, et al. Improving outcomes in mechanically ventilated adult ICU patients following implementation of the ICU liberation (ABCDEF) bundle across a large healthcare system. Crit Care Explor. 2024;6(1):e1001. https://doi.org/10.1097/CCE.0000000000001001. PMID: 38250248
35. Chanques G, Nelson J, Puntillo K. Five patient symptoms you should assess every day. Intensive Care Med. 2015;41(7):1347–50.
36. Inoue S, Hatakeyama J, Kondo Y, Hifumi T, Sakuramoto H, Kawasaki T, et al. Post-intensive care syndrome: its pathophysiology, prevention, and future directions. Acute Med Surg. 2019;6(3):233–46.
37. Thiolliere F, Falandry C, Allaouchiche B, Geofray V, Bitker L, Reignier J, et al. Intensive care-related loss of quality of life and autonomy at 6 months post-discharge: does COVID-19 really make things worse? Crit Care. 2022;26(1):94.
38. Jones C, Bäckman C, Capuzzo M, Flaatten H, Rylander C, Grifths RD. Precipitants of post-traumatic stress disorder after intensive care: a hypothesis-generating study of diversity in care. Intensive Care Med. 2007;33(6):978–85.
39. Vincent JL, Shehabi Y, Walsh TS, Pandharipande PP, Ball JA, Spronk P, et al. Comfort and patient-centered care without excessive sedation: the eCASH concept. Intensive Care Med. 2016;42(6):962–71.
40. Pallanch O, Ortalda A, Pelosi P, Latronico N, Sartini C, Lombardi G, et al. Effects on health-related quality of life of interventions that affect survival in critically ill patients: a systematic review. Crit Care. 2022;26(1):126.
41. Chanques G, Ely EW, Garnier O, Perrigault F, Eloi A, Carr J, et al. The 2014 updated version of the intensive care unit confusion assessment method compared to the 5th version of the diagnostic and statistical manual of mental disorders and other current methods used by intensivists. Ann Intensive Care. 2018;8(1):33.

42. Cavallazzi R, Saad M, Marik PE. Delirium in the ICU: an overview. Ann Intensive Care. 2012;2(1):49.
43. Indovina P, Barone D, Gallo L, Chirico A, De Pietro G, Giordano A. Virtual reality as a distraction intervention to alleviate pain and suffering during medical procedures: a comprehensive review of the literature. Clin J Pain. 2018;34(9):858–77.
44. Merliot-Gailhoustet L, Raimbert C, Garnier O, Carr J, De Jong A, Molinari N, et al. Improving discomfort for critically ill patients using electronic relaxation devices: results from the E-CHOISIR randomized controlled crossover trial (Electronic-CHOIce of a system for intensive care relaxation). Crit Care. 2022;26(1):263.
45. Wolf G, Bruno RR, Reiter M, Kantzow B, Kelm M, Jung C. Virtual reality device training for extracorporeal membrane oxygenation. Crit Care. 2020;24(1):390.
46. Haley AC, Wacker DA. Cinematic virtual reality for anxiety management in mechanically ventilated patients: feasibility and pilot study. Acute Crit Care. 2022;37(2):230–6.
47. Lee SY, Kang J. Effect of virtual reality meditation on the sleep quality of patients in an intensive care unit: a randomized clinical trial. Intensive Crit Care Nurs. 2020;59:1–7.
48. Jawed YT, Golovyan D, Lopez D, Khan SH, Wang S, Freund C, et al. Feasibility of a virtual reality intervention in the intensive care unit. Heart Lung. 2021;50(6):748–53.
49. Naef AC, Erne K, Exl MT, Nef T, Jeitziner MM. Visual and auditory stimulation for patients admitted to an intensive care unit: a mixed method study. Intensive Crit Care Nurs. 2022;73:1–7.
50. Fiani B, Figueras RA, Samones P, Lee C, Castillo A, Sangalang B, et al. Long-term stays in intensive care units (ICU) can lead to long-term cognitive impairment (LTCI): neurosurgery nursing strategies to minimize risks. Cureus. 2022;14(9):e28967.
51. Turon M, Fernandez-Gonzalo S, Jodar M, Gomà G, Montanya J, Hernando D, et al. Feasibility and safety of virtual reality-based early neurocognitive stimulation in critically ill patients. Ann Intensive Care. 2017;7(1):81.
52. Navarra-Ventura G, Gomà G, de Haro C, Jodar M, Sarlabous L, Hernando D, et al. Virtual reality-based early neurocognitive stimulation in critically ill patients: a pilot randomized clinical trial. J Person Med. 2021;11(12):1260.
53. Vlake JH, Van Bommel J, Wils EJ, Korevaar TIM, Hellemons ME, Schut AFFC, et al. Effect of intensive care unit-specific virtual reality (ICU-VR) to improve psychological Well-being and quality of life in COVID-19 ICU survivors: a study protocol for a multicenter, randomized, controlled trial. Trials. 2021;22(1):328.

Chapter 23
Chronically Critically Ill Patients on Prolonged Mechanical Ventilation and Unweanable Patients

Dario S. Villalba and Gustavo A. Plotnikow

23.1 Chronically Critically Ill Patients

Advances in knowledge and technology in intensive care units (ICUs) have significantly improved the survival of critically ill patients worldwide. However, these advances have also led to the emergence of a new category of patients: the chronically critically ill [1, 2]. Although there is no universally accepted definition, Khan et al. propose that these patients have one or more of the following clinical conditions: mechanical ventilation (MV) for more than 96 h, tracheostomy, ischemic or hemorrhagic stroke, traumatic brain injury, sepsis, or severe wounds, combined with an ICU stay of at least 8 days [3]. Mechanical ventilation (MV) is a cornerstone of ICU care, and prolonged dependence after the acute phase is widely regarded as an indicator of chronic critical illness [4].

Various studies have estimated that the incidence of chronic critical illness ranges from 5% to 10% among ICU patients requiring invasive MV during the acute episode [3, 5–8]. This patient population is characterized not only by MV dependence, but also by critical illness-related weakness, including myopathy and neuropathy, with marked changes in body composition (loss of lean mass, increased adiposity, and anasarca); neuroendocrine changes that impair anabolism; susceptibility to infection; cerebral dysfunction with prolonged delirium and/or coma; and skin damage resulting from nutritional deficits, edema, incontinence, and prolonged

D. S. Villalba (✉)
Hospital "Santiago Fornos", Chivilcoy, Buenos Aires, Argentina

Santa Catalina Neurorehabilitación Clínica, Buenos Aires, Argentina

G. A. Plotnikow
Hospital Británico de Buenos Aires, Buenos Aires, Argentina

Facultad de Medicina y Ciencias de la Salud, Universidad Abierta Interamericana, Buenos Aires, Argentina

A. R. Baptistella et al. (eds.), *Weaning from Mechanical Ventilation*,
https://doi.org/10.1007/978-3-032-01145-9_23

Table 23.1 Mortality at 1 year, mortality at hospital discharge, discharged to home from the hospital, and patients successfully liberated from the ventilator in the hospital[a]

	Total	ICUs in acute care hospitals	Weaning units in acute care hospitals	Post-acute care hospitals
Mortality at 1 year	59% (56–62)	58% (54–61)	48% (36–60)	67% (60–73)
Mortality at hospital discharge	29% (26–32)	29% (24–35)	–	29% (26–33)
Proportion of patients discharged to home from the hospital	19% (16–24)	13% (8–21)	–	21% (17–27)
Proportion of patients successfully liberated from the ventilator in the hospital	50% (47–53)	50% (46–56)	57% (45–68)	49% (44–53)

[a]Adapted from Damuth [4]

immobility. In addition, patients report distressing symptoms such as pain, thirst, dyspnea, depression, anxiety, and communication difficulties [2, 9, 10]. Persistent inflammation, immunosuppression, and catabolism syndrome (PICS) has also been described in chronically critically ill patients [11].

Outcomes for this patient population were analyzed by Damuth et al. in a systematic review and meta-analysis of 124 studies involving 318,621 patients from 16 countries. They reported a one-year mortality rate of 59% (95% CI: 56–62), an ICU discharge mortality rate of 26% (95% CI: 24–28), and a home discharge rate of 22% (95% CI: 19–25) compared with those discharged to another facility or dying in the hospital. Successful freedom from MV was achieved in 57% (95% CI: 55–60) of cases (see Table 23.1) [4]. In addition, this patient population incurs significant healthcare costs; in the United States, the annual cost of care exceeds $25 billion [3]. Persistent physical impairment and diminished quality of life often persist for years after ICU discharge [9].

23.2 Prolonged Mechanical Ventilation

Dependence on mechanical ventilation is a central feature of patients with chronic critical illness. A consensus led by MacIntyre defined prolonged mechanical ventilation (PMV) as the need for MV for more than 21 days, with use exceeding 6 h per day. The same consensus defined successful weaning as the absence of ventilatory support for more than 7 days, taking into account the underlying cause of MV reinitiation [12].

A systematic review, which excluded meta-analysis due to heterogeneity in patient populations and definitions, identified several risk factors for PMV. These included comorbidities (chronic obstructive pulmonary disease, renal failure, heart failure, and previous stroke), site of intubation and MV initiation, laboratory values (low platelet count, elevated creatinine, low serum albumin, hyperglycemia, and/or hypernatremia), acid-base status on ICU admission (low pH and bicarbonate, elevated CO2), MV settings (high FiO2, high PEEP, low PaO2/FiO2), and ICU admission severity score [13].

Heunks and Van Der Hoeven [14] describe the pathophysiology of PMV dependence as complex and often multifactorial. Therefore, treatment of this condition requires identification of the underlying causes of dependence and development of a targeted treatment strategy. This approach requires a highly specialized multidisciplinary team with expertise in managing this complex patient population. They propose to analyze possible respiratory, neurological, cardiac, respiratory muscle, and endocrine dysfunction and offer tailored solutions for successful weaning in PMV patients.

Despite the extensive literature on PMV, there is no precise definition or universally accepted criteria for determining successful weaning from MV [15].

23.3 Care and Rehabilitation Alternatives for Patients Receiving Prolonged Mechanical Ventilation: A Global Analysis of Options

Although clinical outcomes for patients on prolonged mechanical ventilation (PMV) are often discouraging and associated with high healthcare costs, there is an opportunity to refer selected patients to specialized care and rehabilitation centers. These units may be integrated into acute care hospitals or operate as stand-alone facilities in other healthcare settings.

The PMV consensus recommended that "*for ICU patients who are difficult to wean from mechanical ventilation, care settings should be considered from the perspective of the patients and the care demands of each case. Comorbidities that often accompany the need for MV may prevent transfers to facilities without a level of ICU or acute care capacity. The critical care team must assess the efficacy and safety of all available facilities before discharging patients to specialized centers*" [12].

In countries such as the United States, these facilities vary depending on patient conditions, insurance coverage, and state regulations. Options include:

- *Inpatient rehab programs*, which provide intensive rehabilitation with several hours of therapeutic care per day, typically for 1–2 weeks
- *Skilled nursing facilities*, which focus on recovery but are less intensive, with stays of 2–4 weeks
- *Long-term acute care hospitals*, designed for extended care with no set length of stay and advanced support systems

Some facilities will admit MV-dependent patients for gradual weaning, provided there are adequately trained staff. Skilled nursing facilities often have the largest number of ventilator-dependent patients, although they often face vacancy shortages due to high demand.

Ambrosino and Vitacca highlight the existence of *respiratory intermediate intensive care units (RIICUs)* in countries such as Italy, Canada, the United Kingdom, Germany, Israel, Australia, and Taiwan. These units, located within acute care hospitals, are less costly than ICUs, provide appropriate multidisciplinary support and rehabilitation, and can serve as a bridge to other rehabilitation facilities or home care [9]. They also mention *specialized regional long-term ventilation units (LWUs)*, typically located within rehabilitation hospitals, which provide comprehensive rehabilitation at a lower cost than ICUs [9]. In Argentina, specialized centers for weaning and comprehensive rehabilitation are generally located near Buenos Aires. These facilities admit tracheostomized patients dependent on PMV with the goal of achieving ventilator weaning and decannulation (tracheostomy tube removal) while striving for functional independence. These are referred to as "*centros de desvinculación de la ventilación mecánica y rehabilitación*" (CDVMR, in Spanish) [16–18].

Transfer from the ICU to a specialized center is often driven by clinical assessments demonstrating stability and reduced need for acute ICU care (e.g., absence of vasopressors or inotropes, evidence of stabilization or reversal of acute illness). This is often associated with the performance of a tracheostomy, typically performed between 16 and 20 days after endotracheal intubation. After tracheostomy, transfer to weaning centers may require an additional 1–2 weeks for coordination [12].

23.4 Organization of Specialized Rehabilitation Centers (Facilities)

While there are variations around the world, specialized rehabilitation centers share a common focus on patient recovery rather than life-support care as in the ICU.

Patient recovery at these centers is anchored by strong rehabilitation teams that typically include, in varying degrees, rehabilitation physicians, respiratory therapy, physical therapy, occupational therapy, speech therapy, psychology, nutrition, music therapy, and neuropsychology. In addition, nursing teams with expertise in caring for patients with these characteristics are essential, as are specialty consultants to address diverse patient needs. Access to laboratory services, arterial blood gas analysis, imaging, and endoscopy is also important, depending on the patient's condition.

Outcomes depend on experienced multidisciplinary teams, rehabilitation equipment, patient- and family-centered protocols, and transdisciplinary work with a perspective different from that of the ICU (Table 23.2).

Rehabilitation centers use a range of ventilatory support devices tailored to the patient's stage of recovery. These include CPAP and BiPAP devices, as well as intermediate and life-support systems often used in intensive care units. These devices provide both invasive and non-invasive mechanical ventilation.

Table 23.2 Comprehensive transdisciplinary rehabilitation approach

Prioritization of rehabilitation goals over discipline-specific boundaries
Goals collaboratively defined by all team members
Simultaneous and coordinated interventions
Integration in shared spaces
Elimination of barriers between specialties

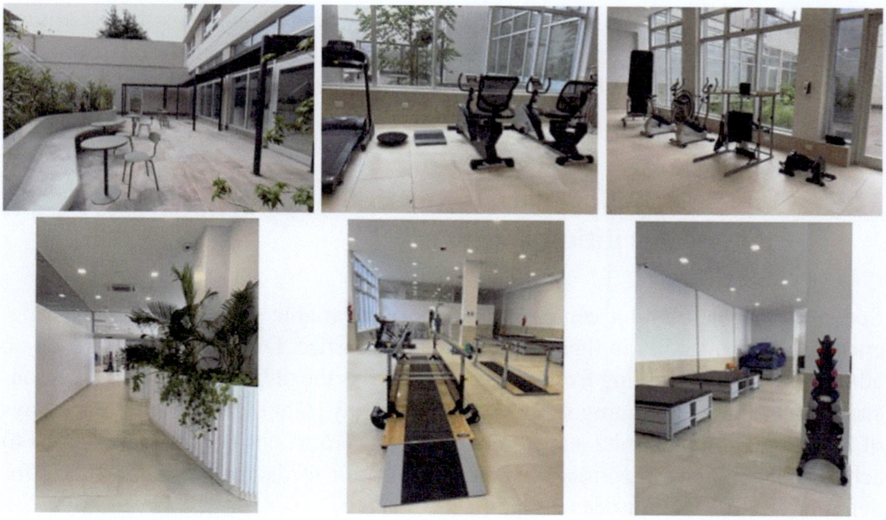

Fig. 23.1 Expansive rehabilitation and recreation areas; Azurduy-Santa Catalina Neuro Rehabilitation Clinic, Argentina

Rehabilitation rooms are typically designed with large areas equipped with equipment such as mats, standing tables, pulleys, ergometers, treadmills, parallel bars, weights, and elastic bands. These facilities must include supplemental oxygen and secretion suction systems. Ideally, they should also provide common areas and green space for recreation (Fig. 23.1).

Despite the increasing incidence of post-ICU patients requiring specialized rehabilitation, there is limited scientific evidence regarding optimal approaches to their care [10]. For critically ill patients, daily implementation of a multicomponent bundle targeting pain, agitation, sedation, delirium, weakness, and weaning from mechanical ventilation by an interprofessional ICU team has been shown to be feasible, safe, and effective in improving patient-centered outcomes [19, 20].

In this context, Balas et al. propose adapting the ABCDEF bundle for the recovery of chronically critically ill patients with severe post-ICU sequelae (Table 23.3)

Table 23.3 Components of the evidence-based ABCDEF bundle

Assessing, preventing, and managing pain
Spontaneous awakening and breathing trials
Optimal choice of analgesia and sedation
Delirium assessment, prevention, and management
Early mobility and exercise
Family engagement and empowerment

[10]. Similarly, Kahn and Carson advocate the transfer of evidence-based critical care practices and professional expertise to specialized rehabilitation centers to improve outcomes for patients with post-ICU sequelae [21].

23.5 Outcomes in Specialized Rehabilitation Centers (Facilities)

Specialized rehabilitation centers have reported variable outcomes, largely influenced by heterogeneity in their operation and expertise. Differences exist based on admission criteria (ranging from clinical stability as the only requirement to demonstrated potential for weaning success), length of stay (ranging from temporary stays of 2–3 months to indefinite stays), goals (ranging from ventilator weaning alone to achieving maximum functional independence prior to discharge), and criteria for defining weaning and/or decannulation success [16].

More than 50% of patients considered "unweanable" in the ICU have been successfully weaned from mechanical ventilation in specialized rehabilitation centers after the acute phase [7]. However, literature reviews indicate a wide range of weaning success rates in PMV patients, ranging from 30% to 70%, especially by tracheostomy [22].

23.5.1 Weaning Methods in PMV Patients

The evidence for PMV weaning methods is largely based on the landmark studies by Brochard and Esteban in the 1990s [23, 24]. In COPD patients requiring more than 15 days of MV, T-piece trials and pressure support yielded similar results [25]. Jubran et al. compared progressive incremental T-piece trials with decremental pressure support in PMV patients who failed their initial T-piece trial. The study showed that T-piece weaning shortened weaning times without affecting other outcomes [26].

Despite the variable percentage of successful weaning cases, one in five patients successfully liberated from MV requires reintubation or reconnection to MV within 28 days of their first night off the ventilator [27].

23.5.2 *Decannulation*

This process represents the final step in the respiratory recovery of PMV-dependent patients. In Argentina and worldwide, approximately 22% of ICU patients undergo tracheostomy due to extubation failure or prolonged MV [28–31]. Despite its prevalence, there is insufficient scientific evidence to establish standardized protocols for decannulation. Two primary factors should be assessed during this process: airway patency and the ability to manage bronchial and salivary secretions. However, comparative studies of variables observed prior to decannulation in different care settings have reported inconsistent results [32].

23.5.3 *Unweanable Patients*

A proportion of patients cannot be weaned or successfully decannulated from MV despite rehabilitation efforts due to comorbidities, underlying disease, or post-ICU sequelae. Weaning efforts should continue until the interdisciplinary team, together with the well-informed patient and family, agrees that such attempts should be discontinued. For patients who cannot be weaned, transparent discussions with the patient and family about prognosis and realistic long-term options are essential. Involvement of palliative care services can add significant value to the patient and family experience in managing PMV care [12].

23.6 Conclusion

Chronically critically ill patients and those with prolonged mechanical ventilation dependency present multidimensional challenges in the ICU. Implementation of evidence-based strategies that include specialized multidisciplinary teams and rehabilitation centers tailored to the needs of these patients is critical. Future research should prioritize the standardization of criteria for the management, weaning, and rehabilitation of these patients to improve their quality of life while reducing associated costs.

References

1. Girard K, Raffin TA. The chronically critically ill: to save or let die? Respir Care. 1985;30(5):339–47.
2. Nelson JE, Cox CE, Hope AA, Carson SS. Chronic critical illness. Am J Respir Crit Care Med. 2010;182(4):446–54.
3. Kahn JM, Le T, Angus DC, Cox CE, Hough CL, White DB, et al. The epidemiology of chronic critical illness in the United States*. Crit Care Med. 2015;43(2):282–7.
4. Damuth E, Mitchell JA, Bartock JL, Roberts BW, Trzeciak S. Long-term survival of critically ill patients treated with prolonged mechanical ventilation: a systematic review and meta-analysis. Lancet Respir Med. 2015;3(7):544–53.
5. Iwashyna TJ, Hodgson CL, Pilcher D, Bailey M, van Lint A, Chavan S, et al. Timing of onset and burden of persistent critical illness in Australia and New Zealand: a retrospective, population-based, observational study. Lancet Respir Med. 2016;4(7):566–73.
6. Estenssoro E, Reina R, Canales HS, Saenz MG, Gonzalez FE, Aprea MM, et al. The distinct clinical profile of chronically critically ill patients: a cohort study. Crit Care. 2006;10(3):R89.
7. Dolinay T, Hsu L, Maller A, Walsh BC, Szűcs A, Jerng JS, et al. Ventilator weaning in prolonged mechanical ventilation-A narrative review. J Clin Med [Internet]. 2024;13(7) Available from: https://doi.org/10.3390/jcm13071909
8. Hill AD, Fowler RA, Burns KEA, Rose L, Pinto RL, Scales DC. Long-term outcomes and health care utilization after prolonged mechanical ventilation. Ann Am Thorac Soc. 2017;14(3):355–62.
9. Ambrosino N, Vitacca M. The patient needing prolonged mechanical ventilation: a narrative review. Multidiscip Respir Med. 2018;26:6.
10. Balas MC, Devlin JW, Verceles AC, Morris P, Ely EW. Adapting the ABCDEF bundle to meet the needs of patients requiring prolonged mechanical ventilation in the long-term acute care hospital setting: historical perspectives and practical implications. Semin Respir Crit Care Med. 2016;37(1):119–35.
11. Chadda KR, Puthucheary Z. Persistent inflammation, immunosuppression, and catabolism syndrome (PICS): a review of definitions, potential therapies, and research priorities. Br J Anaesth. 2024;132(3):507–18.
12. MacIntyre NR, Epstein SK, Carson S, Scheinhorn D, Christopher K, Muldoon S, et al. Management of patients requiring prolonged mechanical ventilation: report of a NAMDRC consensus conference. Chest. 2005;128(6):3937–54.
13. Trudzinski FC, Neetz B, Bornitz F, Müller M, Weis A, Kronsteiner D, et al. Risk factors for prolonged mechanical ventilation and weaning failure: a systematic review. Respiration. 2022;101(10):959–69.
14. Heunks LM, van der Hoeven JG. Clinical review: the ABC of weaning failure–a structured approach. Crit Care. 2010;14(6):245.
15. Rose L, McGinlay M, Amin R, Burns KE, Connolly B, Hart N, et al. Variation in definition of prolonged mechanical ventilation. Respir Care. 2017;62(10):1324–32.
16. Villalba D, Plotnikow G, Feld V, Rivero Vairo N, Scapellato J, Díaz NE. Weaning from prolonged mechanical ventilation at 72 hours of spontaneous breathing. Medicina (B Aires). 2015;75(1):11–7.
17. Hannun M, Villalba D, Díaz Ballve L, Matesa A, Pedace P, Tocalini P, et al. Predictors of weaning and mortality in prolonged mechanical ventilation – surviving survival. Rev Fac Cien Med Univ Nac Cordoba. 2022;79(2):162–7.
18. Villalba D, Navarro E, Matesa A, Brusco A, Morales V, Morel Vulliez GG, et al. Epidemiology of tracheostomized adult patients admitted to specialized weaning centers after acute COVID-19. Respir Care. 2024;69(2):202–9.
19. Balas MC, Vasilevskis EE, Olsen KM, Schmid KK, Shostrom V, Cohen MZ, et al. Effectiveness and safety of the awakening and breathing coordination, delirium monitoring/management, and early exercise/mobility bundle. Crit Care Med. 2014;42(5):1024–36.

20. Pun BT, Balas MC, Barnes-Daly MA, Thompson JL, Aldrich JM, Barr J, et al. Caring for critically ill patients with the ABCDEF bundle: results of the ICU liberation collaborative in over 15,000 adults. Crit Care Med. 2019;47(1):3–14.
21. Kahn JM, Carson SS. Generating evidence on best practice in long-term acute care hospitals. JAMA. 2013;309(7):719–20.
22. Scheinhorn DJ, Chao DC, Stearn-Hassenpflug M. Liberation from prolonged mechanical ventilation. Crit Care Clin. 2002;18(3):569–95.
23. Esteban A, Frutos F, Tobin MJ, Alía I, Solsona JF, Valverdú I, et al. A comparison of four methods of weaning patients from mechanical ventilation. Spanish Lung Failure Collaborative Group. N Engl J Med. 1995;332(6):345–50.
24. Brochard L, Rauss A, Benito S, Conti G, Mancebo J, Rekik N, et al. Comparison of three methods of gradual withdrawal from ventilatory support during weaning from mechanical ventilation. Am J Respir Crit Care Med. 1994;150(4):896–903.
25. Vitacca M, Vianello A, Colombo D, Clini E, Porta R, Bianchi L, et al. Comparison of two methods for weaning patients with chronic obstructive pulmonary disease requiring mechanical ventilation for more than 15 days. Am J Respir Crit Care Med. 2001;164(2):225–30.
26. Jubran A, Grant BJB, Duffner LA, Collins EG, Lanuza DM, Hoffman LA, et al. Effect of pressure support vs unassisted breathing through a tracheostomy collar on weaning duration in patients requiring prolonged mechanical ventilation: a randomized trial. JAMA. 2013;309(7):671–7.
27. Villalba D, Rossetti GG, Scrigna M, Collins J, Rocco A, Matesa A, et al. Prevalence of and risk factors for mechanical ventilation reinstitution in patients weaned from prolonged mechanical ventilation. Respir Care. 2020;65(2):210–6.
28. Abril MK, Berkowitz DM, Chen Y, Waller LA, Martin GS, Kempker JA. The epidemiology of adult tracheostomy in the United States 2002–2017: a serial cross-sectional study. Crit Care Explor. 2021;3(9):e0523.
29. Epidemiology of mechanical ventilation in Argentina. The EpVAr multicenter observational study. Med Intensiva (Engl Ed). 2022;46(7):372–82.
30. Pham T, Heunks L, Bellani G, Madotto F, Aragao I, Beduneau G, et al. Weaning from mechanical ventilation in intensive care units across 50 countries (WEAN SAFE): a multicentre, prospective, observational cohort study. Lancet Respir Med. 2023;11(5):465–76.
31. Website [Internet]. Available from: https://doi.org/10.1164/rccm.201502-0239OC.
32. Diaz-Ballve LP, Villalba DS, Andreu MF, Escobar MA, Morel-Vulliez G, Lebus JM, et al. Respiratory muscle strength and state of consciousness values measured prior to the decannulation in different levels of complexity. A longitudinal prospective case series study. Med Intensiva (Engl Ed). 2019;43(5):270–80.

Chapter 24
Compassionate Extubation

Shaline Ferla Baptistella and Cristina Bueno Terzi

> *... To some of them (elderly patient) the ICU becomes a modern torture chamber, where young physicians consider death their worst enemy and do not appreciate that it may be an old man's friend... The problem is that, in many cases, we are only prolonging the patient's death process.*
>
> *Grenvik [13]*

24.1 Palliative Care

WHO defines palliative care as an approach that improves the quality of life of patients—adults and children—and their families facing problems related to potentially fatal illnesses. It prevents and relieves suffering through early recognition, accurate assessment, and treatment of pain and other problems, whether physical or psychosocial [19, 25, 26].

This care aims to relieve symptoms and improve quality of life, and should be provided in conjunction with curative care, or exclusively when that goal can no longer be achieved [13, 14].

When we analyze patients admitted to the intensive care unit (ICU), the most common reasons for admission are respiratory failure, acute myocardial infarction, intracranial hemorrhage or ischemic stroke, percutaneous cardiovascular procedures, and sepsis. In these settings, mechanical ventilation is the most commonly used life-sustaining measure in 20%–40% of patients admitted to ICUs in the United States [21].

S. F. Baptistella (✉)
Clinical Oncologist, Santa Terezinha University Hospital, Joaçaba, SC, Brazil

Universidade do Oeste de Santa Catarina, Unoesc, Joaçaba, Brazil

C. B. Terzi
Palliative Care Department, State University of Campinas, Campinas, São Paulo, Brazil

A. R. Baptistella et al. (eds.), *Weaning from Mechanical Ventilation*,
https://doi.org/10.1007/978-3-032-01145-9_24

From the above, it is clear that regardless of the reason for admission to the ICU, we are faced with fragile patients at high risk of death with an uncertain immediate prognosis. And in many situations, their family members, already under high levels of stress from the situation, will be asked to make difficult decisions [5].

Providing access to palliative care in these cases allows the patient's and family's preferences regarding the prognosis to become clear, so that the care provided can be aligned with their desires. For example, in end-of-life situations, the goal of care can be reviewed and, if the goal changes from cure to comfort, artificial life-sustaining measures deemed inappropriate can be withheld or withdrawn and symptom control can be prioritized. When in doubt, families usually agree to a time-limited trial of therapy, followed by review and withdrawal of life support if the patient does not improve. This may be a good way to manage some cases.

There is no standardized technique for withdrawing these interventions, and the process must be carefully considered. In general, while some interventions are recommended, others are avoided, in a delicate balance between beneficence and non-maleficence, in an effort to improve what is perceived to be the patient's quality of life.

In this sense, the most frequently discontinued supports and therapies are transfusion of blood products, hemodialysis, use of vasopressors, mechanical ventilation, total parenteral nutrition, antibiotics, intravenous fluids, and enteral nutrition [15].

When these decisions are made without adequate communication with family members, there is also an increase in family demands and a lack of consensus among the team, exposing this patient to more futile treatments [20].

Many studies have documented dramatic geographic variations in the prevalence of withdrawal or non-indication of life-sustaining measures, and some evidence suggests that these decisions are driven more by physician attitudes than by factors such as patient preferences or cultural differences. However, interventions such as palliative care assessment or ethics committee review, family meetings, and standardized protocols for withdrawing life-sustaining measures improve the profile of these decisions [8].

The goal of palliative care is always orthothanasia. In orthothanasia, the disease is the driving force behind death.

Compassionate extubation is the process of withdrawing mechanical ventilation when the goals of patient care have become comfort as the absolute and exclusive priority. The procedure involves a high degree of complexity in terms of communication with the family member and, if possible, the patient, the need for experience in mechanical ventilation, and intensive management and control of symptoms that may occur during the procedure. At this time, understanding the patient's overall clinical condition and defining their prognosis can be challenging [27].

As previously discussed, compassionate extubation validates orthothanasia because it does not aim to artificially prolong life at the expense of suffering, nor does it aim to alter the natural process of death, as the treatments administered no longer interfere with the natural course of the disease [12].

Therefore, withdrawal of mechanical ventilation, otherwise known as compassionate extubation, is not intended to hasten the patient's death and, therefore, should not be confused with euthanasia. On the contrary, it is an action that, when faced with the impossibility of reversing the clinical condition, prioritizes the necessary care so that the patient does not suffer during their death, without engaging in actions whose harm outweighs the benefits to be obtained; in this way, it is a procedure that can be performed in end-of-life care, but requires knowledge and competence [15, 18].

24.2 Protocol

24.2.1 Decision-Making

The process of compassionate extubation must take into account medical, legal, and ethical issues that may vary in different parts of the world [9]. Few healthcare professionals are trained to withdraw life-sustaining measures. The purpose of this chapter is to provide information on best practices for compassionate extubation, thereby improving the quality of end-of-life care for patients.

The process of compassionate extubation begins with consensus among the health care team. To achieve this, professionals must consider the patient's prognosis and whether continued mechanical ventilation will provide opportunities to restore a state of health that is consistent with what the patient and family consider an acceptable quality of life [2, 10]. An important point is that this whole process and approach is interdisciplinary [10].

Although many patients find it threatening to contemplate the circumstances under which a decision to withdraw life support might be considered, advance care planning is critical in this context and allows the patient to plan for future scenarios as the disease progresses. In this discussion, clinicians must address prognostic difficulties and uncertainties, and can use this uncertainty to broaden the discussion beyond an exclusive focus on survival. The emotions underlying patient preferences must also be addressed. From a bioethical perspective, protecting values means giving dignity.

When the patient lacks capacity, surrogate decision-makers need to understand their true role and responsibilities so that they do not feel overwhelmed and pressured. There are two patterns of surrogate decision making. When the patient's wishes are known, the surrogate must carry them out explicitly (substitution judgment). If the patient's wishes are unknown, the surrogate must attempt to make a decision in the patient's best interest.

Once compassionate extubation has been defined, the team and family must be prepared for the procedure.

24.2.2 Family Preparation

First, family members need to understand what the procedure entails and the role of each health care professional involved in the process. In addition, they should be informed about what to expect during the procedure, including possible changes in the patient's appearance, changes in vital signs, noisy breathing, spasms, and/or involuntary movements, along with how these symptoms will be managed, and how, with appropriate treatment, they will not cause distress.

Explain that the time between extubation and patient death can be variable and difficult to predict. Also explain the possibility that the patient may not be able to breathe on their own or survive extubation after the procedure. It is recommended that the family spend time with the patient before the procedure to say goodbye. It is recommended that family members be present during and after the procedure. This may be the last time family members see their loved one alive, so compassion and respect for the patient and family are essential.

Children and adolescents involved in this process need special attention from the team, which may include availability of a psychologist and social worker, if possible. Emphasize that the patient's comfort is the primary concern of all involved [9, 10].

24.2.3 Review Assessments and Supportive Care

Begin by reviewing all interventions the patient is receiving and, if possible, discontinue those that may cause discomfort, such as probes, monitors, and routine laboratory collections. Maintaining intravenous access is important as it may be necessary for symptom control medications.

- It is recommended that tube feedings, parenteral nutrition, and fluids be discontinued 24–48 h prior to extubation.
- It is recommended that vasopressors not be discontinued until after the procedure, as these medications can ensure the circulation of medications used during extubation to control symptoms.
- Patients with automatic implantable cardioverter defibrillators (ICDs) must have the defibrillator function deactivated with a magnetic ring.
- Neuromuscular blocking agents should not be used as a comfort measure during compassionate extubation because they prevent spontaneous breathing. Ethically, they must be discontinued at least 2 h before the procedure, but in patients with multiple organ dysfunction, the effects of these drugs can last up to 18 h. It is recommended to wait the necessary time for the patient to regain voluntary respiratory movement, if possible.
- Intensify respiratory physiotherapy and keep the head elevated at a 35°–45° angle. Prepare suction equipment and medications that may be needed, such as opioids and benzodiazepines.

It is recommended that an experienced physician, nurse or nurse practitioner, and physical therapist be present during the procedure [7, 10, 22, 27].

24.2.4 Weaning from Mechanical Ventilation

There are two approaches to weaning from mechanical ventilation: terminal weaning and immediate extubation.

There is no consensus on which approach is preferred. One study comparing the two did not find a difference in the emotional impact on family members, but immediate extubation put patients at greater risk for airway obstruction and wheezing.

Immediate extubation is the cessation of ventilatory support in a single step with removal of the endotracheal tube. This form requires early and careful dosing of opioids and sedatives. It may be more appropriate for patients who are able to maintain their own ventilation and is a good option for critically ill neurological patients who are already receiving minimal mechanical ventilation support [16].

During terminal weaning, ventilatory support is gradually reduced with the endotracheal tube still in place. This method may be more appropriate for patients with high levels of ventilatory support and those who have difficulty managing secretions or protecting the airway.

To do this, ventilation parameters are gradually reduced and the patient is assessed at each stage, with measures taken to minimize any discomfort. This form of weaning gives the clinician greater control over the process. The following steps are suggested to perform terminal weaning:

- Reduce positive end-expiratory pressure (PEEP) to 5 cm H_2O and FiO_2 to 21%.
- Monitor the patient for 5–10 min and adjust medications for comfort as needed.
- The next steps consist of reducing ventilatory support by 50% each time, observing the patient for 5–10 min, and adjusting symptoms.
- When the patient achieves comfortable spontaneous breathing, the orotracheal cuff is deflated and mechanical ventilation can be withdrawn.

A professional must be responsible for silencing, turning off, and removing the ventilator. Excessive oropharyngeal secretions should be aspirated.

Patients with tracheostomies can be easily disconnected from the ventilator. In patients with bleeding episodes, retention of the orotracheal tube may provide comfort, in which case the patient should simply be disconnected from the ventilator [16].

24.2.5 Assessment and Management of Symptoms During Withdrawal from Mechanical Ventilation

The primary goal during withdrawal of advanced life support is patient comfort, which requires monitoring and prompt treatment of any symptoms that occur. During compassionate extubation, the main symptoms that may occur are dyspnea, anxiety, pain, and delirium.

- Dyspnea and Respiratory Discomfort

It is suggested to observe the ventilation pattern and possible clinical instability, as well as the use of accessory muscles, fear or anxiety facies, paradoxical breathing, in addition to parameters such as increase or decrease in respiratory or heart rate and tidal volume. Based on these observations, we can predict the measures and medications necessary for the patient's comfort before the procedure, allowing us to anticipate the needs of the moment [27].

Standardized tools can be used to assess dyspnea, such as the Respiratory Distress Observation Scale—RDOS (Table 24.1).

The RDOS is an objective, evidence-based tool that helps validate the need for titration of comfort medications during compassionate extubation and end-of-life care. It validates the need for comfort measures or medications to reduce respiratory distress while preventing under- or over-medication of patients.

Using the RDOS guidelines, the critical care nurse and physical therapist can work together in a standardized manner to gradually reduce ventilatory support while maintaining the target RDOS of less than 4 to prevent and minimize patient suffering [6].

Note that RDOS does not apply to neonates, young children, patients with cervical spinal cord injury resulting in quadriplegia, or patients with bulbar amyotrophic lateral sclerosis [6].

Opioids are the cornerstone of the management of dyspnea and respiratory distress in the context of compassionate extubation.

- Premedication: Even if the patient is comfortable before the extubation procedure, it is recommended that an additional dose of opioid be administered to prevent discomfort caused by the procedure, especially in patients who are uncomfortable with routine procedures such as aspiration [11].
- Morphine is the preferred opioid.
- If the patient has no history of opioid or benzodiazepine use, give 2–10 mg intravenously as a bolus. Then give an additional intravenous infusion of 1–5 mg associated with lorazepam or midazolam 1–2 mg intravenously, also as a bolus.
- Continue the IV infusion at 1–2 mg per hour.
- If the patient is already on continuous opioids and benzodiazepines, it may be necessary to increase the above dose by 30%. After 10 min of administration (necessary for peak drug effect), extubate if the patient is comfortable [23].

Table 24.1 Respiratory Distress Observation Scale (RDOS): a validated tool for assessing the severity of respiratory distress in patients unable to self-report, based on observable clinical signs

Respiratory Distress Observation Scale (RDOS)

Purpose

This tool is used for assessing the intensity and distress of patients unable to report dyspnea during monitoring for palliative sedation therapy [4, 28]

Variable	**0 points**	**1 point**	**2 points**	**Sub-total**
Heart rate per min (beats/min = bpm)	Less than 90 bpm	90–109 bpm	Greater than or equal to 110 bpm	
Respiratory rate per minute (auscultated) (breaths/min)	Less than 19 breaths	19–30 breaths	Greater than 30 breaths	
Restlessness: nonpurposeful movements	No	Yes—occasional, slight movements	Yes—frequent movements	
Paradoxical breathing pattern: abdomen moves in or inspiration	No		Yes	
Accessory muscle use: rise in clavicle during inspiration	No	Yes—slight rise	Yes—pronounced rise	
Grunting at end-expiration: guttural sounds	No		Yes	
Nasal flaring: involuntary movement of nares	No		Yes	
Look of fear: ☐ → eyes wide open ☐ → facial muscles tense ☐ → brow furrowed ☐ → mouth open ☐ → teeth together	No		Yes	
			Total	

Instructions for use

Count respiratory and heart rates for one full minute

Grunting may be audible with or without auscultation

An RDOS score of less than 3 indicates respiratory comfort [4]

An RDOS score greater than or equal to 3 signifies respiratory distress and need for palliation [4, 28]

Higher RDOS scores signify a worsening condition [4, 28]

The guidelines and algorithms help the team maintain a coordinated and structured end-of-life (EOL) process and create a less stressful environment for the patient, family, and healthcare team.

Therefore, if the RDOS is still greater than 3, it is recommended to repeat the morphine dose, reassess the RDOS after 10 min, and titrate the morphine dose according to the patient's tolerance. The need for benzodiazepines in conjunction with opioids is generally dictated by the patient's underlying medical condition: most cancer patients require both drugs, whereas patients with a reduced level of consciousness due to the underlying medical condition may not require either two drugs. Note that deep sedation requires two classes of medications: opioids for analgesia (but not loss of consciousness) and sedatives to induce unconsciousness and amnesia [6].

Oxygen and Noninvasive Mechanical Ventilation

- Determine the patient's oxygen requirements for comfort after extubation, considering the goals of extubation and room air maintenance.
- If the oxygen saturation is less than 85% and the RDOS is greater than 4, it is suggested that a low flow of O_2 through the nasal cannula be considered.
- There is no data in the literature to support the use of oxygen to relieve dyspnea in patients without hypoxemia.
- The use of a high-flow catheter may improve oxygenation and relieve dyspnea in selected patients. However, it is not associated with a reduction in the need for opioids or anxiolytics. Its use may prolong the process of death while improving dyspnea.
- In addition, once started, weaning is uncommon and all these aspects need to be discussed in the goals of care before its installation [3].

Noninvasive positive pressure ventilation can be used in specific circumstances:

- In patients who want life-prolonging measures but with restrictions (order not to intubate)
- In those with the intention of reducing respiratory effort and the need for opioids/anxiolytics, in an attempt to prolong survival for a short period of time to achieve a specific goal (for example, to allow a family visit)

It must be remembered that noninvasive ventilation can be uncomfortable, cause anxiety, make sleep difficult, limit communication, and, if not discussed, can confuse the goal of care [1].

- Laryngeal Stridor

The most common risk factors for the occurrence of laryngeal stridor are: traumatic intubation, history of self-extubation, prolonged intubation, and elevated SAPS II (simplified acute physiology score). It is more likely to occur up to 1 h after extubation.

To reduce the risk, methylprednisone 100 mg can be used, one dose 6 h before and one dose 30 min before extubation. If the patient develops stridor, it can be treated with racemic epinephrine aerosol, 2.5 mg in 3 ml of saline solution [10]:

- Anxiety and Restlessness

These symptoms require treatment with benzodiazepines. For delirium in critically ill patients, the drug of choice is haloperidol, which has a peak effect 30 min after intravenous administration and can be repeated every 15 or 30 min as needed.

- Respiratory Secretion

To control and reduce respiratory secretions, the following medications are recommended:

- Scopolamine, 20 milligrams intravenously, started 12–48 h before extubation, administered every 6 h
- Atropine, 0.5% (eye drops) one to two drops sublingually also every 6 h [10]

24.3 Action and Care After Mechanical Ventilation

It is recommended that a team member remain with the patient and family for 30–60 min after the condition has stabilized. This allows for rapid adjustment of medications, if needed, and helps the family remain calm as they adjust to the patient's condition.

- Monitor Symptoms

An experienced physician and nurse (or nurse practitioner) should be available to assess and adjust symptom control shortly after extubation [10].

It is important to document all steps of the above procedure in the medical record, as well as the patient's immediate post-extubation outcome (instabilization, death) [5, 10, 17].

Always keep medications such as opioids and benzodiazepines at the bedside, ready to use if needed. The most severe respiratory distress occurs in the first few hours after extubation. Additional doses of opioids and benzodiazepines can and should be given at this time.

More important than dose titration is symptom relief. It is recommended to aim for a respiratory rate of less than 30 breaths per minute in a patient without signs of pain, respiratory effort, or agitation. We emphasize that studies show that using these medications to relieve patients' symptoms does not shorten their lives [24].

For patients whose discomfort cannot be controlled after extubation, palliative sedation may be necessary to provide adequate comfort.

- Family Support

It is recommended that family members remain at the bedside during the procedure. Encourage them to ask for clarification of any questions that may arise after extubation. Multidisciplinary grief support for family members (chaplain, psychologist) is very important. During this time, family members can communicate through talking, playing music, and using visual resources such as photos or pictures that they find valuable for the situation [9].

- Time of Death and Transfer from the ICU

Most patients die in the ICU within a short period of time. Patients who are stable for 24–48 h after extubation can be transferred, ideally to a room where the family can be present and close by. This transfer must be discussed with the family in advance, as the realization that the outcome of extubation is death may cause a great deal of anxiety. If transfer is performed, ensure that the receiving team is prepared to maintain care and control symptoms [7, 10].

24.4 Final Considerations

Compassionate extubation is a procedure that is already well established as an ethical option for patients with irreversible disease and suffering. However, its poor performance, both technically and in communication with the patient and family, can lead to even greater suffering. Therefore, a technically rigorous execution will reduce stress for patients and families, as well as misunderstandings, discomfort, and additional suffering for everyone involved in the process.

Begin with a decision involving professionals, family members, and, if possible, the patient. Make it clear that the goal of the process is to withdraw mechanical ventilation from a patient who no longer benefits from this support, remembering that end-of-life care in the ICU is both an art and a science.

Once the decision has been made, the involved professionals and family members need to be prepared and aware of the procedure to be performed. Evaluate and prepare the environment in which the procedure will take place, as well as anticipate and separate the materials needed to control symptoms.

Mechanical ventilation is then withdrawn, and the focus is on symptom control with opioids and benzodiazepines. Always consider the predicted dose of these medications. After the procedure, the patient should be closely monitored to ensure symptom stability. At this time, as at all times, family support is essential [10]. Emphasize that withdrawing life support is not withdrawing care, by saying, "The focus of care has changed, but we continue to provide care."

More recently, simulation labs have been used to improve understanding and learning of these and other palliative care procedures, promoting a safe environment for practice without compromising patient care [27]. Expanding access to education and training is critical and fundamental.

References

1. Azoulay E, Kouatchet A, Jaber S, et al. Non-invasive ventilation for end-of-life oncology patients. Lancet Oncol. 2013;14:e200–1. https://doi.org/10.1016/S1470-2045(13)70141-4.
2. Bandrauk N, Downar J, Paunovic B. Withholding and withdrawing life-sustaining treatment: the Canadian Critical Care Society position paper. Can J Anesth/J Can Anesth. 2018;65:105–22. https://doi.org/10.1007/s12630-017-1002-1.
3. Bramati PS, Azhar A, Khan R, et al. High flow nasal cannula in patients with cancer at the end of life. J Pain Symptom Manag. 2023;65:e369–73. https://doi.org/10.1016/j.jpainsymman.2022.12.141.
4. Campbell ML, Templin TN. Intensity cut-points for the respiratory distress observation scale. Palliat Med. 2015;29(5):436–42.
5. Cherny IN, Fallon MT, Kaasa S, et al. Oxford textbook of palliative medicine. Oxford University Press; 2021.
6. Cooney-Newton K, Hare EC. Palliative care and population management compassionate Extubation of the ICU patient and the use of the respiratory distress observation scale. Crit Care Nurs Clin North Am. 2022;34:67–78. https://doi.org/10.1016/j.cnc.2021.11.004.

7. Coradazzi AL, Inhaia CL, Santana MT, et al. Palliative withdrawal ventilation: why, when and how to do it? Hospice and palliative medicine. Int J. 2019;3 https://doi.org/10.15406/hpmij.2019.03.00141.
8. Curtis JR. Interventions to improve care during withdrawal of life-sustaining treatments. J Palliat Med. 2005;8:S116–31. https://doi.org/10.1089/jpm.2005.8.s-116.
9. Downar J, Delaney JW, Hawryluck L, Kenny L. Guidelines for the withdrawal of life-sustaining measures. Intensive Care Med. 2016;42:1003–17. https://doi.org/10.1007/s00134-016-4330-7.
10. Elio Barbosa Raimondi Belfiori JHZJVSS. Cuidados Paliativos: da clínica a bioetica. São Paulo: CREMESP; 2023.
11. EPERC. End of life. Palliative Education Resource Center; 2024.
12. Fukumitsu KO. Vida, morte e luto. Atualidades Brasileiras. São Paulo: Summus; 2018.
13. Grenvik A. "Terminal weaning"; discontinuance of life-support therapy in the terminally ill patient. Crit Care Med. 1983;11:394–5. https://doi.org/10.1097/00003246-198305000-00019.
14. NIH. What are palliative care and hospice care? National Institute on Aging. 2024. https://www.nia.nih.gov/health/hospice-and-palliative-care/what-are-palliative-care-and-hospice-care#. Accessed 17 Mar 2024.
15. Ortega-Chen C, Van Buren N, Kwack J, et al. Palliative extubation: a discussion of practices and considerations. J Pain Symptom Manag. 2023;66:e219–31. https://doi.org/10.1016/j.jpainsymman.2023.03.011.
16. Prendergast TJ, Puntillo KA, McPhee SJ, et al. Withdrawal of life support: intensive caring at the end of life. In: Care at the close of life: evidence and experience. New York; 2011.
17. Robert R, Le Gouge A, Kentish-Barnes N, et al. Terminal weaning or immediate extubation for withdrawing mechanical ventilation in critically ill patients (the ARREVE observational study). Intensive Care Med. 2017;43:1793–807. https://doi.org/10.1007/s00134-017-4891-0.
18. Sanchez y Sanches KM, Seidl EMF. Ortotanásia: uma decisão frente à terminalidade. Interface - Comunicação, Saúde, Educação. 2013;17:23–34. https://doi.org/10.1590/S1414-32832013000100003.
19. Shah N, Mehta Z, Mehta Y. High-flow nasal cannula oxygen therapy in palliative care. 2019. https://www.mypcnow.org/fast-fact/high-flow-nasal-cannula-oxygen-therapy-in-palliative-care/. Accessed 4 Aug 2024.
20. Sibbald R, Downar J, Hawryluck L. Perceptions of "futile care" among caregivers in intensive care units. Can Med Assoc J. 2007;177:1201–8. https://doi.org/10.1503/cmaj.070144.
21. Society of Critical Care Medicine. Critical care statistics. SCCM. 2024. https://www.sccm.org/Communications/Critical-Care-Statistics. Accessed 6 Mar 2024.
22. Sprung CL, Cohen SL, Sjokvist P, et al. End-of-life practices in European intensive care units. JAMA. 2003;290:790. https://doi.org/10.1001/jama.290.6.790.
23. Timothy E. Quill. Primer of palliative care. Timothy E. Quill; 2007.
24. von Gunten C, Weissman D. Ventilator withdrawal protocol. 2019. https://www.mypcnow.org/fast-fact/ventilator-withdrawal-protocol/. Accessed 4 Aug 2024.
25. WHO. Palliative care. 2020. https://www.who.int/news-room/fact-sheets/detail/palliative-care. Accessed 6 Mar 2024.
26. WHO. Palliative care. 2024. https://www.who.int/europe/health-topics/palliative-care#tab=tab_1. Accessed 4 Aug 2024.
27. Yeow M-E, Chen E. Ventilator withdrawal in anticipation of death: the simulation lab as an educational tool in palliative medicine. J Pain Symptom Manag. 2020;59:165–71. https://doi.org/10.1016/j.jpainsymman.2019.09.025.
28. Zhang, et al. Validity, reliability, and diagnostic accuracy of the respiratory distress observation scale for assessment of dyspnea in adult palliative care patients. J Pan Symptom Manage. 2019;57(2):304–10.

Index

A. R. Baptistella et al. (eds.), *Weaning from Mechanical Ventilation*,
https://doi.org/10.1007/978-3-032-01145-9

E

MIX
Papier aus verantwortungsvollen Quellen
Paper from responsible sources
FSC® C105338

If you have any concerns about our products,
you can contact us on
ProductSafety@springernature.com

In case Publisher is established outside the EU,
the EU authorized representative is:
Springer Nature Customer Service Center GmbH
Europaplatz 3, 69115 Heidelberg, Germany

Printed by Libri Plureos GmbH
in Hamburg, Germany